Penguin Education

Skills

Edited by David Legge

WITHDRAWN

Penguin Modern Psychology Readings

General Editor
B. M. Foss

Skills

Selected Readings

Edited by David Legge

Penguin Books

Penguin Books Ltd, Harmondsworth,
Middlesex, England
Penguin Books Inc., 7110 Ambassador Road,
Baltimore, Md 21207, U.S.A.
Penguin Books Ltd, Ringwood,
Victoria, Australia

First published 1970
This selection copyright © David Legge, 1970
Introduction and notes copyright © David Legge, 1970

Made and printed in Great Britain by
Richard Clay (The Chaucer Press) Ltd,
Bungay, Suffolk
Set in Monotype Times

Contents

Introduction

This book is concerned with perceptual–motor skill. As Welford (1958) has pointed out, psychologists use the word skill in a broader sense than do trade unionists or sportsmen. Man's everyday activities demand the exercise of countless perceptual–motor skills – many of which go totally unremarked. The simple acts of walking, picking up a cup or articulating words are all skills. They require the co-ordinated integration of sensory information and muscular responses to attain some specifiable goal. More complex skills such as driving a car or operating a lathe make similar but greater demands on man's central nervous system.

It might be thought that the ubiquitous role of perceptual–motor skills in behaviour would have put the analysis of skill high on the list of priorities for research. In fact studies of thinking, learning, perception and individual differences have taken precedence in research effort. This picture was radically altered by the Second World War when practical considerations focused attention on man's capacities and limitations, particularly in relation to his role as an operator of complex machinery. Perhaps the earlier lack of interest was due to the fact that there is seldom an informative verbal correlate of skilled performance. Few can say much about how they perform a skill, and what they do say may have only passing relevance to the actual operation of the mechanisms underlying the skill.

With the notable exceptions of Woodworth's (1899) thesis on the control of voluntary movement and Bryan and Harter's (1899) classic paper on the acquisition of skill by morse code telegraphists, nearly all the work on skill before 1939 was dominated by the S–R theory of learning as proposed by Thorndike (1913, 1932) and Hull (1943, 1952). The acquisition of skill was described simply as the formation of a stimulus–response chain similar to the making of connexions through a telephone exchange. This view was challenged by Tolman (1932) who proposed that behaviour was governed by goals in an apparently teleological manner rather than pushed from behind by states of deprivation. The inadequacy of the Hullian (S–R) approach to skill was exposed by Lashley (1951) and as skills research gathered momentum a new basis for analysis emerged.

The new approach placed great weight on the concept of feedback; a concept borrowed from control engineering (Wiener, 1948). The term feedback denotes information about the output of a system which is fed back into the system. In a sense, feedback tells a mechanism what it is doing. Feedback can provide the basis for a self-adjusting system which maintains its output in dynamic equilibrium. A primitive device dependent upon negative feedback is exemplified by the governor on a steam engine, or by a thermostat. The flexible nature of skilled behaviour, described by Bartlett (1947), demanded a more dynamic system than Hull's theory envisaged. A system that is sensitive to its own product – that is, one with feedback – has the necessary degree of flexibility and furthermore appears to act in a teleological manner. Many of the ideas that have advanced our understanding of skill in the last twenty years may be traced back to engineering and computer technology.

When performing a skill man fills the role of an information processing device. To function effectively he must register and interpret information, and compute and execute responses in accord with some strategy or programme which guides him towards success. This aspect of man's behaviour may be mimicked by a model drawn from control engineering. Man is more flexible than even the most sophisticated machines and appears to have the capacity to acquire an almost unlimited variety of guiding programmes. However, the machine analogy is a fruitful one because it provides an opportunity to apply the methods of assessment of inanimate information processing devices to the analysis of mechanisms underlying behaviour.

A successful model of perceptual–motor behaviour would be most unlikely to emerge without consideration of the physiology and structure of man. In this field of research there is a reciprocal interaction between the psychologist, engineer and physiologist. The ideas of the one help to direct the thoughts of the others, and vice versa. One example of this interaction may be found in the analysis of the role of proprioception in the performance of perceptual–motor skills. Proprioception provides information about the state of one's muscles and joints without looking at them.

Initially emphasized by Sherrington (1906) as an essential component of the integration of motor behaviour at spinal level, the role played by proprioception in the control of skilled movements has been increasingly recognized (Bahrick, 1957; Fitts, 1951; Gibbs, 1954; Legge, 1965). The use of proprioceptive information has the great advantage of freeing vision for monitoring more distant events. However, although considerable strides have been made towards understanding the physiology of skill at a peripheral level, the central control mechanisms remain obscure. It is here that engineering models are again valuable since they suggest particular kinds of organization for the psychologist and physiologist to try to identify.

An engineering model of the mechanisms underlying skill is inevitably inadequate not only because it fails to describe the organic structure of the mechanisms but also because it omits certain essential variables. The human operator's performance is affected by emotion and stress and in addition there are large individual differences both in performance under optimal conditions and in response to stress. The concept of level of arousal has been a fruitful one in providing a description of these phenomena. The relation between performance and arousal is a complex one – such that as arousal increases performance initially improves and then later deteriorates. In addition, the general level of arousal varies from task to task, a lower level being optimal for more complex tasks (Colquhoun and Corcoran, 1964; Hebb, 1955; Malmo, 1959). Furthermore this theory also provides a plausible account of some aspects of individual differences in skill and response to stress (Broadbent, 1963; Corcoran, 1965).

The articles in this book illustrate the kind of research and conceptual analysis that have been used in the analysis of perceptual–motor skill. Areas of research which fall outside the definition of perceptual–motor skill have been omitted. However, references to work on vigilance, two-channel listening, complex sensory detection and the design of displays and controls are included in the Further Reading list which will be useful in directing the reader to a fuller study of the literature.

In order to provide a methodological background to reported results experimental papers have generally been included in full. There are one or two exceptions to this principle where certain passages containing technical detail have been omitted in order to save space.

This book of readings has been divided, perhaps somewhat arbitrarily, into seven parts. Part One is basically introductory and describes some of the approaches that have been adopted to the problem of analysing perceptual–motor skill.

Part Two contains four articles about laboratory investigations of particular components of skill. A great deal of the work on reaction time, the control of movements and continuous tracking has been developed on the basis of the theoretical structure provided by the statistical theory of information (Shannon and Weaver, 1949). In these papers are examples of how information theory can provide a valuable index of performance and a means of assessing the capacity of a particular man–machine system. The tasks used in many of these experiments appear to be very simple and to bear little resemblance to the everyday situations in which skills are manifested, but they represent attempts to capture in the laboratory essential components of more complex skills.

Part Three contains three articles concerning the fundamental nature of movement and response modulation. Two important concepts that are developed in this section are those of 'ballistic' movements and the intermittent character of the central response computing mechanism. These three papers provide a historical context for more recent developments in this field which may be followed up in the list of suggestions for further reading. The basic model implied by these analyses is a cybernetic one but clearly, as Craik (1947) stressed, there are critical differences between the ideal system borrowed from engineering and the human operator.

The role of proprioception in perceptual–motor skill is developed in Part Four. The plight of patients with reduced or absent proprioceptive feedback from their limbs illustrates the importance of this sense for motor control (Gibbs, 1954;

Wiener, 1948). However, the precise way in which proprioception contributes to skill is still to be determined. Evidence points to an increasing dependence upon proprioception as a skill improves (Fitts, 1951; Fleishman and Rich, 1963) and decreasing trust in proprioception with increasing age (Welford, 1958). Logically, proprioception can provide some information that might otherwise demand the use of vision and thus to some extent reliance on proprioception reduces the visual load. However, evidence indicates that this load-shedding function introduces other difficulties. Proprioception is basically less precise than vision and, in addition, direct integration of visual and proprioceptive spatial information seems to be impossible (Legge, 1965). Proprioception may also be valuable in other ways. Notterman and Page (1962) have examined the effects of withdrawing augmented proprioceptive feedback from the controls of a complex tracking task while maintaining a complex relation between the controls and the visual display. They show how proprioception provides important intermediate information to the subject which tells him what kinds of response he has made before the delayed change to the visual display has occurred. Removing this information markedly impaired performance.

Proprioception may also help the temporal co-ordination of responses (Adams and Creamer, 1963). It has been suggested that if the speed of proprioceptive feedback is altered then motor performance will be upset. Dinnerstein, Frigyesi and Lowenthal (1962) have developed an explanation of Parkinsonian tremor on the basis of a reduction in the velocity of proprioceptive feedback.

In Part Five there are three articles describing models of the mechanisms underlying perceptual–motor skill. There is a continuing trend for models of this kind to include both physiological and engineering concepts. Some models emphasize the physiological components, others the engineering components. Engineering models tend to be expressed in the form of flow diagrams often with a mathematical specification of the functioning of the system, and the complexity of these models depends upon the kind of skill being modelled. Physiological models are often basically cybernetic models with an explicit attempt to specify the anatomical and physiological identity of the constituents of the cybernetic model. Ultimately a physiologically valid description will be required, but at present it is often more fruitful to approach that goal via the intermediate description provided by the language of cybernetics and information theory

Part Six contains four papers on the acquisition of skill. This topic was one of the earliest to be submitted to experimental study, and Bryan and Harter's (1899) paper influenced a great deal of later work. They believed that as a man's skill at a task improved, it passed through a number of stages characterized by increasing size of the units of organization of the skill. Their evidence implied that improvement was not continuous, but proceeded in discrete steps. Each new improvement was followed by a plateau, perhaps allowing consolidation at that level. Then before the next upward surge in performance there was a decrement that could indicate a reorganization of the underlying mechanisms in a potentially more efficient way, but which temporarily was less effective than the previous kind of organization. Taylor (1943), however, has questioned the generality of plateau phenomena and Crossman (1959) has collated evidence showing continuous improvement for a large number of tasks, and has presented a theory to describe the relationship between performance and degree of practice.

Part Seven is devoted to the breakdown of skill. There are two main reasons for studying decrements in skill. First, it may be important to establish the variety of conditions under which a skill can be performed and this necessitates altering the conditions until the skill shows a decrement. Secondly, by studying the way a skill deteriorates, clues may be obtained showing how it is organized during performance under optimal conditions. Frequently experiments are performed with both aims in view. Some experiments have been carried out in which the essential question was to discover the relation between two or more underlying processes. Legge (1965, 1966) has adopted this approach using nitrous oxide and alcohol, two central nervous depressant drugs, to impair performance. The relative effects of these drugs on different tasks reflect the nature of the underlying processes. In one such experiment (Legge, 1966) alcohol and fatigue (produced by continuous performance) were both shown to affect handwriting (a well-practised skill). Handwriting increased in size. However, the effects of depressant drugs on handwriting can most parsimoniously be accounted for in terms of an effect on perception. Depending upon the way fatigue acts, different patterns of effects of the two variables applied jointly would be predicted. The data showed them to be independent. The drugs decrease the efficiency of the proprioceptive monitoring system demanding an increase in size to compensate for this effect. Fatigue affects responses, making them less discriminable, and this too may be compensated for by an increase in size. This experiment therefore established that depressant drugs and fatigue produce the same observable effect, but act in different ways. It also confirmed that in this kind of skill psychologically meaningful responses (e.g. letters) are more or less continuously monitored by proprioception.

This book presents a number of articles illustrating particular ideas about perceptual–motor skills. It is hoped that the reader will obtain the flavour of research into this field of psychology and, perhaps, develop a taste for reading more.

This book of readings was initiated by Professor G. C. Drew, University College, London. It was a great privilege for me to be asked to edit this selection and I have been most fortunate to have had Professor Drew's advice, support and encouragement throughout. I would like to thank Miss G. R. Hardy for her help with the collection of copy. I am indebted to Miss J. E. Stockdale who assisted with the final preparation of the book for publication.

References

ADAMS, J. A., and CREAMER, L. R. (1963), 'Proprioception variables as determiners of anticipatory timing behaviour', *Human Factors*, vol. 4, pp. 217–22.

BAHRICK, H. P. (1957), 'An analysis of stimulus variables influencing the proprioceptive control of movements', *Psychol. Rev.*, vol. 64, pp. 324–8.

BARTLETT, F. C. (1947), 'The measurement of human skill', *Brit. med. J.*, vol. 1, pp. 835–8, 877–80.

BROADBENT, D. E. (1963), 'Possibilities and difficulties in the concept of arousal', in *Vigilance: a Symposium*, McGraw-Hill.

BRYAN, W. L., and HARTER, N. (1899), 'Studies in the telegraphic language: the acquisition of a hierarchy of habits', *Psychol. Rev.*, vol. 6, pp. 345–75.

COLQUHOUN, W. P., and CORCORAN, D. W. J. (1964), 'The influence of time of day and social isolation on the relationship of temperament to performance', *Brit. J. soc. clin. Psychol.*, vol. 3, pp. 226–31.

CORCORAN, D. W. J. (1965), 'Personality and the inverted-U relation', *Brit. J. Psychol.*, vol. 56, pp. 267–73.

CRAIK, K. J. W. (1947), 'Theory of the human operator. I. The operator as an engineering system', *Brit. J. Psychol.*, vol. 38, pp. 56–61.

CROSSMAN, E. R. F. W. (1959), 'A theory of the acquisition of speed-skill', *Ergonomics*, vol. 2, pp. 153–66.

DINNERSTEIN, A. J., FRIGYESI, T., and LOWENTHAL, M. (1962), 'Delayed feedback as a possible mechanism in Parkinsonism', *Percept. mot. Skills*, vol. 15, pp. 667–80.

FITTS, P. M. (1951), 'Engineering psychology and equipment design', in S. S. Stevens, (ed.), *Handbook of Experimental Psychology*, Wiley.

FLEISHMAN, E. A., and RICH, S. (1963), 'Role of kinaesthetic and spatial–visual abilities in perceptual–motor learning', *J. exp. Psychol.*, vol. 66, pp. 6–11.

GIBBS, C. B. (1954), 'The continuous regulation of skilled responses by kinaesthetic feedback', *Brit. J. Psychol.*, vol. 45, pp. 24–39.

HEBB, D. O. (1955), 'Drives and the C.N.S. (Conceptual Nervous System)', *Psychol. Rev.*, vol. 62, pp. 243–54.

HULL, C. L. (1943), *Principles of Behavior*, Yale University Press.

HULL, C. L. (1952), *A Behavior System*, Yale University Press.

LASHLEY, K. S. (1951), 'The problem of serial order in behavior', in L. A. Jeffress, (ed.), *Cerebral Mechanisms in Behavior: The Hixon Symposium*, Wiley.

LEGGE, D. (1965), 'Analysis of visual and proprioceptive components of motor skill by means of a drug', *Brit. J. Psychol.*, vol. 56, pp. 245–54.

LEGGE, D. (1966), 'Attention, drugs and skill', *Proc. XVIII Int. Cong. Psychol., Moscow*.

MALMO, R. B. (1959), 'Activation: a neuropsychological dimension', *Psychol. Rev.*, vol. 66, pp. 367–86.

NOTTERMAN, J. M., and PAGE, D. E. (1962), 'Evaluation of mathematically equivalent tracking systems', *Percept. mot. Skills*, vol. 15, pp. 683–716.

SHANNON, C. E., and WEAVER, W. (1949), *The Mathematical Theory of Communication*, University of Illinois Press.

SHERRINGTON, C. S. (1906), 'On the proprioceptive system, especially its reflex aspect', *Brain*, vol. 29, pp. 467–82.

TAYLOR, D. W. (1943), 'Learning telegraphic code', *Psychol. Bull.*, vol. 40, pp. 461–87.

THORNDIKE, E. L. (1913), *Educational Psychology. Vol. II. The Psychology of Learning*, Teachers College, Columbia University.

THORNDIKE, E. L. (1932), *The Fundamentals of Learning*, Teachers College, Columbia University.

TOLMAN, E. C. (1932), *Purposive Behavior in Animals and Man*, Appleton-Century-Crofts.

WELFORD, A. T. (1958), *Ageing and Human Skill*, Oxford University Press.

WIENER, N. (1948) *Cybernetics*, Wiley.

WOODWORTH, R. S. (1899), 'The accuracy of voluntary movement', *Psychol. Rev. Monogr. Suppl.*, vol. 3, whole no. 13.

Part One The Nature and Assessment of Skill

The layman tends to reserve the term skill for performance that demands respect and is frequently only attained after a long period of practice. The psychologist uses the word in a wider sense. Welford (Reading 1) discusses the psychological usage of the word skill and stresses the flexible nature of the mechanisms underlying behaviour. In so doing, he describes a basic model of the underlying processes. The modern views about these processes owe much to the radical views advanced by Lashley (Reading 2) who was instrumental in breaking the research traditions based upon classical S–R chain theories of behaviour.

Two very different approaches to the analysis and assessment of skill are represented by Fleishman (Reading 3) and Fitts and Posner (Reading 4). Using factor analysis Fleishman shows a way of determining the basic units of skill, while Fitts and Posner show how information theory provides a means of quantifying skilled behaviour.

1 A. T. Welford

On the Nature of Skill

Excerpt from chapter 2 of A. T. Welford, *Ageing and Human Skill*, Oxford University Press for the Nuffield Foundation, 1958, pp. 17–27.

The term 'skill' is used somewhat differently in industry and in psychology. In the former a man is regarded as skilled when he is qualified to carry out trade or craft work involving knowledge, judgement, accuracy and manual deftness usually acquired as the result of a long training, whereas an unskilled man is not expected to do anything which cannot be learnt in a relatively short time. Semi-skilled jobs are regarded as intermediate, involving the characteristics of skilled work but to an extent which demands a training extending over weeks or months rather than years. The fundamental questions of interest to those concerned with industry are: 'What characteristics in a job will make it easy or difficult for any given man to learn it?' and 'Which jobs will require a man who has been through an apprenticeship and which will require a shorter training?' In other words, one asks what is it that differentiates between work which makes greater and lesser demands for training. The picture is not, of course, in practice quite as simple as this. Industrial organizations show, as do all social institutions, a degree of inertia so that in the course of time jobs may change in character but not in grading as regards skill. In these cases, the skill-demands of a job may be largely a matter of its history. Again, classification in terms of training is clearly too narrow, as some recent attempts to give a skill-rating to *responsibility* have recognized.

A psychologist's approach is to ask the question: 'When we look at a man working, by what criteria in his performance can we tell whether he is skilled and competent or clumsy and ignorant?' In other words, he asks: 'How is complex performance organized and what is it that differentiates between more and less trained or expert levels?' The psychological concept of skill is thus wider than the industrial in two ways. Firstly, skill in the psychological sense can exist in the performance of many jobs which in industry would be graded as semi-skilled or unskilled. Secondly, and more important, the psychological use of the term covers so-called 'mental' operations as well as manual. Indeed, from the psychological standpoint, the distinction between manual and mental skill is difficult to maintain in any absolute sense. All skilled performance is mental in the sense that knowledge and judgement are required, and all skills involve some kind of co-ordinated overt activity by hands, organs of speech or other effectors. In manual skills the overt actions clearly form an essential part of the activity and without them the purpose of the skill as a whole would disappear. In mental skills the overt actions play a more incidental part, serving rather to give expression to a skill than forming an essential part of it. They thus may be varied within fairly wide limits without destroying the nature of the underlying skill.

In spite of these differences all skills, industrial and psychological, motor and mental, appear to possess three characteristics[1] which provide us with a convenient framework for discussion:

1. They consist essentially of the building of an organized and co-ordinated activity in relation to an object or a situation and thus involve the whole chain of sensory, central and motor mechanisms which underlie performance.

2. They are learnt in that the understanding of the object or situation and the form of the action are built up gradually in the course of repeated experience.

3. They are serial in the sense that within the over-all pattern of the skill many different processes or actions are ordered and co-ordinated in a temporal sequence.

Within any skilled performance these characteristics are closely bound together, and in order to gain an adequate view of the nature of skill all must be considered.

1. Discussions of parts 2 and 3 are not included in this excerpt.

A. T. Welford

The Receptor–Effector Aspect of Skill

We may think of the chain of processes which leads from stimulation falling on the sense organs to the resulting behaviour as being in three parts. First, there are what may be called *receptor* processes which have to do with the reception of the incoming signals by the sense organs and their interpretation. At the opposite end of the chain are what may be called *effector* processes which shape and carry out the resulting action. Between these there occur what may be termed *translation* processes which relate perception to action. It is not always easy to decide in a particular case where the line should be drawn between receptor and translation processes or between translation and effector, but many cases seem clear enough to show that the distinction ought to be made.

We shall consider these three types of processes in turn.

The receptor side

Skilled performance would seem in the first instance to depend upon two important principles of what may be broadly termed perception: first, that perception is essentially an *organizing process*, and second that in this process *past actions and experience* play a leading role.

Organization in perception. Between the receipt of stimuli by the sense organs and the attainment of meaningful perception it seems that a chain of processes occur which are of considerable complexity, although often they take place so quickly that they are quite unconscious and perception appears to be 'immediate'. The broad fact that these are organizing processes is obvious enough. For instance, in visual perception the incoming data from the eyes are integrated, grouped and ordered so that normally we see not just a mosaic of more and less stimulated points, but coherent objects which have form and structure. It is also obvious that normally we do not perceive with only one sense at a time, but that data from different senses are organized together, and that the resulting perception, although it is predominantly, say, visual or auditory, has been partly shaped by stimuli coming through other sensory channels. A well-known

23

example is the fact that it seems easier to hear what a man is saying if we can also see him speaking.

The process of grouping and organizing may be thought of as consisting essentially of the *abstraction of constants* from the total mass of data presented in space and over time, together with the selection of some data as dominant and important while the rest are relegated to the background and more or less neglected. This process makes perception substantially independent of the precise details of stimulation – words are, in an important sense, the same whether written, printed or spoken. Data thus organized are no longer treated as complexes compounded out of a multitude of separate elements, but as *single units*. The perceived wholes are thus in a very real sense 'simpler' than the stimuli giving rise to them. Psychological simplicity is, in fact, not the same thing as objective simplicity, but is essentially dependent upon the degree to which the data can be organized into larger units of this kind.

It appears that such a treatment of the data is by no means the end of the perceptual process but that it is often – probably typically – followed by one or more of three further types of organizing activity. Firstly, a unitary whole which has been built up may be analysed into parts, as when we examine an object in detail. This analysis, although it involves breaking up a whole into smaller units, is not simply the reverse of the unifying process: each of the parts is itself a unified whole and each is still recognized as belonging within the framework of the larger whole out of which it has been analysed. Secondly, certain features of the whole may be further abstracted and become perceptual units on their own: for instance, when reading a passage of prose we may become aware of features such as style. Thirdly, a number of unitary wholes may themselves be subjected to further processes of selection and integration which result in the formation of still larger units, as when reading we integrate words into sentences, sentences into paragraphs and so on.

Although perceptual units built up in these ways may appear in consciousness as being present 'all at once', they often result from the integration of data which are not all present at the same instant, but which extend over a considerable period of time.

When reading, for instance, the material organized into a paragraph has taken an appreciable time to observe. In perceiving an object which is too large to observe at a single glance, we are putting together data from many individual glances which may have taken place over several seconds or even minutes. Some perceptual units, such as musical themes or visually seen movement, have indeed an essentially temporal character, the perceived wholes being by their very nature configurations in which time is a necessary dimension.

The number of stages passed through on the way to full meaningful perception probably tends to vary somewhat between individuals and within the same individual according to circumstances. The same is true of the time taken: often they occur, as we have already said, very rapidly; often, however, they take a considerable time, so that it is impossible to draw a hard and fast line between perception and thinking.

Whether rapid or slow, perception seems to involve mental activity and effort by the observer, so that the attainment of meaningful perception is not a mere process of 'registration', but is essentially a kind of *response* to the material presented. We may conveniently call this a *perceptual response* to distinguish it from the overt action which may be taken in dealing with the presented material once it has been perceived.

The role of past experience. Some of this organization is doubtless the result of the hereditary constitution of the organism. Certainly hereditary constitution sets some *limits* to the organization which takes place in the sense that we cannot do what we have no inherited potentiality for doing. But it is clear that for almost all important purposes organization at each stage of the perceptual process represents the application to the incoming sense data of material brought by the observer to the present situation from the past. In precisely what form this 'past' is available for use in the present is not known, but a number of important principles of the *manner in which it is used* are known with fair certainty. This fitting of terms from past experience to incoming data is part of the process of giving them 'meaning'. The word is confusing, however, because it is used to cover three rather different types of process, namely *identification*, *setting in a*

25

context and *significance for ensuing action.* It is the first two that concern us here, the last belonging more properly to a discussion of the translation process.

As regards identification, perception is, as we have seen, essentially an integrative process if it is considered in terms of incoming data, but in terms of the results achieved it is a matter of discriminating or differentiating one object from another, of recognizing similarities and differences. The process of identification involves placing the object presented to our senses in one of a number of categories provided by our past experience. The categories may be broad and general or narrow and precise and it would seem that the amount of data required and of 'perceptual work' increases as the categories become more specific. Thus when crossing a road, the identification of an on-coming vehicle as a car rather than a lorry, omnibus, etc., is easier and quicker than if we have to specify the make, colour, style and other details of the car.

The progressive, hierarchical nature of the classification by which objects are identified in perception is shown by the fact that often an object is specified as belonging to a particular major class with some extra detail which enables it to be placed in a subclass. For example, we may say a vehicle is an *omnibus* painted *red.* The classes and subclasses appear to behave as unitary 'codes' applied to incoming material in such a way that it is invested with all the characteristics normally associated with the class or subclass concerned. In this way a great deal of 'perceived' detail is not really perceived but inferred, in the sense not only that some detail not actually present is believed to be so, but also that some detail in fact present is not observed. Usually, although not always, the inference is either correct or not in serious error, and this fact results in a substantial economy of effort in perception. The concept of 'economy of effort' or 'economy of specification' appears to be of widespread application to perception and to hold out important possibilities of quantitative treatment (Attneave, 1954; Hochberg and McAlister, 1953).

While identification may be thought of as the aligning of present data with past experience similar to them, placing presently perceived objects into a context or 'framework' involves setting them in relation to other things very unlike themselves. This framework or setting is both spatial and temporal, so that an object is perceived as located in space, for example in a room or in relation to other objects such as the controls of a machine; and events are perceived as localized in time, and series of events can be perceived as forming sequences and rhythms. Some kind of simultaneous spatial and temporal reference enables movement and causal relationships to be perceived.

The relating of data to past material does not always take place after the data have been received: some of the perceptual 'work' involved is often, indeed usually, done beforehand and this enables identification to be made more easily and quickly when the data actually arrive. It seems that this can be done in one of three ways. Firstly, we may know definitely that certain major categories of possible identifications are excluded. Thus, we find it easier to identify a series of pictures if we know in advance that they will all be of, say, animals than if they may also include buildings, scenery and various other types of object. We shall even find it easier if we know that *most* of the pictures will belong to a particular category so that there is a bias in favour of one category as opposed to others. Secondly, terms from past experience having an essentially sequential character will imply future events as soon as the initial member of the sequence is identified. Thus, for instance, having identified a tune by the first few bars, we are expecting the remainder. Thirdly, we seem able to use the various present data and material from past experience to, as it were, 'compute' predictions of future events and by doing so we are able to expect sequences we have never experienced before.

It would seem that in everyday perception we unconsciously use these various methods to build up a kind of running hypothesis constantly predicting a little ahead of events. The accuracy attained is usually sufficient to effect a very considerable saving of time in dealing with moment-to-moment events, and indeed renders us unaware of most of them, leaving only the rare, unexpected events to engage our conscious attention. This constant prediction enables action to be taken which has reference not to the state of affairs immediately present, but to a state that is expected to exist in the future, as for instance when, in driving a car, adjustments of the controls are made not to the present positions of vehicles on the road, but to the positions they will occupy a few seconds hence.

The result of this continual short-term prediction is that when incoming data are familiar they are identified and fitted into context *immediately* and without any intervention of consciousness. When, however, data are novel or unexpected, there seems to be an active search for terms of past experience which are 'fitting' or 'appropriate', and there may be use of images, searching for analogies, and a considerable amount of trial and rejection before satisfaction is reached.

Each new perceptual response leaves the observer different from what he was before, so that the 'past' which he brings to deal with any new data is in some way changed. The amount of change may, of course, be either small or large and will depend to some extent on the time scale involved – a series of small changes from second to second may add up to a large change over a longer period. Whether small or great, however, it appears not to be due to the mere addition of another experience to a 'stock' already existing. The past experience brought to deal with any incoming signal seems not to consist of an aggregate of past impressions, but appears to be in an organized or *schematized* form which is affected by each new impression in a manner which can be compared to the *modification* of a 'plastic' model.

The translation process

The relating of perception to action is a process which is often thought of as an aspect of perception, constituting the forward-looking part of 'meaning' in the sense that it confers upon perception significance for subsequent action. Alternatively, it might be regarded as a preliminary stage of the effector process. It would seem, however, to be sufficiently distinct from both to be considered separately as a link between the two.

A good example, as the term implies, is translation from one language to another: material perceived in the one language must be converted into the other to make a verbal or written response. Other examples are contained in the use of codes of various kinds. Most important for skilled performance are relationships between display and control studied under that title by many authors (e.g. Garvey *et al.*, 1954, 1955), under the heading of 'stimulus–response compatibility' by Fitts *et al.* (1953, 1954) and under the title of 'transformations' by Crossman (1956).

When lifting an object by hand from one position and putting it down in another the relationship between what is seen and what is done is straightforward. The actions of the hand are closely related to the perceived positions and movements of the object. Similarly direct relationships between what is seen and done obtain when using hand tools. With machine tools and other mechanical and electronic devices, however, the relationship between perception and action may be complicated in several ways. For instance, a side-to-side motion of a pointer on a scale may result from a rotary motion of a control knob. Or again, the force required on a control lever may bear no directly linear relationship to the force it controls.

Many translations seem to be, as it were, ready to hand or 'built into' the repertoire that a man can bring to bear upon a task. This is obviously so in the case of direct hand movements, and, for most people, of such basic educational attainments as reading. It also applies to machine controls with which certain 'expected' relationships between actions and their effects have been demonstrated. Thus, for instance, clockwise rotation of a knob is expected to make the pointer of a horizontal scale above it move from left to right. Or to take a more homely illustration, most people would be confused by a tap that had to be rotated anti-clockwise to turn it off. These display–control relationships are learnt in the course of experience and their precise form is thus more a matter of individual experience channelled by social convention than of any fundamental characteristic of the organism. Doubtless almost any set of relationships could be learnt in time. They seem to be much easier to master, however, if those in any one set are all consistent according to a single rule than if different rules apply to different displays and controls. It thus appears that, like perception, the translation process works on an economy principle in the sense that if a single translation can be applied to all display–control relationships, or at least all in a given task, less data have to be carried by the subject's memory and less uncertainty arises when any control has to be used.

In a task for which no translation has already been built up the subject has to construct one *ad hoc*. An elaborate case of this would arise in the breaking of an unknown code. A very simple case is that of making movements when all we can see of what we are doing is in a mirror. Left–right movements are normally not affected and cause little difficulty. Back and forth movements are, however, reversed and make it surprisingly (to most people) difficult to trace a design seen in a mirror. It frequently seems possible to analyse these translations into one or more specifiable stages of spatial, symbolic or other transformation. Thus, in the mirror case we have to make a single spatial transformation of the far–near dimension.

Once a rule of translation has been built up, putting it into use can often precede the signal which would normally initiate it. When a particular signal or type of signal is expected we can often carry out the translation process and prepare responding action before it arrives so that when it does, it, as it were, triggers off a pre-formed response.

The effector side

The translation process may be thought of as a response to perception and in turn as a stimulus to effector action, initiating a chain of events containing a series of stages which are, in an important sense, the reverse of those leading from an external stimulus to perception. That is to say, there is a transition from a unitary integrated process to a series of detailed muscular movements. The nature of the events on the effector side is not at all well known – no doubt because they are usually unconscious – but it seems clear that they involve a progressive differentiation and particularization.

The first of them is probably some kind of general *orientation* or *attitude* which determines in broad outline what is to be done. Next, perhaps, come what may be called *general methods* of dealing with the object or situation concerned, and these are followed by particular *knacks* and *dexterities* which in turn bring into play detailed muscular movements.

It should be noted that throughout the functioning of the effector side there seems again to be an organizational quality which is similar in several important ways to that of the receptor side. In particular:

1. At each stage there is the use of pre-existing patterns of response. As with the receptor side, some of these may be innate; but it again seems clear that, though their limits are set by innate capability, this limitation is in most cases small compared with the influence of past learning and experience.

2. The organization of muscular movements produced by the effector side has a reference which is not only spatial but also temporal, so that movements do not occur as isolated units but are bound into sequences. This is especially noticeable when actions are performed in a rhythmical manner, but is an essential characteristic of all manipulative operations and, indeed, of all bodily movements except the very simplest reflexes. In this connexion it is to be noted that, just as a series of signals may lead to a single perceptual response, so a single translation may lead to a series of actions.

3. The attitudes, methods, knacks and so forth which are brought into play in the building of effector action show a generalized quality in that they do not lead to exact stereotyped muscular movements. The actual movements made on any occasion are adapted to the requirements of that occasion, and, as these requirements are never quite the same twice, the precise way in which the actual movements occur varies from one occasion to the next, even when a performance is nominally repeated exactly.

Human performance appears to be almost infinitely variable. It is often assumed that we achieve this variation because we acquire in the course of time a very large number of pre-formed responses which can be put to use as occasion requires. The variability of the performance seems, however, too great to be reasonably accounted for in this way except in a few very special cases. It would appear better to think of the central mechanisms as capable of producing a response which is formed *ad hoc* by a kind of 'calculation' based on many influences derived from the present aims and past experience of the subject and the sensory data of various kinds available at the time. We should, in other words, think, as Craik (1943) urged, of the whole receptor, translatory and effector system as a kind of calculating machine capable of receiving several different inputs and producing an output which is derived from the various input parameters acting in concert. Such a system results in a response which is unique on each occasion, although it is determinate and based on constants which are, at least in principle, discoverable.

References

ATTNEAVE, F. (1954), 'Some informational aspects of visual perception', *Psychol. Rev.*, vol. 61, pp. 183–93.

CRAIK, K. J. W. (1943), *The Nature of Explanation*, Cambridge University Press.

CROSSMAN, E. R. F. W. (1956), 'The information capacity of the human operator in symbolic and non-symbolic control processes', in Ministry of Supply Publication WR/D 2/56, *Information Theory and the Human Operator*.

FITTS, P. M., and DEINIGER, R. L. (1954), 'S–R compatibility: correspondence among paired elements within stimulus and response codes', *J. exp. Psychol.*, vol. 48, pp. 483–92.

FITTS, P. M., and SEEGER, C. M. (1953), 'S–R compatibility: spatial characteristics of stimulus and response codes', *J. exp. Psychol.*, vol. 46, pp. 199–210.

GARVEY, W. D., and KNOWLES, W. B. (1954), 'Response time patterns associated with various display–control relationships', *J. exp. Psychol.*, vol. 47, pp. 315–22.

GARVEY, W. D., and MITNICK, L. L. (1955), 'Effects of additional spatial references on display–control efficiency', *J. exp. Psychol.*, vol. 50, pp. 276–82.

HOCHBERG, J., and McALISTER, E. (1953), 'A quantitative approach to figural "goodness"', *J. exp. Psychol.*, vol. 46, pp. 361–4.

2 K. S. Lashley

The Problem of Serial Order in Behaviour

Excerpt from K. S. Lashley, 'The problem of serial order in behavior', in L. A. Jeffress (ed.), *Cerebral Mechanisms in Behavior: The Hixon Symposium*, Wiley and Chapman & Hall, 1951, pp. 122–30. (Page references of Wiley edition.)

A consideration of the control of extent and rate of movement supports the view that sensory factors play a minor part in regulating the intensity and duration of nervous discharge; that a series of movements is not a chain of sensory–motor reactions. The theory of control of movement which was dominant at the turn of the century assumed that, after a movement is initiated, it is continued until stopped by sensations of movement and position, which indicate that the limb has reached the desired position. This theory was opposed by a good bit of indirect evidence, such as that accuracy of movement is increased rather than diminished with speed. I had opportunity to study a patient who had a complete anesthesia for movements of the knee joint, as a result of a gunshot wound of the cord (Lashley, 1917). In spite of the anesthesia, he was able to control the extent and speed of movements of flexion and extension of the knee quite as accurately as can a normal person.

The performance of very quick movements also indicates their independence of current control. 'Whip-snapping' movements of the hand can be regulated accurately in extent, yet the entire movement, from initiation to completion, requires less than the reaction time for tactile or kinesthetic stimulation of the arm, which is about one-eighth of a second, even when no discrimination is involved. Such facts force the conclusion that an effector mechanism can be pre-set or primed to discharge at a given intensity or for a given duration, in independence of any sensory controls.

Central Control of Motor Patterns

This independence of sensory controls is true not only of intensity and duration of contraction of a synergic muscle group but is true also of the initiation and timing of contraction of the different muscles in a complex movement. The hand may describe a circular movement involving coordinated contractions of the muscles of the shoulder, elbow and wrist in about one-tenth of a second, and the stopping of movement at a given position, of course, is only a small fraction of that time. The finger strokes of a musician may reach sixteen per second in passages which call for a definite and changing order of successive finger movements. The succession of movements is too quick even for visual reaction time. In rapid sight reading it is impossible to read the individual notes of an arpeggio. The notes must be seen in groups, and it is actually easier to read chords seen simultaneously and to translate them into temporal sequence than to read successive notes in the arpeggio as usually written.

Sensory control of movement seems to be ruled out in such acts. They require the postulation of some central nervous mechanism which fires with predetermined intensity and duration or activates different muscles in predetermined order. This mechanism might be represented by a chain of effector neurons, linked together by internuncials to produce successive delays in firing. In some systems the order of action may be determined by such a leader or pace setter. Buddenbrock (1921) has shown for the stick insect, and Bethe (1931) for a number of animals from the centipede to the dog, that removal of one or more legs results in a spontaneous change in the order of stepping. Thus, for the insects, the normal order is alternate stepping of the first pair of legs with right first, left second, right third leg advancing together. With removal of the left first leg, the right first and left second alternate and the order becomes right first, left third, right third stepping together, with left second and right second advancing together, instead of alternately. These investigators were interested in spontaneity of reorganization, rather than in the mechanism of coordination, and did not propose any theory for the latter. They did show, however, that it is necessary to remove the leg completely to get the change in pattern of movement; sensory impulses from a limb stump would prevent it. Such coordination might be explained, perhaps, by a combination of loss of excitability in the centers of the absent limb, by the excitation of the remaining anterior center as a leader or pace setter, and the spread of alternate waves of inhibition and excitation from the more anterior to the more posterior limb centers. The spontaneous change in coordination shows, however, that the coordination is not due to the action of predetermined anatomic paths but is the result of the current physiological state of the various limb centers.

Such an hypothesis implies also the assumption of a polarization of conduction along the neuraxis, with the order of excitation determined by the spatial arrangement of the centers of the legs. I see no other possibility of accounting for the facts. The examples of circular movement and of finger coordination, involving temporal integration of movements, seem to call for a similar hypothesis. They might be ascribed to an habitual linkage of the movements through a simple chain of internuncials but for two facts. First, such series are usually reversible at any point or can be started from any point. This would require the assumption of a second set of internuncials habituated to conduct in the opposite direction, and this in turn leads to the further assumption of a polarization of conduction. Second, such patterns of coordinated movement may often be transferred directly to other motor systems than the ones practiced. In such transfer, as to the left hand for writing, an analysis of the movements shows that there is not a reduplication of the muscular patterns on the two sides, but a reproduction of movements in relation to the space coordinates of the body. Try upside-down mirror writing with the left hand and with eyes closed for evidence of this. The associative linkage is not of specific movements but of directions of movement. An analysis of systems of space coordinates suggests mechanisms which may contribute to production of such series of movements in a spatial pattern.

Space Coordinate Systems

The work of Sherrington, Magnus and others on postural tonus and reflexes has defined one level of spatial integration rather fully, yet it is doubtful if these studies have revealed the effective neural mechanism. The work has shown that the tonic discharge to every muscle in the postural system is influenced by afferent impulses from every other muscle, toward increased or decreased activity, according to its synergic or antergic action. To these influences are added vestibular and cerebellar effects. Diagrammatically these mutual influences of the muscular system may be represented by separate reflex circuits from each receptor to every muscle, as Sherrington (1906, p. 148) has done. But no neuroanatomist would, I am sure, maintain that such separate circuits or paths exist. What the experiments on posture actually show is a correlation of sensory stimulation and of tonic changes in a network of neurons whose interconnexions are still undefined. The reactions isolated experimentally have the characteristics of simple directly conducted reflexes, but their combination results in patterns of movement and posture which have definite relations to the axes of the body and to gravity.

This postural system is based on excitations from proprioceptors. The distance receptors impose an additional set of space coordinates upon the postural system, which in turn continually modifies the coordinates of the distance receptors. The dropped cat rights itself, if either the eyes or the vestibular senses are intact, but not in the absence of both. The direction of movement on the retina imposes a directional orientation on the postural system. Conversely, the gravitational system imposes an orientation on the visual field. Upright objects such as trees or the corners of a room appear upright, at no matter what angle the head is inclined. Derangement of the vestibular system can disturb the distance orientation or the orientation of the receptors, as in the apparent swaying of the vertical as a result of the after-images of motion following hours of rocking in a small boat.

There are other, still more generalized systems of space coordinates. We usually keep track of the compass points or of some more definite index of direction by a temporal summation of the turns made in walking, though not always with success. Finally, there is a still more plastic system in which the concepts of spatial relations can be voluntarily reversed, as when one plays blindfold chess alternately from either side of the board.

Explanation of these activities, these complex interactions, in terms of simple isolated interconnexions of all the sensory and motor elements involved seems quite improbable on anatomic grounds and is ruled out by results of our experiments on sectioning of the spinal cord. Ingebritzen (1933) studied rats with double hemisection of the cord; one-half of the cord cut at the second, the other at the fifth cervical segment. In the best case only a small strand of the spinocerebellar tract of one side remained intact. These rats were able to balance in walking, oriented to visual stimuli, scratched with the right or left hind foot according to the side of the face stimulated, were able to run mazes correctly, and even learned to rise on the hindfeet and push down a lever with the forepaws in opening a box.

The alternative to the isolated-path theory of the space coordinates is that the various impulses which modify postural tonus are poured into a continuous network of neurons, where their summated action results in a sort of polarization of the entire system. I shall consider later the integrative properties of such a net. For the moment I wish to emphasize only the existence of these systems of space coordinates. Their influences pervade the motor system so that every gross movement of limbs or body is made with reference to the space system. The perceptions from the distance receptors, vision, hearing and touch are also constantly modified and referred to the same space coordinates. The stimulus is *there*, in a definite place; it has definite relation to the position of the body, and it shifts with respect to the sense organ but not with respect to the general orientation, with changes in body posture.

Memories of objects usually give them position in the space system, and even more abstract concepts may have definite spatial reference. Thus, for many people, the cardinal numbers have definite positions on a spiral or other complicated figure. What, if anything, such space characters can contribute to temporal integration is an open question. They provide a possible basis for some serial actions through interaction of postural and timing mechanisms.

Rhythmic Action

The simplest of the timing mechanisms are those controlling rhythmic activity. T. Graham Brown (1914) first showed by his studies of deafferented preparations that the rhythmic movements of respiration and progression are independent of peripheral stimulation and are maintained by a central nervous mechanism of reciprocal innervation. He suggested that this mechanism of reciprocal innervation, rather than the simple reflex, is the unit of organization of the whole nervous system. He thus foreshadowed, in a way, the conception of reverberatory circuits which is coming to play so large a part in neurological theory today. Holst (1937) has recently shown that the rhythmic movement of the dorsal fin of fishes is a compound of two superimposed rhythms, that of its own innervation and that of the pectoral fins. These two rhythms are centrally maintained.

Musical rhythms seem to be an elaboration of the same sort of thing. The time or beat is started and maintained at some definite rate, say 160 per minute. This rate is then imposed upon various activities. The fingers of the musician fall in multiples of the basic rate. If the leader of a quartet speeds up the time or retards, all the movements of the players change in rate accordingly. Not only the time of initiation but also the rate of movement is affected. The violinist, in a passage requiring the whole bow, will draw the bow from frog to tip at a uniform rate for the required number of beats, whether the tempo is fast or slow. With practiced violinists, the rate of movement is extremely accurate and comes out on the beat at the exact tip of the bow.

Superimposed on this primary rhythm is a secondary one of emphasis, giving the character of 3/4, 4/4, 6/4, or other time. The mechanism of these rhythms can be simply conceived as the spread of excitation from some centers organized for reciprocal innervation; as a combination of the principles of Brown and of Holst. There are, however, still more complicated rhythms in all music. That of the melodic line is most uniform. In much music, the melodic progression changes in two, four, or some multiple of four measures. In improvisation, the performer keeps no count of measures, yet comes out almost invariably in a resolution to the tonic of the key after some multiple of eight measures.

Here a generalized pattern is impressed on the sequence, but it is a simpler pattern than that of grammatical structure. It only requires the recurrence of a pattern at certain rhythmic intervals; a pick-up of a specific pattern after so many timed intervals.

There are, in addition, still less regular rhythms of phrasing and emphasis. Parallels to these can be found in speech. The skilled extemporaneous speaker rounds his phrases and speaks with a definite though not regular rhythm.

The rhythms tend to spread to almost every other concurrent activity. One falls into step with a band, tends to breathe and even to speak in time with the rhythm. The all pervasiveness of the rhythmic discharge is shown by the great difficulty of learning to maintain two rhythms at once, as in three against four with the two hands. The points to be emphasized here are the widespread effects of a rhythmic discharge indicating the involvement of almost the entire effector system, the concurrent action of different rhythmic systems, and the imposition of the rate upon both the initiation and speed of movement. Consideration of rhythmic activity and of spatial orientation forces the conclusion, I believe, that there exist in the nervous organization, elaborate systems of interrelated neurons capable of imposing certain types of integration upon a large number of widely spaced effector elements; in the one case transmitting temporally spaced waves of facilitative excitation to all effector elements; in the other imparting a directional polarization to both receptor and effector elements. These systems are in constant action. They form a sort of substratum upon which other activity is built. They contribute to every perception and to every integrated movement.

Interaction of Temporal and Spatial Systems

Integration ascribed to the spatial distribution of excitations in the nervous system has been much more intensively studied than the temporal aspects of nervous activity. Theories of integration are based almost exclusively upon space properties, time entering only in theories of facilitation, inhibition and after-discharge. In cerebral functions, however, it is difficult to distinguish between spatial and temporal functions. The eye is the only organ that gives simultaneous information concerning space in any detail. The shape of an object impressed on the skin can scarcely be detected from simultaneous pressure, but the same shape can readily be distinguished by touch when traced on the skin with a moving point or when explored by tactile scanning. The temporal sequence is readily translated into a spatial concept. Even for vision it might be questioned whether simultaneous stimulation gives rise directly to space concepts. The visual object is generally surveyed by eye movements, and its form is a reconstruction from such a series of excitations. Even with tachistoscopic exposures, the after-discharge permits a temporal survey, and, with visual fixation, shifts of attention provide an effective scanning.

Since memory traces are, we believe, in large part static and persist simultaneously, it must be assumed that they are spatially differentiated. Nevertheless, reproductive memory appears almost invariably as a temporal sequence, either as a succession of words or of acts. Even descriptions of visual imagery (the supposed simultaneous reproductive memory in sensory terms) are generally descriptions of sequences, of temporal reconstructions from very fragmentary and questionable visual elements. Spatial and temporal order thus appear to be almost completely interchangeable in cerebral action. The translation from the spatial distribution of memory traces to temporal sequence seems to be a fundamental aspect of the problem of serial order.

I spoke earlier of the probability of a partial activation or priming of aggregates of words before the sentence is actually formulated from them. There is a great deal of evidence for such preliminary facilitation of patterns of action in studies of reaction time and of word association. Reaction time, in general, is reduced by preliminary warning or by instructions which allow the subject to prepare for the specific act required. In controlled association experiments, the subject is instructed to respond to the stimulus word by a word having a certain type of relation to it, such as the opposite or a part of which the stimulus is the whole; black–white, apple–seed. The result is an attitude or set which causes that particular category to dominate the associative reaction. Whether such preliminary reinforcement is to be ascribed to accumulation of excitatory state, as defined by Sherrington (1906), or to some other physiological process, the facts of behavior assure that it is a genuine phenomenon and plays a decisive role in determining the character of the response.

Once the existence of such states of partial activation is recognized, their possible role in temporal integration must be considered. There are indications that one neural system may be held in this affair of partial excitation while it is scanned by another. Here is an example. A series of four to six numbers is heard: 3–7–2–9–4. This is within the attention or memory span and is almost certainly not remembered in the sense in which one's telephone number is remembered, for memory of it is immediately wiped out by a succeeding series of numbers. While it is retained in this unstable way, subject to retroactive inhibition, the order of the numbers can be reassorted: 3–7–2–9–4, 3–2–7–9–4, 4–9–2–7–3 and the like. It is as if, in this case, a rhythmic alternation can suppress alternate items, or a direction of arousal can be applied to the partially excited system. Another example which illustrates even more clearly the spatial characteristics of many memory traces is the method of comultiplication, used in rapid mental calculation. In attempts to play a melody backward, we have a further illustration. I find that I can do it only by visualizing the music spatially and then reading it backward. I cannot auditorily transform even 'Yankee Doodle' into its inverse without some such process, but it is possible to get a spatial representation of the melody and then to scan the spatial representation. The scanning of a spatial arrangement seems definitely to determine, in such cases, the order of procedure. Two assumptions are implied by this. First, the assumption is that the memory traces are associated, not only with other memory traces, but also with the system of space coordinates. By this I do not mean that the engram has a definite location in the brain; our experiments show conclusively that such is not the case. Rather, when the memory trace is formed it is integrated with directional characters of the space system, which give it position in reference to other associated traces. Second, the assumption is that these space characters of the memory trace can be scanned by some other level of the coordinating system and so transformed into succession.

This is as far as I have been able to go toward a theory of serial order in action. Obviously, it is inadequate. The assumption concerning spatial representation and temporal representation may even beg the question, since no one can say whether spatial or temporal order is primary. Furthermore, such determining tendencies as the relation of attribute to object, which gives the order of adjective and noun, do not seem to be analysable into any sort of spatial structure or for that matter, into any consistent relationship. I have tried a number of assumptions concerning the selective mechanism of grammatical form (spatial relations, the relative intensity or prominence of different words in the idea and so on) but I have never been able to make an hypothesis which was consistent with any large number of sentence structures. Nevertheless, the indications which I have cited, that elements of the sentence are readied or partially activated before the order is imposed upon them in expression, suggest that some scanning mechanism must be at play in regulating their temporal sequence. The real problem, however, is the nature of the selective mechanism by which the particular acts are picked out in this scanning process, and to this problem I have no answer.

Such speculations concerning temporal and spatial systems do little more than illustrate a point of view concerning nervous organization which is, I believe, more consistent both with what is known of the histology and elementary physiology of the brain and also with behavior phenomena than are the more widely current theories of simple associative chains of reactions.

References

BETHE, A. (1931), 'Plastizität und Zentrenlehre', *Handb. d. norm. u. path. Physiol.*, 15 (zweite H), pp. 1175–220.

BROWN, T. G. (1914), 'On the nature of the fundamental activity of the nervous centers', *J. Physiol.*, vol. 48, pp. 18–46.

BUDDENBROCK, W. V. (1921), 'Die Rhythmus der Schreitbewegungen der Stabheuschrecke Dyxippus', *Biol. Centralb.*, vol. 41, pp. 41–8.

HOLST, N. V. (1937), 'Vom Wesen der Ordnung im Zentralnervensystem', *Die Naturwissenschaften*, vol. 25, pp. 625–31, 641–7.

INGEBRITZEN, O. C. (1933), 'Coordinating mechanism of the spinal cord', *Genet. Psychol. Monogr.*, vol. 13, pp. 485–555.

LASHLEY, K. S. (1917), 'The accuracy of movement in the absence of excitation from the moving organ', *Amer. J. Psychol.*, vol. 43, pp. 169–94.

SHERRINGTON, C. S. (1906), *The Integrative Action of the Nervous System*, Constable.

3 E. A. Fleishman

Dimensional Analysis of Movement Reactions

Excerpts from E. A. Fleishman, 'Dimensional analysis of movement re-actions', *Journal of Experimental Psychology*, vol. 55, 1958, pp. 438–53.

In previous studies the interrelationships among performances on a wide range of psychomotor tasks have been investigated (2, 7, 8, 11, 12). A primary concern has been to provide a functional classification of abilities accounting for individual differences in such skills.

The present study is concerned with a class of psychomotor skills which is probably the most important and contains the most numerous and complex kinds of human movements. These fall under the general heading of *movement reactions*, as defined earlier by Brown and Jenkins (1). In movement reactions one is interested in such things as the ability to make smooth or coordinated control movements, to move a body member or control at a given rate, in a rhythmical fashion, in a certain sequence, or along specified pathways. The distinguishing feature is that skill *during* the movement is of primary interest, as contrasted with *positioning movements*, where terminal accuracy is the primary feature, and *static reactions*, where maintenance of a certain limb position is the central task. Thus, although the act of reaching out to a given position in space to a control lever (positioning reaction) is the first step in operating that lever, the manner in which it is moved is the more significant feature of the reaction.

The classification of motor abilities into static, positioning and movement reactions by Brown and Jenkins (1) is entirely a rational classification. Each of these areas, in turn, they subdivided into more restricted motor-response categories. A recent study (5) has investigated the utility of the rational distinctions made among static and positioning reactions through an analysis of intercorrelations among performances on representative tasks of these skills. The general finding was that from the point of view of individual differences, static reactions are usefully considered as involving different abilities from positioning reactions, but that different positioning tasks involve highly specific skills with little generality from one task to another. On the other hand, in another study involving movement reactions (11), broad group factors were found which contributed to skill on many superficially diverse kinds of tasks.

These group factors, empirically derived from the intercorrelations among tasks, did not conform in any simple manner to the subcategories of movement reactions outlined by Brown and Jenkins (1). For example, movement reactions are categorized by them into discrete, repetitive, serial and continuous types. Our results indicated that performance on tasks representing these 'subcategories' grouped into somewhat different kinds of categories which cut across those provided by Brown and Jenkins.

The present study is a more definitive follow-up of the previous study involving movement reactions. The earlier study was based on the intercorrelations among performances on twenty-four psychomotor tasks, originally administered to over 1000 Navy pilot candidates in 1947. In the present study, tasks were specifically selected or designed around certain hypotheses derived from the earlier study. These tasks were administered in the laboratory, under controlled conditions, to an unselected sample of basic trainee airmen in 1954.

The objectives of this study were: (a) to replicate the earlier study under more controlled conditions, (b) to obtain more precise definitions of the factors identified through the inclusion of certain additional tasks and (c) to investigate the relationships between the factors identified and performance on a complex task performed under different conditions of difficulty.

Hypothesized Factors

The tasks were selected or constructed with a view to certain of the factors identified in the previous analysis of complex psychomotor tasks (11). These factors and their tentative definitions from this previous study are as follows:

1. Fine control sensitivity. The ability to make fine, highly controlled limb adjustments in movements of moderate scope (labeled Psychomotor Coordination I in previous study, 11).

2. Multiple limb coordination. The ability to coordinate more gross movements, where the use of more than one body member simultaneously is required (labeled Psychomotor Coordination II in previous study, 11).

3. Rate control. The ability to make continuous anticipatory motor adjustments relative to changes in speed and direction of a continuously moving target or object.

4. Response orientation. The ability to make rapid discriminations as to direction and choice of movements.

On the basis of the previous analysis (11), at least three tasks were included to sample each of these ability categories. Certain tasks in the previous analysis as well as new ones were included in order to clarify the generality of these factors and to sharpen the original definitions. For example, tasks thought to represent the fine control sensitivity factor were, Rotary Pursuit, Complex Coordination and Rudder Control, Pursuit Confusion and Two-Hand Coordination. The task called Control Adjustment was a new device constructed with the definition of the fine control sensitivity factor in mind and will be described later. The Dial Setting Test was included, since this seemed to require highly controlled wrist–finger movements and its possible loading (or lack of loading) on fine control sensitivity would help determine the generality of this factor.

Three tasks which measured multiple limb coordination in the previous study were Plane Control, Two-Hand Coordination and Complex Coordination. The Two-Hand Pursuit Task, and the two Rudder Control scores were added in the present study as possible measures of this factor.

Tasks assumed to measure the rate control factor were the Single Dimension Pursuitmeter, Two-Hand Pursuit and Rate Control Tasks. The task called Motor Judgement was added since it appeared to involve a greater degree of rate judgement and anticipation than other tests of this factor. If our original definition

45

of this factor was correct, then this test should be among the better measures of this factor. The Visual Coincidence Test, which requires only a button-pressing response, was included to see if emphasis in this factor is mainly in judgement of rate of the stimulus rather than the response.

The response orientation factor was thought to be represented by the Discrimination Reaction Time, Printed Discrimination Reaction Time and Dial Setting Tests.

Tasks representative of three other factors were also included in the study. Tasks in the present study, which have loadings on these factors in previous studies in our series, are indicated in parentheses.

5. *Reaction time.* The speed with which an individual is able to respond to a stimulus when it appears (see 2, 10). (Visual, Auditory, Jump Visual and Jump Auditory Reaction Time Tests.)

6. *Arm–hand steadiness.* The extent to which an individual is able to make steady, restricted arm–hand movements of the type which minimize strength and speed (2, 6, 7). (Track Tracing and Steadiness-Precision Tests.)

7. *Speed of arm movement.* The speed with which gross arm movements, of limited scope, can be made (2, 9, 10). (Rotary Aiming, Jump Visual Reaction Time and Jump Auditory Reaction Time Tests.)

Method

Description of the experimental tasks

Brief descriptions of the thirty-one task variables follow. References to more detailed descriptions are given where available:

1. *Two-hand coordination.* (See 13 and Figure 1.) The *S* attempts to keep a target-follower on a small target disk as the target moves irregularly and at varying rates. In the present study the target was reduced to 0·5 in diameter. Movement of the target-follower to the right and left is controlled by one lathe-type handle; movement to and from is controlled by the other handle.

Consequently, simultaneous rotation of both handles moves the follower in any resultant direction. Score was the total time on target during four 1-min trials separated by 15-s rests.

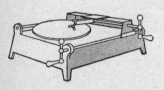

Figure 1 Two-hand coordination

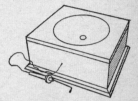

Figure 2 Rotary pursuit

2. Rotary pursuit. (See 12 and Figure 2.) The *S* attempts to keep a prod-stylus in contact with a small metallic target, set in a rapidly revolving phonograph-type disk. Score was the total time on target during five 20-s trials separated by 10-s rests.

3. Complex coordination. (See 13 and Figure 3.) Patterns of lights are presented whose positions are to be matched by appropriate adjustments of stick and rudder controls. A correct response is accomplished only when both the hands and feet have completed and maintained the appropriate adjustments, at which point a new pattern of lights to be matched is presented. Score is the number of completed matchings during two 2-min test periods separated by a 30-s rest.

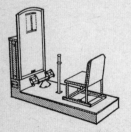

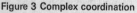

Figure 3 Complex coordination

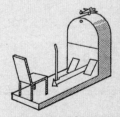

Figure 4 Plane control

4. Plane control. (See 14 and Figure 4.) The attitude of a model airplane is varied irregularly in its roll, pitch and yaw axes by a motor-driven cam system. The *S* attempts to keep the airplane in

47

a straight-and-level attitude by making compensatory adjustments of stick and pedal controls. Score is the amount of time S keeps the plane straight and level (on target in all three components) during four 1-min test periods, separated by 15-s rests.

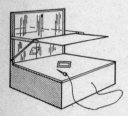

Figure 5 Pursuit confusion

5. *Pursuit confusion* (*time on target*). (See 11 and Figure 5.) The S attempts to keep a stylus on a variable-speed target as it moves through a diamond-shaped slot. The task is complicated by the fact that the entire target area is visible only by mirror vision. Score is the time on target during four 1-min test periods separated by 15-s rests.

6. *Pursuit confusion* (*errors*). Same as above, but score is the amount of time S is in contact with the sides of the slot.

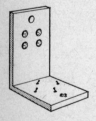

Figure 6 Discrimination reaction time

7. *Discrimination reaction time*. (See 12 and Figure 6.) The S manipulates one of four toggle switches as quickly as possible in response to a series of visual stimulus patterns differing from one another with respect to the spatial arrangement of their component parts (e.g. position of a lighted red lamp relative to a

lighted green lamp). Score is the cumulated times of response for a series of forty reactions for each stimulus pattern (S must respond within 3 s). Each set of twenty reactions was separated by a 35-s rest.

8. Motor judgement. (See 12 and Figure 7.) The S is confronted by two adjacent disks rotating at a constant speed. Each disk has black and white sections on its perimeter. Between these disks is a pointer, whose speed of rotation S can control. A forward movement of this stick slows the pointer and a backward movement speeds up the pointer. The S cannot stop the rotation of this pointer completely and he can exert no control over the two rotating disks. The S is required to manipulate the control stick so as to make as many revolutions of the pointer as possible without crossing the black areas on the rotating disks. To do this properly he must integrate his estimates of the speed of each disk, the pointer and his own control movements. Score is the ratio of number of pointer revolutions to number of errors (crossings of black areas) during four 1-min trials separated by 15-s rests.

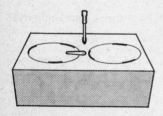

Figure 7 Motor judgement

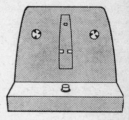

Figure 8 Visual coincidence

9. Visual coincidence. (See 13 and Figure 8.) The S must react to a thin bar of light which moves from top to bottom behind a curved, translucent vertical screen. When the position of the moving light passes exactly between a pair of adjacent, stationary lights, S responds by pushing a button. If the reaction of S occurs at the exact point of coincidence, two red signal lamps at the sides of the screen flash. If S presses the button too soon or too late, no correct response is recorded (even if S holds the button down).

49

For each of sixteen stimulus presentations, the reference lights may appear at different places on the screen and the bar of light may move at different rates. Score is the number of correct responses for sixty-four stimulus presentations, with a 10-s rest between each series of sixteen presentations. Each series of sixteen presentations comprised 100 s.

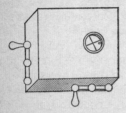

Figure 9 Two-hand pursuit

10. Two-hand pursuit. (See 12 and Figure 9.) This is similar in its response aspects to variable 1, except this task involves compensatory rather than following pursuit. The *S* is required to coordinate the movements of two control handles to keep a small target under a cross-hair as it deviates from a null position. Score is the time the target is kept 'on target' during four 1-min trials separated by 15-s rests.

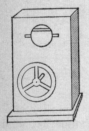

Figure 10 Single dimensional pursuit

11. Single dimension pursuitmeter. (See 12 and Figure 10.) The *S* makes compensatory adjustments (in and out movements) of a control wheel, in order to keep a horizontal line in a null position as it deviates from center in irregular fashion. The control wheel is dampened pneumatically, introducing a lag into the system. Score is the time the horizontal line is held in a null position during four 1-min trials separated by 15-s rests.

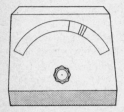

Figure 11 Rate control

12. Rate control. (See 12 and Figure 11.) A vertical target line moves back and forth across a curved scale, with frequent changes in direction and rate of movement. The *S* attempts to keep a thin pointer in coincidence with this line by adjustive rotary manipulations of a knob control. Score is total time the pointer and target line are in coincidence during four 1-min trials, separated by 15-s rests.

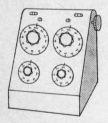

Figure 12 Dial setting

13. Dial setting. (See 12 and Figure 12.) The *S* is required to set four dials to the exact numbered positions indicated in four stimulus apertures, one of which corresponds to each dial. When all four dials are set exactly according to the indicated numbers, four new stimulus numbers appear in the apertures. Score is the number of settings completed in three 2-min trials, separated by 15-s rests.

14. Control adjustment. (See Figure 13.) The *S* is required to match the position of a red light with a corresponding green light. The position of the lighted green light is controlled by a highly sensitive control stick. A slight movement of the stick to the right displaces the lighted green light to the right and a slight movement of the stick to the left displaces the green light to the left. When *S* has matched the two lights and held this position for 0·5 s, the red light moves to a new position and *S* proceeds to match it. Score is the number of completed matches in four 1-min trials separated by 20-s rests.

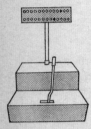

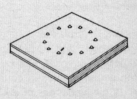

Figure 13 Control adjustment   Figure 14 Rotary aiming

15. Rotary aiming. (See 2 and Figure 14.) The task is to strike at a series of buttons arranged in a circular pattern on a horizontal panel going from one button to the next as rapidly as possible. Score is the number of strikes in four 30-s trials separated by 25-s rests.

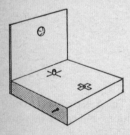

Figure 15 Reaction time

16. Visual reaction time. (See 2 and Figure 15.) The *S* keeps his finger on a button, depressing it ($\frac{1}{8}$ in) as rapidly as possible in response to a single amber light before him. A click provides him with a ready signal before each light stimulus is presented with the foreperiod (between click and light) varying in a random order from 0·5 and 1·5 s. Score is the cumulated reaction time for a series of twenty reactions.

17. Auditory reaction time. (See 2 and Figure 15.) Same procedure and scoring as Visual Reaction Time except that *S* responds to buzzer when it sounds instead of a light.

18. Jump visual reaction time. (See Figure 15.) Same procedure and scoring as Visual Reaction Time except *S* does not keep his finger on the response button, but keeps it on a cross 6 in from the response button. He must move his hand to the button as rapidly as possible as each light stimulus appears.

19. Jump auditory reaction time. (See Figure 15.) Same as Jump Visual Reaction Time except response is to buzzer instead of light.

20. Track tracing. (See 2 and Figure 16.) The *S* is required to negotiate an irregular slot pattern with a T-shaped stylus held at arm's length. Score is the number of errors (contacts with the back, top and sides of slot) during four attempts. No time limits.

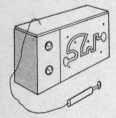

Figure 16 Track tracing

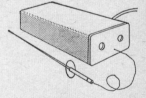

Figure 17 Steadiness-precision

21. Steadiness-precision. (See 2 and Figure 17.) The *S* moves a long stylus forward, slowly and steadily, away from his body, trying not to hit the sides of a cylindrical passage. Score is the number of errors (contacts with sides) during eight attempts, four through each of two passageways. No time limits.

22. Rudder control – center target. (See 13 and Figure 18.) The *S* sits in a mock airplane cockpit, which he attempts to keep lined up steadily with one of three target lights as they come on in front of him. His own weight throws the seat off balance unless he applies and maintains proper correction by means of foot pedals. During this condition, only the center target was used. Score was the total time the cockpit is held lined up with the center light during three 30-s trials separated by 15-s rests.

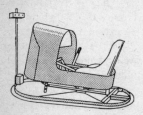

Figure 18 Rudder control

23. Rudder control – triple target. (See Figure 18.) Same apparatus as 22 above, but in this condition *S* must utilize appropriate pedal control to shift the cockpit from one light to the other as these come on at random intervals. Score is the total time the cockpit is lined up with the proper light during three 112-s trials separated by 30-s rests.

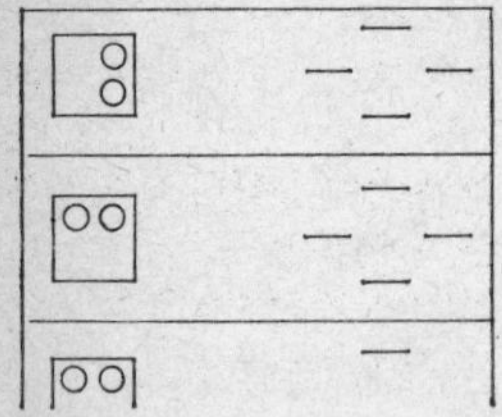

Figure 19 Printed discrimination reaction time

24. Printed discrimination reaction time. (See 2 and Figure 19.) Going from item to item as rapidly as possible, the *S* makes a check mark in one of four slots (arranged in an up–down, right–left pattern), according to the configuration of black and white dots. Score is the number of corrects minus twice the number wrong for one continuous 100-s trial.

Variables 25–31 represent different conditions administered on the Multidimensional Pursuit Apparatus (14 and Figure 20). In the original version of this apparatus, S is confronted with four dials representing airspeed, altitude, bank and turn indicators. Pointers on each of these dials vary irregularly, continuously and independently of one another. The S attempts to keep all the

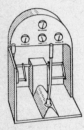

Figure 20 Multidimensional pursuit

pointers in the center of their respective scales by compensatory adjustments of simulated stick, rudder and throttle controls. Score is the amount of time the pointers on all four dials are lined up *simultaneously* in a zero position. In the present study, seven different tasks were performed on this apparatus. The apparatus was modified in order to allow S to practice on single components or on combinations of components. The following conditions were administered to S in the order described. Within each condition S received four 1-min trials, separated by 15-s rests. Between conditions, S received a 5-min rest, during which he was given instructions for the condition to follow.

25. Multidimensional pursuit – bank. All dials were covered, except the lower center dial indicating 'Bank'. The S attempted to keep the pointer centered on this one dial through right and left compensatory movements of the stick control only. Score was the amount of time the pointer was 'on target'.

26. Multidimensional pursuit – heading. All dials were covered, except upper center dial indicating 'Heading'. The *S* attempted to keep the pointer on this dial centered through compensatory right and left foot adjustments on the rudder pedals. Score was the amount of time the pointer was 'on target'.

27. Multidimensional pursuit – air speed. All dials were covered, except the extreme right dial indicating 'Air Speed'. The *S* attempted to keep this pointer centered by compensatory forward and backward movements of the small 'throttle control' handle manipulated by his left hand. Score was the amount of time this pointer was 'on target'.

28. Multidimensional pursuit – bank and altitude. Two dials were uncovered and *S* had to keep both pointers centered through coordinated use of the stick in two dimensions. Forward and backward stick movement controlled the pointer on the altitude dial, while right and left movement controlled the pointer on the bank dial. Score was the amount of time *both* pointers were 'on target' simultaneously.

29. Multidimensional pursuit – bank and heading. The two dials indicating Bank and Heading were uncovered and *S* had to keep both pointers centered through simultaneous stick (right and left movement only) and foot pedal adjustments. Score was amount of time *both* pointers were 'on target' simultaneously.

30. Multidimensional pursuit – bank and air speed. Two dials were uncovered and *S* had to keep their respective pointers centered through simultaneous movements of the right hand (control stick right and left) and the left hand (throttle control handle to forward and back). Score was amount of time *both* pointers were 'on target' simultaneously.

31. Multidimensional pursuit – bank, heading and air speed. Three dials were uncovered and *S* had to keep their respective pointers centered through simultaneous adjustments of both hands as well as both feet. Score was amount of time *all three* pointers were 'on target' simultaneously.

The reader will note the subtasks were administered in an assumed order of difficulty. It should be noted that the 'Bank' component is involved in each of the complex conditions. In turn, these involved one hand in two dimensions, one hand and feet, two hands, and finally both hands and feet. [. . .]

Administrative procedure

The complete battery of tasks was administered to 204 basic trainee airmen at Lackland Air Force Base. Half the Ss were administered the seven subtasks of the Multidimensional Pursuit Apparatus (variables 25–31 above) before receiving the remaining tasks, while the other half received the Multidimensional Pursuit Tasks last. In the administration of these other experimental tasks (variables 1 to 24) a rotational procedure was used in which the order of occurrence of each task in the series was fixed (in the order listed above), but different Ss started at different points in the series. Two models of each apparatus were used in order to test two Ss simultaneously. In each case, the two test models were wired into a single scoring and control console monitored by E.

Data analysis procedures

For each task the obtained distributions of raw scores were transformed to normalized distributions of standard scores (stanines), each with a range from 1 to 9, a mean of 5 and SD of 2. Conversions were made so that the 9 end of the scale was always indicative of 'good' performance (e.g. low errors, high time-on-target and low reaction time). [. . .]

Results and Discussion

Pearson product-moment correlations among the thirty-one variables were obtained. Factors were extracted from this matrix by Thurstone's Centroid Method (15). Extractions were continued beyond the point where the product of the two highest centroid loadings became less than the standard error of the original correlation of the same two variables. Ten centroid factors were extracted. Orthogonal rotations of the primary axes were made by means of Zimmerman's graphical method (16) using the

Table 1

Rotated Factor Loadings[1]

Variable	I RO	II FS	III RT	IV SAM	V AHS	VI MLC	VII RC	VIII D	IX WT	X Res	h²
1. Two-Hand Co-ordination	15	25	13	02	06	33	32	18	-12	-09	37
2. Rotary Pursuit	-09	50	-08	17	18	00	05	26	08	28	48
3. Complex Co-ordination	09	35	06	21	27	30	07	21	19	08	43
4. Plane Control	12	02	-01	11	25	41	19	21	03	25	40
5. Pursuit Con-fusion – T.O.T.	23	12	-04	01	11	-07	37	24	02	04	28
6. Pursuit Con-fusion – Errors	-04	04	05	06	36	11	19	31	-07	18	31
7. Discrimination Reaction Time	67	19	11	03	19	09	03	18	01	18	61
8. Motor Judgement	07	40	03	01	11	03	40	15	06	06	37
9. Visual Coincidence	36	12	14	-03	08	12	12	15	-10	01	23
10. Two-Hand Pursuit	18	13	07	18	26	32	37	00	-07	26	47
11. Single Dimension Pursuit	24	27	-02	23	05	25	-06	-09	14	26	37
12. Rate Control	-03	30	29	-16	-02	17	30	06	14	08	35
13. Dial Setting	43	40	-03	05	08	-06	27	-08	-03	13	45
14. Control Adjust-ment	14	46	-12	24	06	18	22	-11	-04	17	43
15. Rotary Aiming	07	26	17	38	08	-22	-02	18	04	10	34
16. Visual Reaction Time	01	15	56	24	02	-08	02	-08	-03	11	42
17. Auditory Reaction Time	06	07	63	18	10	04	06	-08	-11	19	51
18. Jump Visual Reaction Time	12	12	54	54	-01	-10	02	18	-09	-05	66
19. Jump Auditory Reaction Time	13	04	64	44	00	-02	13	27	00	-06	71
20. Track Tracing	00	29	09	24	50	00	-03	-09	-02	00	41
21. Steadiness-Pre-cision	06	10	19	09	43	00	17	-09	-05	-19	32
22. Rudder Control – Single Target	08	44	06	01	03	52	19	44	-13	-09	73
23. Rudder Control – Triple Target	04	48	08	-06	-03	48	20	46	-13	-09	75
24. Printed Discrimi-nation Reaction Time	52	24	01	24	21	-08	-04	06	-02	19	48
25. MP – Bank	24	07	10	12	02	21	-12	17	51	05	45
26. MP – Heading	24	27	20	-14	10	10	-10	11	61	02	60
27. MP – Air Speed	23	18	22	-19	13	-11	17	12	64	04	65
28. MP – Bank and Altitude	32	15	02	24	00	26	37	09	56	-03	71
29. MP – Bank and Heading	41	11	02	13	-02	08	22	02	75	-15	84
30. MP – Bank and Air Speed	31	24	15	09	15	19	14	09	72	04	79
31. MP – Bank, Heading and Air Speed	33	17	10	-01	05	05	23	21	66	08	69

1. Decimals omitted.

2. Factors are identified as follows: I, response orientation; II, fine control sensitivity; III, reaction time; IV, speed of arm movement; V, arm–hand steadiness; VI, multiple limb coordination; VII, rate control; VIII, doublet; IX, within task factor; X, residual.

criterion of simple structure and positive manifold. The accuracy of the rotational procedure was checked through reproduction of original correlation coefficients and through a comparison of communalities in the centroid and rotated matrixes.

Interpretation of factors

Factors were interpreted for psychological meaningfulness from the projections of the task variables on the rotated axes. The ten factors identified will be described in turn. Tasks with loadings of 0·30 or higher are listed under each factor.

Factor I appears to be the response orientation factor previously identified (5, 6, 11). It has been found general to visual-discrimination reaction psychomotor tasks involving rapid directional discrimination and orientation of movement patterns.

No.	Variable	Loading
7	Discrimination Reaction Time	0·67
24	Printed Discrimination Reaction Time	0·52
13	Dial Setting	0·43
29	Multidimensional Pursuit – Bank and Heading	0·41
9	Visual Coincidence	0·36
31	Multidimensional Pursuit – Bank, Heading, and Air Speed	0·33
28	Multidimensional Pursuit – Bank and Altitude	0·32
30	Multidimensional Pursuit – Bank and Air Speed	0·31

This factor has been found distinct from the factor called spatial orientation, which represents the ability to comprehend the arrangement of a visual stimulus pattern. The present factor appears to involve the ability to make the correct movement in relation to the correct stimulus. In other words, 'Given this stimulus, which way should I move?' The Discrimination Reaction Time Tests were among the best measures of this factor in previous studies (5, 6, 11). In the Dial Setting Test, critical features involve moving the correct one of four knobs in correct relation to the four stimulus windows, but even more crucially turning the knobs in the correct direction so as to achieve a match more quickly.

The lower loading (0·23) of the Pursuit Confusion Test on this factor may at first appear disturbing. This test involves mirror tracing, and the 'which way do I move' question would certainly appear critical. Similarly, the Two-Hand Coordination and Two-Hand Pursuit Tests involve such response decisions. The distinction between these three tests and those on the factor appears to be that these involve continuous responses to continuous stimuli. Tests on the factor involve discrete reponses to successive stimuli.

The presence of the Visual Coincidence Test on this factor implies that this factor may extend to situations in which the choice is whether to respond or not. Of special interest is the presence of four subtasks of the Multidimensional Pursuit Task on this factor. It is to be noted that these are the subtasks involving more than one component at a time. Here associating the correct control with the correct dial is especially critical in obtaining a score. The three subtasks involving no choice of control did not load on this factor.

Factor II is defined as fine control sensitivity.

No.	Variable	Loading
2	Rotary Pursuit	0·50
23	Rudder Control – Triple Target	0·48
14	Control Adjustment	0·46
23	Rudder Control – Single Target	0·44
13	Dial Setting	0·40
8	Motor Judgement	0·40
3	Complex Coordination	0·35
12	Rate Control	0·30

All of these tasks involve the ability to make fine, highly controlled (but not overcontrolled) adjustments at some critical stage of performance. These results confirm previous indications (11), that this ability extends to arm–hand as well as to leg movements. The presence of Dial Setting and Rate Control suggests the extension to wrist–finger movements as well. Of special interest is the substantial loading of the Control Adjustment task on this factor. This device was specifically constructed as a measure of this hypothesized factor. On the negative side, Pursuit Confusion, originally hypothesized as a measure of this factor, loaded on another factor.

Factor III is restricted to the four reference measures of reaction time.

No.	Variable	Loading
19	Jump Auditory Reaction Time	0·64
17	Auditory Reaction Time	0·63
16	Visual Reaction Time	0·56
18	Jump Visual Reaction Time	0·54

None of the more complex tasks appear on this factor. This factor has been defined simply as the speed with which S can react to a stimulus when it appears. These results agree with previous indications (2, 3, 10) that individual differences in this ability are independent of whether the stimulus is auditory or visual. These results also confirm that this reaction time factor does not contribute to individual differences in the Discrimination Reaction Time task briefly practiced. Reaction Time does contribute variance, however, after considerable practice is given on this task (see 10).

Factor IV is restricted to those tasks in the present analysis which have previously identified a speed of arm movement factor. This represents simply the speed with which S can make a gross, discrete arm movement.

No.	Variable	Loading
18	Jump Visual Reaction Time	0·54
19	Jump Auditory Reaction Time	0·44
15	Rotary Aiming	0·38

The distinction between this factor and the reaction time factor is again brought out. For example, this speed of arm movement contributes variance in those reaction-time tasks which require a 6-in arm movement to the response button (variables 18, 19) but not in those reaction time tests requiring only a button-pressing response. The Rotary Aiming Task involves no sudden onset of stimuli but does involve a series of rapid, discrete arm movements. This factor is not found in any of the complex tasks as represented in the present study. Previous work has shown that this factor does not contribute variance in performance on the Complex Coordination, Discrimination Reaction

Time, Plane Control and Rotary Pursuit Tasks, but only at high levels of proficiency achieved after continued practice on these tasks (3, 5, 9, 10).

Factor V is identified as arm–hand steadiness, and defined as the ability to make precise and steady arm–hand movements of the type which minimize strength and speed.

No.	Variable	Loading
20	Track Tracing	0·50
21	Steadiness-Precision	0·43
6	Pursuit Confusion (Errors)	0·36

This factor has appeared in a number of our studies. It has been found to extend to tasks requiring maintenance of a steady arm position, to tasks requiring steadiness during an arm movement, and to various planes of movement, etc. (2, 7, 12). However, in no previous study has it been found to extend to more complex psychomotor performances. Of interest in the present study is the loading of Pursuit Confusion (Errors) on this factor. It will be recalled that this score represents hits against the sides of a depressed slot.

Factor VI includes tasks, all of which involve simultaneous manipulation of multiple limbs.

No.	Variable	Loading
22	Rudder Control – Single Target	0·52
23	Rudder Control – Triple Target	0·48
4	Plane Control	0·41
1	Two-Hand Coordination	0·33
10	Two-Hand Pursuit	0·32
3	Complex Coordination	0·30

This confirms previous indications (11) that the ability represented by this factor is general to tasks requiring coordination of two feet (e.g. Rudder Control), two hands (Two-Hand Pursuit, Two-Hand Coordination), and hands and feet (Plane Control and Complex Coordination). This factor is labeled multiple limb coordination. These are the only tasks in the study which require multiple limb involvement, except for certain subtasks on the Multidimensional Pursuit Apparatus. It should be noted that all the tasks loaded on this factor present a display which allows S to assess the degree to which he is 'coordinating'. In the Multi-dimensional Pursuit task there is no single indication of this, but instead S must divide his attention between spatially separate dials. It is possible that these differences in control–display characteristics are of consequence with respect to the abilities measured by such tasks.

Factor VII appears the same as that called rate control in one of our recent studies (11). Since loadings are low, this must be regarded as our most tentative interpretation. However, all these loadings are consistent with our interpretation.

No.	Variable	Loading
8	Motor Judgement	0·40
5	Pursuit Confusion (Time on Target)	0·37
10	Two-Hand Pursuit	0·37
28	Multidimensional Pursuit – Bank and Altitude	0·37
1	Two-Hand Coordination	0·32
12	Rate Control	0·30

The common feature of all these tasks is that there is an element of pursuit involved. Each task requires the examiner to make anticipatory adjustments relative to changes in speed and/or direction of a continuously moving object. All compensatory and following pursuit tasks in the present study, with the exception of the Single Dimension Pursuitmeter, are located on this factor. These results confirm our previous indications that this factor cuts across the traditional categorization of pursuit tasks into 'following pursuit' (e.g. Rate Control and Two-Hand Coordination) and compensatory pursuit (e.g. Two-Hand Pursuit). These results suggest that from the point of view of individual differences, this distinction may be arbitrary, and the nature of such tasks may better be thought of in terms of a third underlying variable. Our previous study showed this factor to be general to tasks other than those traditionally called pursuit. The presence of the Motor Judgement Task on this factor in the present analysis is further evidence of this. This task was included specifically to test the original definition of this factor. This is not a typical pursuit task, but there is considerable involvement of rate judgement and adjustment. The S must consider the rate of movement of two different disks, a pointer, and of his own control movement to make an adequate response. It will be noted that the task, Visual Coincidence, does not load on this factor. This task was included to see if judgement of stimulus rate as opposed to response rate was the key to this factor. It will be recalled that only a button-pressing response is required in this task. The absence of this task from factor VII suggests that this factor represents skill in the motor aspects of the response rather than skill in the purely interpretational aspects of the rate of the stimulus.[1]

Factor VIII is a doublet factor confined to the subtasks on the Rudder Control Task and is of doubtful psychological significance.

Factor IX is confined to the seven subtasks administered on the Multidimensional Pursuit device and does not extend to the other ability measures. Moreover, there is no consistent patterning of these loadings from one such task to another (see Table 1). It is possible that this 'within-task' factor represents specific or spurious variance due to experimental dependence of an unknown source. Although scores on each condition were obtained independently at successive stages, they were obtained on the same apparatus in the same order and during a single testing period for each S. It is not known, for example, to what extent positive or negative transfer effects might be represented in the intercorrelations among these subtasks. Whatever the nature of factor IX, it is clear that we cannot define it in terms of the more general ability measures included in the present study.

It was hoped that inclusion of the several scores on the Multidimensional Pursuit Apparatus would yield information on the relation between task complexity (in terms of number of display-control components involved) and factorial complexity (number of abilities required). As indicated earlier, the main conclusion possible from these data is that response orientation is involved when the task is complicated by the requirement that two or three controls be operated, but that this factor is not involved in the single component subtasks. Perhaps just as important is the finding that these results are independent of the particular con-

1. This has been confirmed in a recent study in which we obtained only insignificant correlations between psychomotor pursuit tasks and motion picture tests of rate judgement and discrimination.

trol used or combination of controls (two feet, two hands, hand and feet, etc.) involved. The critical skill appears to be that of associating the correct control movement with the various display variations.

It should also be pointed out that a large portion of the variance in the other experimental tasks remains specific to individual tasks. However, this should not minimize the importance of discovering whatever common variance there is. Generalization of experimental results from one task to another might well depend on this common variance. However, this remains to be evaluated in other laboratory contexts.

The importance of discovering this common variance certainly applies to the kind of predictions one may be able to make about individual differences in psychomotor performances. For a recent review of the utility of these concepts to the description and prediction of individual differences of practical consequence, the reader is referred elsewhere (4).

It is not possible here to review the place and limitations of factor analysis in experimental psychology. It would seem, however, that results of such studies can provide a set of working dimensions for conceptualizing task variables in terms of common ability requirements. The utility of the descriptive models provided by this approach needs to be assessed by nonfactorial investigations.

Summary

The study confirms previous indications that movement reaction tasks of the kinds investigated may be grouped into several broad classes representing common ability requirements. The ability categories inferred from the factor analysis results were labeled fine control sensitivity, multiple limb coordination and response orientation. A factor called rate control was considered more tentative. Definitions of these factors and the diverse kinds of tasks to which they apply are described. Three other factors were identified as arm–hand steadiness, reaction time and speed of arm movement, but these did not contribute to performance in the more complex movement reaction tasks under the present conditions of administration.

References

1. J. S. BROWN and W. O. JENKINS, 'An analysis of human motor abilities related to the design of equipment and a suggested program of research', in P. M. Fitts (ed.), *Psychological Research on Equipment Design*, U.S. Government Printing Office, 1947. (AAF Aviat. Psychol. Res. Rep. no. 19.)

2. E. A. FLEISHMAN, 'Dimensional analysis of psychomotor abilities', *J. exp. Psychol.*, vol. 48 (1954), pp. 437–54.

3. E. A. FLEISHMAN, 'Predicting advanced levels of proficiency in psychomotor skills', in G. Finch and F. Cameron (eds.), *Symposium on Air Force Human Engineering, Personnel, and Training Research*. National Academy of Sciences, Washington, 1956, pp. 142-51. (National Research Council Publ. 455.)

4. E. A. FLEISHMAN, 'Psychomotor selection tests: research and application in the U.S. Air Force', *Personnel Psychol.* vol. 9 (1956), pp. 449–67.

5. E. A. FLEISHMAN, 'A comparative study of aptitude patterns in unskilled and skilled psychomotor performances', *J. appl. Psychol.*, vol. 41 (1957), pp. 263–72.

6. E. A. FLEISHMAN, 'Factor structure in relation to task difficulty in psychomotor performance', *Educ. psychol. Measmt*, vol. 17 (1957), pp. 522-32.

7. E. A. FLEISHMAN, 'An analysis of positioning movements and static reactions', *J. exp. Psychol.*, vol. 55 (1958), pp. 13–24.

8. E. A. FLEISHMAN and W. E. HEMPEL, JR, 'A factor analysis of dexterity tests', *Personnel Psychol.*, vol. 7 (1954), pp. 15–32.

9. E. A. FLEISHMAN and W. E. HEMPEL, JR, 'Changes in factor structure of a complex psychomotor test as a function of practice', *Psychometrika*, vol. 19 (1954), pp. 239–52.

10. E. A. FLEISHMAN and W. E. HEMPEL, JR, 'The relation between abilities and improvement with practice in a visual discrimination reaction task', *J. exp. Psychol.*, vol. 49 (1955), pp. 301–12.

11. E. A. FLEISHMAN and W. E. HEMPEL, JR, 'Factorial analysis of complex psychomotor performance and related skills', *J. appl. Psychol.*, vol. 40 (1956), pp. 96–104.

12. W. E. HEMPEL, JR, and E. A. FLEISHMAN, 'A factor analysis of physical proficiency and manipulative skill', *J. appl. Psychol.*, vol. 39 (1955), pp. 12–16.

13. A. W. MELTON (ed.), *Apparatus Tests*, U.S. Government Printing Office, 1947. (AAF Aviat. Psychol. Program Res. Rep. no. 4.)

14. A. W. MELTON, (ed.) *Apparatus Tests (Supplement)*, U.S. Government Printing Office, 1947. (AAF Aviat. Psychol. Program Res. Rep. no. 4 Supplement.)

15. L. L. THURSTONE, *Multiple-Factor Analysis*. University of Chicago Press, 1947.

16. W. S. ZIMMERMAN, 'A simple graphical method for orthogonal rotation of axes', *Psychometrika*, vol. 11 (1946), pp. 51–5.

4 P. M. Fitts and M. I. Posner

The Measurement of Skills

Excerpts from chapter 5 of P. M. Fitts and M. I. Posner, *Human Performance*, Brooks/Cole, 1967, pp. 83–92.

Types of Tasks

A distinction may be made between three different temporal patterns of stimulus events. Events are said to be *discrete* if they have a clearly defined beginning and end. Much of the knowledge available in experimental psychology concerns discrete stimulus events, such as the presentation of a single light or tone and discrete responses, such as the press of a lever or a single word.

Even discrete events have dynamic aspects. Stimuli always occur in some kind of context both spatial and temporal. Responses to new stimuli are always superimposed upon ongoing behaviour – the basic bodily processes, postural adjustments, etc. Thus, even in discrete tasks, 'stimulus' and 'response' are convenient abstractions from and simplifications of the real world of dynamic events and ongoing behavior. Judged by the neural and muscular activity involved, even so simple a response as a lever push is a complex pattern never exactly reproduced.

Stimulus or response events are said to be *serial* when the beginning and ending of units can be identified but events follow each other in rapid sequence. Reading is a serial task when viewed in terms of eye movements. In reading, the eye remains fixed for periods of 200 ms or longer, and these periods are separated by short, saccadic movements lasting less than 40 ms. If the subject receives information about future events, a serial task allows for the preparation of the next movement to be made while the last movement is being executed.

Finally, stimulus events may be *continuous*. A moving object, for instance, presents continuous information. In most studies of tracking behavior the subject is presented with a stimulus course which varies continuously. In these tasks the subject is required to make corrections so as to keep the system in a balanced state. Driving an automobile is a familiar tracking task. [. . .] Man is limited in his ability to respond to rapidly occurring signals. Tasks which present continuous information place severe demands upon this ability.

Optimal Measures

An experimental analysis of skills depends upon the method chosen to measure performance. Consider the skill of the baseball batter. No single measure captures all aspects of his performance in that skill. The batting average is the most frequently used measure, but a clean-up hitter might be selected because of his ability to hit a long ball. This ability might be reflected in a relatively low batting average but a large number of total bases per hit. Or a good batter might be one who hits frequently with men on base, giving a high number of runs batted in. A leadoff hitter might be selected who walks frequently, perhaps scoring a large number of runs but having a low batting average.

The psychologist is often characterized as having a 'black-box' or stimulus–response approach to behavior, in that his observations are restricted to sequences of events in the individual's environment and to observable response sequences. However, as is evident from the case of the batter, there are many ways to characterize such input–output relations, and some of these are much more valuable than others in revealing important aspects of human skills.

Among the more valuable characteristics of a system of measurement adequate to the investigation of skills is sensitivity to input, output and the relation or balance between input and output. The only reason that the batting average is a useful measure is that over the course of a season each batter faces a large number of the available pitchers. A batter may have a wonderful average, but if he has yet to face strong pitching it is meaningless. In order to understand the meaning of the output (batting average) we must understand the meaning or quality of the input (quality of pitching faced). In order to describe the course of improvement in skills and to compare skills, it is necessary to capture the degree to which the output reflects the stimulus input.

A second criterion for a system of measurement is that it should be appropriate to the three types of tasks outlined above – discrete, serial and continuous. It should also allow meaningful comparisons between performances in these situations.

Next, the measure should be sensitive to the accuracy of the responses made by the subject. The batting average, for example, is sensitive only near the region of the criterion. That is, it is sensitive to hits as opposed to outs but is not sensitive to the difference between a strikeout and a well-hit line drive that is caught. To be appropriate for all levels of skill, a measure should be sensitive to different aspects of performance even when these are far from the criterion used to define success.

The measure should take into account the length of time taken to perform a skill as well as the accuracy with which it is performed. Most skills depend at least partly on timing. In addition, time is a continuous measure and can discriminate between performances, even when a skill is so poorly performed as to give 0 per cent correct responses or so well learned as to give 100 per cent. More important, a measure must be sensitive to time because man is often able to vary his accuracy in proportion to the amount of time he takes to perform a task. A typist can go fast and make many errors or go more slowly and reduce error. Neither time nor accuracy alone can be used to compare the performance of two typists, but the two together can be.

Finally, the measure must be very general if it is to be useful in both perceptual–motor and language skills. Such generality may be somewhat at a disadvantage in particular cases but it allows for the broadest investigation of human skills.

Information Transmission

No single measure can meet all the criteria perfectly. In earlier chapters, many different types of measurement were introduced for the purpose of analysing specific problems. These measures are as different from each other as, on the one hand, the time it takes to roll a cigar and, on the other, the number of digit series reproduced correctly 50 per cent of the time. Each of these measures is appropriate within the context in which it was used. This chapter develops the concept of the rate of information transmission as a means of measuring skills. Like all measures, it summarizes certain aspects of performance and ignores others. In recent years, however, it has proved to be useful for comparing a variety of skills and has provided us with a more general picture of man's abilities and limitations.

The idea of man as a transmitter of information has already been introduced a number of times in this book. Up to this point, however, the ideas used have been mostly in accord with common-sense notions of what information is and how man uses it in making responses. It is now necessary to present in a more detailed manner a system for the measurement of information. The development here is intuitive rather than rigorous. More complete treatments of the subject are available in Attneave (1959) and Garner (1962).

Amount of information

'Information' implies a gain in knowledge in some manner. A technical definition of the term, as developed in communication engineering (Shannon and Weaver, 1949), is both more precise and less general. In order for information to be conveyed, there must be uncertainty. The amount of information potentially available increases with the amount of uncertainty in the situation. The statement that 2 plus 2 equals 4 conveys no information to most of us because there is no uncertainty about the relation to begin with. The assertion that the result of a coin flip was 'either heads or tails' conveys no information, because it does not reduce our genuine uncertainty about the outcome. However, the simpler statement 'it is tails' does convey information.

How much information is there in a statement? The amount of information increases with the number of possible things which might have occurred. Thus there is more information in a statement that a die came up four than that a coin came up tails, because six things could have occurred with the die and only two with the coin. There was, to begin with, more uncertainty with respect to the die. The amount of uncertainty then increases with N, where N is the number of possible things which might have occurred.

Consider the case of coin flipping. If one coin is flipped, either of two things can occur; with two coins any of four things; with three coins any of eight things. As the number of coins increases by one, the number of alternatives multiplies in powers of two. Since one coin flip is like another, it is convenient to define information in a way which allows each flip to contribute equal information. The function which increases by equal amounts while N multiplies is called the logarithm of N. It is useful, therefore, to define information as the logarithm of N. The base of the logarithm is purely arbitrary. However, if information is to increase by one unit each time N doubles, the base 2 is proper. Since many systems have only two states, like coin flips or truth values or lights, the base 2 is convenient. Information (H), as defined in equation 1, is measured in units called bits (abbreviated from binary digits):

$$H = \log_2 N. \qquad \qquad 1$$

In our examples so far, all the alternatives (N) in a given situation were equally probable. What happens when they are not? The statements that it will be cold in Alaska in January and that it will be warm in Alabama in August convey little information because they are virtually certain to be true. However, the reverse suggestion would convey much more information, since it is so improbable. Information should reflect the probability (p) as well as the number of alternatives (N). When the alternatives are equally likely, $p = 1/N$ or $N = 1/p$ and equation 1 may be made to read as follows:

$$H = \log_2 1/p. \qquad \qquad 2$$

Notice that this equation is identical to equation 1 when it is the case that all events are equally likely.

In skills it is often the average information in a series of events which is desired. Each event contributes information in accordance with its probability. The amount of information contributed by each occurrence of an event is given by equation 2. However, any event occurs only as often as its probability (p). Thus, its weighted contribution to the total uncertainty is $p \log_2 1/p$. To calculate the average uncertainty (H) in the sequence, all these values are added together for each event (i), which gives equation 3:

$$H = \sum_{i=1}^{N} p_i \log_2 1/p_i. \qquad \qquad 3$$

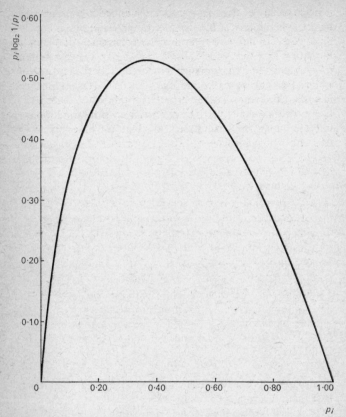

Figure 1 The curve shows $p_i \log_2 1/p_i$ for each value of p_i. It may be used in the computation of information (see text). (After Garner, 1962)

For example, consider a situation in which there are four lights with probabilities 0·1, 0·2, 0·3 and 0·4. Since one, and only one, light occurs on any trial, the probabilities add to 1. The average uncertainty about which event will occur in a sequence of such light flashes is shown below.

$$H = 0{\cdot}1 \log_2 1/0{\cdot}1 + 0{\cdot}2 \log_2 1/0{\cdot}2 + 0{\cdot}3 \log_2 1/0{\cdot}3 + \\ + 0{\cdot}4 \log_2 1/0{\cdot}4. \qquad \textbf{4}$$

Figure 1 may be used for calculating the amount of information from equation **4**. The figure gives the values of $p_i \log_2 1/p_i$ for all values of p_i. In order to solve equation **4** you first look up the value 0·1 on the x-axis of the figure. Follow the line through 0·1 vertically until you come to the curve and then read off the corresponding value (0·32) on the y-axis. The same is done for the other possible values of i (0·2, 0·3 and 0·4). These values are then added to yield the average information in the sequence, which is about 1·84 bits. Of course, Figure 1 is approximate. More exact calculation may be made from a table of logarithms.

Information transmitted

The information transmitted is that amount of the stimulus information which is represented in the subject's response. Information transmission will be maximum when one, and only one, response always occurs when a given stimulus is presented. If any other response occurs, the amount of information transmitted will be reduced.

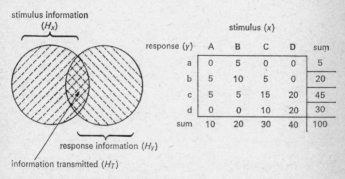

response (y)	A	B	C	D	sum
a	0	5	0	0	5
b	5	10	5	0	20
c	5	5	15	20	45
d	0	0	10	20	30
sum	10	20	30	40	100

Figure 2 The diagram portrays the relationship between stimulus, response and transmitted information. The matrix in Table 1 illustrates hypothetical data which might be obtained from an experiment

To get a feeling for the calculation of information transmitted, look at Figure 2. In this Venn diagram the left circle represents the information in the stimulus, and the right represents the information in the response. In any example, the stimulus and response information can be calculated by use of equation **3** and Figure

1. If these two values are added, the sum includes all the information in the two circles: this includes the overlap of the two circles twice. The overlap information is represented twice in the sum since both circles include it.

One method of calculating information transmitted is illustrated in Table 1, using the example shown in Figure 2. The

Table 1

H_x = stimulus information
  = $0{\cdot}1 \log_2 1/0{\cdot}1 +0{\cdot}2 \log_2 1/0{\cdot}2 +0{\cdot}3 \log_2 1/0{\cdot}3 +$
    $+0{\cdot}4 \log_2 1/0{\cdot}4$
  = $0{\cdot}33+0{\cdot}46+0{\cdot}52+0{\cdot}53$
  = $1{\cdot}85$ bits

H_y = response information
  = $0{\cdot}05 \log_2 1/0{\cdot}05 +0{\cdot}2 \log_2 1/0{\cdot}2 +0{\cdot}45 \log_2 1/0{\cdot}45 +$
    $+0{\cdot}3 \log_2 1/0{\cdot}3$
  = $0{\cdot}22+0{\cdot}46+0{\cdot}42+0{\cdot}52$
  = $1{\cdot}62$ bits

$H_{x,y}$ = cell information
  = $5(0{\cdot}05 \log_2 1/0{\cdot}05)+2(0{\cdot}1 \log_2 1/0{\cdot}1)+0{\cdot}15 \log_2 1/0{\cdot}15+$
    $+2(0{\cdot}2 \log_2 1/2)$
  = $5(0{\cdot}22)+2(0{\cdot}33)+0{\cdot}41+2(0{\cdot}46)$
  = $3{\cdot}09$ bits

H_T = information transmitted
  = $H_x+H_y-H_{x,y}$
  = $1{\cdot}84+1{\cdot}62-3{\cdot}09$
  = $0{\cdot}37$ bits

---

figures in the cells represent the number of times each response occurs to each stimulus. Entries along the diagonal are correct responses. Table 1 shows first how to calculate the stimulus and response information for this example. Then the information in the cells $H_{x,y}$ which is the total area of the two circles of the Venn diagram, is computed. Finally, this value is subtracted from the sum of the stimulus and response information to obtain the information transmitted, which is represented by the doubly shaded area of the Venn diagram.

For any situation in which a stimulus–response matrix of the type shown in Figure 2 can be developed, it is possible to calculate the information transmitted. Experiments on reaction time, absolute judgement and memory are among those for which information transmitted can be calculated.

Information-transmission rate

The measures that have been derived so far have a number of important properties. They are sensitive to the number of alternative items which might occur on any trial. They reflect the degree to which the response is related to the stimulus. Finally, they are general, since they can be calculated whenever a set of events, each with a probability, can be specified. Moreover, they can be extended easily to take into consideration the speed as well as the information in the response.

When the information transmitted per response is divided by the time it takes to respond, the rate at which information is transmitted is obtained. The rate of information transmission is useful for all tasks which place emphasis upon speed. It can be used for discrete, serial or continuous tasks. For the mathematics of information involving continuous input, see Shannon and Weaver (1949).

The amount of information transmitted and the rate of information transmission are measures which have most of the desirable properties listed earlier.

Two disadvantages of these measures should be noted. First, these measures are not very useful when errors are of differential significance. The information measures do not differentiate between near misses and far misses. As long as one response always occurs to a given stimulus, information transmitted will be maximal and *any* departure will affect the measure equally. Second, information is defined only for a series of events where the probabilities governing the events are not changing. Since information is a function of the probability of events, it is usually necessary for the subject to have some knowledge of these probabilities. This knowledge may be obtained from instruction or from learning. Only when the subject's experience mirrors the objective probabilities can it be expected that information will be related to performance.

Information measures have many uses and are readily adapted

to different aspects of performance. As the book progresses, some new applications will be considered and methods of calculating information provided.

Redundancy

The measure of *redundancy* is one of the most useful provided by information theory. Redundancy (R) is calculated by means of equation **5**:

$$R = 1 - \frac{H_{\text{actual}}}{H_{\text{max}}}. \qquad\qquad 5$$

H_{max} is the maximum value of information which that sequence of events can give. H_{actual} signifies the actual amount of information derived from a sequence of events. The maximum value always occurs when the elements in a sequence of N events are all equally likely to occur and when the occurrence of one event cannot be predicted from any previous event. When either of these requirements is violated, the actual information falls below the maximum, and the sequence is said to be redundant. The English language is redundant for two reasons. First, the probability of occurrence is not equal for all the letters: E, for example, is much more likely to occur than Q. Second, the probability of a letter's occurring is greatly affected by the letters which occurred previously. The redundancy of English has been computed (Shannon and Weaver, 1949) and the amount of redundancy of a language has been shown to be related to the rate of learning.

Noise

In human behavior there is a great amount of apparently spontaneous variability. Engineers and information theorists call such variability, when it has to do with communication systems, *noise*. The amount of noise in a system can be specified in a statistical sense. In Figure 2, $H_y - H_T$ represents the amount of noise added to the response by the subject.

Just as it can be used to specify the amount of noise contributed by the subject, information theory can be used to show that there is additional information embedded in the noise. Errors made by man almost never are random; they are instructive for illustrating properties of his information-processing system. For example, when the letter *P* is forgotten in a memory experiment, there is a high likelihood that *B*, *T*, or another letter which sounds like *P* will have been substituted for it. The error contains information about the way in which man's memory system codes these items.

Information coding

Codes, as illustrated by various natural and artificial languages, are not peculiar to information theory. Nevertheless, information theory has brought added rigor to the study of codes. A code consists of a population or alphabet of symbols and a system of rules or constraints among them. Codes are simple if they have no redundancy and the order of symbols to be presented to a subject is random. When rules are introduced which govern the order of symbols, such as in English, the code becomes redundant. Natural languages, which have many rules or constraints, are highly redundant. The linguist seeks to understand the rules, in the form of unit sequences and grammar, which produce the redundancy.

The idea of a code has wide application in the study of human information processing. Man has great ability in learning the rules of complex codes. More and more, biological and behavioral scientists are couching their theories in the terms of coding processes. We hear about the genetic code, a highly redundant code which determines inheritance. Theories of hearing are often expressed as a process by which physical signals are recorded by the ear into neural activity, the code of the nervous system. The study of codes and coding processes bridges the gap between many formerly unrelated areas, each attempting to describe an aspect of the living system.

Channel capacity and human limitations

The theory of information published by Shannon and Weaver (1949) set forth and elaborated upon the concept of the capacity of an information channel perturbed by noise. Three aspects of this development should be noted. First, the concept of channel capacity is a formal theoretical concept. Channel capacity is not something one measures directly but it is inferred as the maximum possible rate at which a channel can transmit information. Second, the idea of a channel includes a specification of the information code to be employed. If the code is changed, the capacity of the channel may change also. Third, the term channel capacity refers to the rate at which information is transmitted and not to the amount of information per response.

The concept of channel capacity as employed in information theory should not be confused with concepts regarding man's capacities and limitations. Man does have a limited capacity for many tasks. Some of man's capacities can be discussed in terms of the amount or rate of information transmission. However, there is not a single human channel capacity for all tasks and codes. It is not possible to predict on purely rational grounds the limits to the rate at which human beings process information. Instead, the limitations on many different aspects of processing have been analysed from empirical studies.

References

ATTNEAVE, F. (1959), *Applications of Information Theory to Psychology*, Holt.

GARNER, W. R. (1962), *Uncertainty and Structure as Psychological Concepts*, Wiley.

SHANNON, C. E., and WEAVER, W. (1949), *The Mathematical Theory of Communication*, University of Illinois Press.

Part Two
Laboratory Studies of the Components of Skill

One attribute of skilled performance is the production of appropriate responses to deal with a particular problem. Sometimes these responses are discrete and do not have to meet rigorous limits of accuracy – for example, typing on an electric machine. Other responses, to be successful, have to be very precisely executed in time and space – for example, returning a serve in lawn tennis. This is essentially a contrast between selecting among a number of pre-programmed alternative responses and generating what is tantamount to a unique response.

Tasks have been developed in the laboratory for studying these processes experimentally. The study of choice reactions described by Welford (Reading 5) and Brainard *et al.* (Reading 6) throws light on the time it takes to decide among different numbers of alternatives, and a variety of models have been developed to account for this aspect of behaviour. Audley and Pike (1965) have examined several models of choice behaviour and categorized them in terms of the underlying mechanisms they imply. It is now clear that the early enthusiasm with which information theory was greeted was misplaced and that other theoretical approaches provide as good a description of choice behaviour. Nevertheless information theory provides a valuable approximation and a basis for quantifying the difficulty of choice situations which is pragmatically useful.

The performance of continuous skills requiring precise movements such as driving a car or playing ball games has been studied in the laboratory through a task called 'tracking'. The subject is required to modulate his response according to a continuously varying signal. Poulton (Reading 7) describes this task and also stresses the dependence of skilled performance upon a number of predictor mechanisms. The use of information theory to quantify performance in a tracking task is described by Crossman (Reading 8). Crossman's analysis depends upon the assessment of the control of redundant voluntary movements and in particular the way in which the time to complete a movement varies as a function of its amplitude and accuracy. This relation is known as Fitts' Law (Fitts, 1954; Fitts and Peterson, 1964). These papers show that the speed and accuracy of a subject's performance are limited by his capacity to take in information, to take decisions and to control his responses accurately. Within limits, these limitations may be described successfully using the concepts of information theory.

References
AUDLEY, R. J., and PIKE, A. R. (1965), 'Some alternative stochastic models of choice', *Brit. J. math. stat. Psychol.*, vol. 18, pp. 207–25.
FITTS, P. M. (1954), 'The information capacity of the human motor system in controlling the amplitude of movement', *J. exp. Psychol.*, vol. 47, pp. 381–91.
FITTS, P. M., and PETERSON, J. R. (1964), 'Information capacity of discrete motor responses' ,*J. exp. Psychol.*, vol. 67, pp. 103–12.

5 A. T. Welford

The Measurement of Sensory–Motor Performance

Excerpts from A. T. Welford, 'The measurement of sensory–motor performance: survey and reappraisal of twelve years' progress', *Ergonomics*, vol. 3, 1960, pp. 189–230.

Perhaps the most important pioneer break into this problem was made by Hick (1952) who proposed, on the basis of his own data and also those of Merkel (1885), that in making choice reactions the subject gains 'information', in the information-theory sense of the term, at a constant rate.

Merkel had presented his subjects with signals ranging in different trials from one to ten alternatives. The signals consisted of the arabic numerals 1–5 and roman numerals I–V, printed round the edge of a disc. The subject waited for each signal with his fingers pressed on ten keys and, when a number was illuminated, released the corresponding key. The arabic numerals corresponded in order to the fingers of the right hand, and the roman to the left. When less than ten choices were required some of the numerals were omitted.

Hick's own experiments used as a display ten pea-lamps arranged in a 'somewhat irregular circle'. The subject reacted by pressing one of ten morse keys on which his fingers rested. Choices of less than ten were again obtained by omitting some of the lights. The frequencies of the various signals for any given degree of choice were carefully balanced and presented in an irregular order so as to ensure as far as possible that the subject should not be able to predict what signal was coming next. Each light appeared 5 s after the completion of the previous response – an interval too long for the subject to judge accurately when the signal would appear.

Hick found that if the number of possible signals is taken as n and reaction time is plotted against log $(n + 1)$, the observed reaction times for different numbers of signals lie on a straight line which also passes through the origin. We can thus write:

$$\text{choice reaction time} = \text{K} \log(n+1) \qquad \textbf{1}$$

where K is a constant. If we work in logarithms to the base 2, log $(n + 1) = 1$ when $n = 1$ and K is the simple reaction time – a convenient result.

The obvious question arises, why $(n + 1)$ and not n? Hick has pointed out that if the subject is uncertain when a signal will appear he is faced with the task, when it does appear, not only of deciding which it is, but also of deciding that a signal has occurred at all: failure to do so will result in his either reacting when there is no signal present or failing to react when there is one. The additional task of guarding against such errors can be conceived as adding one to the number of possible states of affairs that he has to distinguish – instead of states corresponding to signals 1, 2, 3, . . ., n he has to deal with states corresponding to 0, 1, 2, 3, . . ., n. If the subject were in no doubt when a signal was coming, as, for example, if he were to determine the point of time himself at which the signal light came on, the $+ 1$ in equation would not be required since there would be no temporal uncertainty to be resolved. We may denote the sum of the possibilities including 'no signal' as N, defining N as the *equivalent total* number of equally probable alternatives from which the subject has to choose, and may then rewrite equation 1 as:

$$\text{choice reaction time} = K \log N. \qquad 2$$

This formulation we may call *Hick's Law*. It should be understood that it is an 'ideal' formula and that time lags in the apparatus or in the making of a response may add a constant to the time. [. . .]

Hyman's (1953) and Bricker's (1955) view is that uncertainty about when a signal will come and about which signal has arrived should be treated separately and that we should write instead of equation 2:

$$\text{choice reaction time} = a + b \log n \qquad 3$$

where a and b are constants, and a is equal to the simple reaction time and caters for temporal uncertainty. Again there may be an additional constant due to time lags in the apparatus or in the execution of the response.

Support for this approach appears, at first sight, to come from results by Klemmer (1957) which indicate that information due to temporal uncertainty in a simple reaction time task can be calculated in terms of the variability of the warning period given of a signal's appearance, and of the subject's ability to estimate time. Klemmer's calculations suggest a mechanism different from that involved in making choices, and one which gains information at a much higher rate. The variations in reaction time that he reports between different degrees of temporal uncertainty are, however, small and, as Hick has pointed out in a private communication, should be distinguished from the effects of having to guard against premature or omitted reactions. Hick has further emphasized that since n could in certain circumstances approach 0, equation 3 cannot have general validity since log n would then approach $-\infty$.

Equations 1 and 2 have some intuitive support as well as the theoretical advantage pointed out by Hick: the larger the range of possible signals and responses, the more time the subject is likely to spend scanning them for the occurrence of a signal compared with the time he spends 'wondering when a signal is coming', i.e. in 'scanning' the absence of signal. At the same time it is reasonable to suppose that with practice he might turn his main attention to possible signals or responses and away from the possibility of 'no signal'. The extent to which he did so would be marked by a reduction of the $+1$ in equation 1 and its approach to 0. Again, if the subject's attention were positively deflected away from the possible signal sources, a figure in excess of $+1$ might be needed.

What is clear is that equation 1 gives a better fit than equation 3 to almost all the available data including not only Merkel's and Hick's but also Brown's (1960) and Hyman's own, some of which are shown in Figure 1. Hyman's experiments required the subject to respond verbally to lights which varied from 1 to 8 in different trials. The regression line in Figure 1 has been fitted by eye to pass through the origin. It clearly is a very reasonable fit. The best fit would, however, have been obtained by using a quantity a little less than $+1$ in equation 1. This is perhaps understandable in view of the fact that Hyman's subjects were given a warning 2 s before each signal – a length of time short enough for them to have been able to estimate the time of arrival more accurately than was possible in Hick's experiment.

The only results so far found by the present writer to be fitted better by equation 3 than by equation 1 are from an experiment by Venables (1958) who used a method closely similar to Hyman's in a comparison of schizophrenics and normal subjects. Results from the latter conformed better to equation 1, but those from one of the two groups of schizophrenics were more in line with equation 3. The other group of schizophrenics produced somewhat scattered results which could be fitted equally well by either equation. It should be noted that both groups of schizophrenics differed from normals in the addition of a substantial constant time for all degrees of choice. Their results would seem, therefore, to need special consideration anyway, which would take us into a detailed discussion of changes occurring in schizophrenia and carry us beyond the scope of this paper.

Whichever side is favoured in this controversy, the general line of approach is supported by three further findings:

1. The amount of information conveyed by the signals in a choice reaction task is reduced if they are not all of equal frequency. The amount of information due to uncertainty about which signal will occur can be worked out by summing the amounts of information conveyed by each signal weighted according to the probability of its occurrence. Let us call this $\log n_m$ – the *equivalent* number of equi-probable choices and corresponding to $\log n$ in equation 1. We can thus write:

$$\log n_m = \sum_i \left(p_i \log \frac{1}{p_i} \right) \qquad 4$$

where p_i is the probability of each signal in the set taken in turn. To take account of the requirement to avoid premature or omitted reactions we need to write to place of equation 1:

$$\text{choice reaction time} = K \log (n_m + n_t) \qquad 5$$

where n_t is the addition due to the need to avoid premature or omitted reactions. This is, in fact, the basic form of equation 1 since if all the p_is are equal $n_m = n$ and n_t normally $= +1$.

Hyman (1953) and Crossman (1953) both found reductions of about the expected amounts in the average times required to make choices when the signal frequencies were unequal. Hyman's

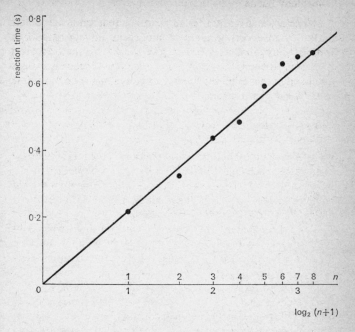

Figure 1 Data from an experiment by Hyman, plotted in terms of equation **1**. The total number of reactions represented is about 20,000 – 5000 from each of four subjects

task has already been briefly described. Crossman's was not, strictly speaking, a reaction time task at all, but involved sorting a pack of cards into various different categories such as picture/non-picture. The times for sorting in these ways were compared with the times for sorting into categories of equal frequency such as red/black or the four suits.

2. Reduction of information also occurs when the signals tend to follow each other in recognizable sequences or when any signal is followed by any other more often than would be expected by chance, even though the over-all signal frequencies are equal. Hyman (1953) also found the expected shortening of average reaction times in these cases.

3. The amount of information gained is reduced if the subject makes errors. A convenient method of calculating the amount of information gained when errors are present is to make a table with, say, a column for each signal and a row for each response, and to enter the responses made to each signal in the appropriate cells. We can then write:

$$\log n_m = \log T + \frac{1}{T} \sum_{\text{SR}} \left(f_{\text{SR}} \log \frac{f_{\text{SR}}}{f_{\text{S}} \times f_{\text{R}}} \right) \qquad 6$$

where T is the total number of readings, f_{S} is the total frequency of signals in each column taken in turn, f_{R} is the total frequency of responses in each row taken in turn, and f_{SR} is the frequency of readings in each cell taken individually. Hick (1952) sets out a practical example from his experiments.

Hick found that the shortening of reaction times when substantial numbers of errors were made was by approximately the amounts expected. This finding is important because it gives us a rational means of combining speed and accuracy of performance into the single score of *amount of information gained*. It also means that times for different tasks can be regarded as comparable only if errors are held constant, and conversely that error rates can be properly compared only if times are held constant.

The same considerations imply that the $+1$ in equation 1 will be reduced if premature responses occur or if responses are omitted.

Hick has noted in a private communication that most, perhaps all, experiments in this area have tacitly assumed that all errors are equally 'bad', and suggests that this may not in fact be correct. Further work would seem to be required on this matter.

References

BRICKER, P. D. (1955), 'Information measurement and reaction time', in H. Quastler (ed.), *Information Theory in Psychology*, Free Press, pp. 350–59.

BROWN, I. D. (1960), 'Many messages from few sources', *Ergonomics*, vol. 3, pp. 159–68.

CROSSMAN, E. R. F. W. (1953), 'Entropy and choice time: the effect of frequency unbalance on choice response', *Quart. J. exp. Psychol.*, vol. 5, pp. 41–51.

HICK, W. E. (1952), 'On the rate of gain of information', *Quart. J. exp. Psychol.*, vol. 4, pp. 11–26.

HYMAN, R. (1953), 'Stimulus information as a determinant of reaction time', *J. exp. Psychol.*, vol. 45, pp. 188–96.

KLEMMER, E. T. (1957), 'Simple reaction time as a function of time uncertainty', *J. exp. Psychol.*, vol. 54, pp. 195–200.

MERKEL, J. (1885), 'Die zeitlichen Verhältnisse der Willensthätigkeit', *Philos. Stud.*, vol. 2, pp. 73–127.

VENABLES, P. H. (1958), 'Stimulus complexity as a determinant of the reaction time of schizophrenics', *Canad. J. Psychol.*, vol. 12, pp. 187–90.

6 R. W. Brainard, R. S. Irby, P. M. Fitts and E. A. Alluisi

Some Variables Influencing the Rate of Gain of Information

R. W. Brainard, R. S. Irby, P. M. Fitts and E. A. Alluisi, 'Some variables influencing the rate of gain of information', *Journal of Experimental Psychology*, vol. 63, 1962, pp. 105–10.

Choice time, or disjunctive reaction time (RT), has been found to be a linear increasing function of the average amount of information transmitted (H_t) per stimulus–response event in a variety of tasks (e.g. Gregg, 1954; Hick, 1952; Hyman, 1953). Hick found that the same function fitted the data when errorless performance was required and also when S speeded up his responses to the point where a substantial number of errors occurred. Hyman, demanding errorless performance, found that RT was a linear function of stimulus information, H_x, (and, therefore, of H_t) when three different procedures for varying average H_x were used: (a) the number of equally probable alternative stimuli was varied, (b) the relative frequency of occurrence of different stimuli was varied and (c) the degree of sequential dependence of stimuli was varied. The mathematical equivalence of these three methods of varying stimulus uncertainty has been shown by Shannon and Weaver (1949); their psychological equivalence can be inferred from the results of Hyman's study.

Similar results have been obtained with the use of self-paced serial-reaction tasks. For example, in a serial card-sorting task Crossman (1953) found choice time to be linearly related to the average information processed per response, and in a serial switch-moving task Archer (1954) found that the average time per response increased as a linear function of the relevant information presented in the stimulus (over the range from 1 to 4 bits/stimulus), but was independent of the irrelevant information presented (over a range from 0 to 2 bits/stimulus).

Although a linear relation between RT and H_t of the form $RT = a + bH_t$ has been consistently obtained, the slopes and intercepts of the functions, i.e. the numerical values of a and b, have varied widely from one task to another. Thus it is clear that parameters other than the informational characteristics of the task are significant in determining RT, specifically in modifying the slope and intercept of the function.

The present study was planned to investigate some of the parameters that may be responsible for the difference in slope and intercept obtained in earlier studies. Specifically, the objective was to determine the effects of (a) two types of stimulus codes (numerals and light patterns), (b) two types of response codes (vocal and finger) and (c) self-paced serial v. discrete-reaction tasks. The four combinations of stimulus and response codes were chosen to provide high and low levels of S–R compatibility. Three levels of stimulus uncertainty (1, 2 and 3 bits/ stimulus) were obtained by varying the number of equally probable alternative stimuli. Only naïve Ss were used, each S serving under only one S–R coding condition and one level of stimulus uncertainty. Thus the experiment also provides further tests of the generality of the linear relation of RT to H_t.

Method

The study was conducted in two parts, which were identical except for the specific S–R pairings used. Pairing of (a) key pressing responses to spatially arranged lights and (b) vocal responses to numerals were used in the first part. It was predicted that these S–R ensembles should show high compatibility, i.e. give relatively high values of H_t per second. Pairings of (c) key pressing responses to numerals and (d) vocal responses to spatially arranged lights were employed in the second part. It was predicted that the latter S–R ensembles would be relatively less compatible since neither physical correspondence nor overlearning operated in its favor. The data of the two parts of the experiment were collected at different times, but the same apparatus and procedures were used throughout and Ss were drawn from the same population of university students.

Stimuli

Two sets of stimuli were used: 0·25-in high arabic numerals and 0·5-in diameter ruby lights. The numerals appeared as projections on the centre of a 10-in diameter circular display of opal glass (brightness of 2·5 ft-L), The lights (440 ft-L) were mounted on a vertically placed panel; they were arranged spatially in two semi-circles to correspond with the placement of the finger tips. Each of the stimulus surfaces was located approximately 28 in directly in front of the seated *S*.

The amount of information characterizing a stimulus event was varied by random selection of stimuli from among two, four or eight equally likely alternatives (1, 2 or 3 bits/stimulus, respectively). One set of conditions consisted of either two, four or eight arabic numerals. At the lowest level of stimulus uncertainty the numerals used were 4 and 7; the numerals 3, 4, 7 and 8 were used at the intermediate level, and all the numerals from 2 through 9 were used at the highest level of uncertainty. The other set of conditions consisted of either two, four or eight ruby-colored lights. For reference purposes the lights, from left to right, were assigned the numbers 2 through 9; the specific lights used in making up the three levels of stimulus uncertainty were those corresponding to the three sets of numeral stimuli. Any light not being used in a specific condition was replaced with a 0·5-in diameter metal cap that was set flush with the plane of the panel.

Mode of information presentation

Stimuli were presented both in a self-paced serial-reaction task and in a discrete-reaction task. In the self-paced task, the first stimulus appeared approximately 3 s after a 'get ready' burst of broad-band noise was presented through the earphones worn by *S*. Each succeeding stimulus appeared 0·15 s after *S* had responded to the previous stimulus. The interval of 0·15 s represents the electromechanical switching time of the experimental apparatus; it was subtracted from the self-paced response times to yield the RTs. (No corrections were made for the rise time of the incandescent lights, lags of the voice key or time clocks, or differential brightness of the ruby lights and projected numerals.)

Discrete stimuli were presented at the rate of one stimulus every 10 s. A red circle in the center of the display screen (or a green light in the center of the array of ruby lights) appeared together with a broad-band noise signal to provide a 'get ready' indication during the 2 s immediately preceding each stimulus presentation. The stimulus remained on for 8 s; it was followed by the 2-s warning for the next stimulus, etc.

Responses

For the key pressing task, a bank of ten keys was arranged horizontally in two semicircles to correspond with a natural placement of the finger tips. These keys were numbered from left to right, 1, 2, 3, ... 10. Wooden blocks were inserted under those keys for which no corresponding stimulus would appear. The fingers used in the key pressing responses for the three levels of stimulus complexity were the two index fingers (4 and 7) for the 1-bit/stimulus level, the middle and index fingers of both hands (3, 4, 7 and 8) for the 2-bits/stimulus level, and all but the little fingers for the 3-bits/stimulus level. When making these motor responses, S's task was to depress the key that corresponded to the stimulus presented. Specific errors were recorded on an 8×8 electromechanical counter matrix.

In making vocal responses S's task was to identify the stimulus by responding with its numerical label. The responses were monitored and errors recorded by E, who had in front of him a list of the series of stimuli being presented to S. The S's responses were also tape recorded so that ambiguities in scoring could be resolved by replaying the record.

Procedure

The study employed a $4 \times 3 \times 2$ factorial design, consisting of the four S–R codes (light and numerical stimuli paired with vocal and key pressing responses), the three levels of stimulus uncertainty (1, 2 and 3 bits/stimulus), and the two task conditions (self-paced and discrete).

Different groups of twenty Ss were assigned to each of the combinations of the four S–R pairings with the three levels of stimulus uncertainty (twelve groups); however each S served under both self-paced and discrete-reaction conditions. Each S

served for five trials lasting somewhat less than an hour in all. Trials 1, 3 and 5 (100 responses per trial) required self-paced serial reactions, whereas Trials 2 and 4 (fifty responses per trial) required discrete reactions. The first self-paced trial was given for purposes of task familiarization and data obtained from it were omitted from analysis.

Each S was seated in a small experimental booth. Ambient lighting was furnished by a single miniature fluorescent light; brightness contrast was high and all stimuli were quite legible. Broad-band noise (approximately 60 dB) was presented continuously to S through their earphones during all self-paced trials in order to mask extraneous sounds. Earphones were also worn during the discrete-reaction trials, but masking noise was presented only during the 2-s interval just prior to the presentation of each stimulus.

Subjects

The Ss were 240 undergraduate students at the Ohio State University, 156 men and eighty-four women. In each part of the study Ss were assigned to one of the six groups used in that part on the basis of order in reporting to E, with the restriction that each group contain thirteen men and seven women.

Results

Three measures of performance were computed: (a) average reaction time (RT, in s/response), (b) average information transmitted per response (H_t, in bits/response) and (c) average rate of information transmission per response (H_t/RT, in bits/s).

Relation between RT and H_t

Average RT and average H_t were computed from the 100 discrete reactions of each S; similar estimates were also computed from the last 200 self-paced serial reactions of each S. Scores for Ss were then averaged to obtain group estimates. The relation between these average RTs and H_ts were examined for each of the eight functions obtained for the different combinations of the two modes of information presentation (discrete and self-paced reactions) and the four S–R pairings. The least-squares linear equations of best fit for the eight conditions are given in Table 1. For none of the conditions was the deviation from linearity statistically significant ($P > 0.05$ in each case).

Table 1

Empirical Linear Equations of Best Fit for Average RT, in s/response, as a Function of Average H_t, in bits/response

S–R Pairing	Task	Equation
N–M	SP	RT = $0.281 + 0.183 (H_t)$
N–M	D	RT = $0.317 + 0.180 (H_t)$
N–V	SP	RT = $0.485 + 0.011 (H_t)$
N–V	D	RT = $0.360 + 0.061 (H_t)$
L–M	SP	RT = $0.229 + 0.111 (H_t)$
L–M	D	RT = $0.182 + 0.136 (H_t)$
L–V	SP	RT = $0.267 + 0.205 (H_t)$
L–V	D	RT = $0.335 + 0.178 (H_t)$

Note.—N=numerals, L=lights, M=motor (key pressing), V=vocal, SP=self-paced, D=discrete.

An average Pearson r between RT and H_t was obtained for all *S*s who used a given S–R code under similar (serial or discrete) conditions. For one of the more compatible conditions (key pressing responses to spatially arranged lights) and for both of the less compatible conditions the correlations were high (the average correlation was $+0.84$). Thus, for these conditions, approximately 70 per cent of the variation in average RT is accounted for by the variations in H_t. However, the average correlation between RT and H_t was only $+0.34$ for the group tested under conditions in which vocal responses were made to numerical stimuli; here the variations in H_t account for only about 10 per cent of the variations in RT.

Effect of mode of information presentation

The two modes of information presentation (discrete *v.* self-paced serial reactions) produced relatively small differences in performance. The linear relations between RT and H_t were nearly identical within each of the four S–R pairings and the differences between the four pairs of discrete and self-paced conditions in terms of the correlations of RT and H_t were in no case statistically significant ($P > 0.05$ in each case). There were small differences between the discrete and self-paced serial reactions in both RT and H_t, however, as shown in Figure 1.

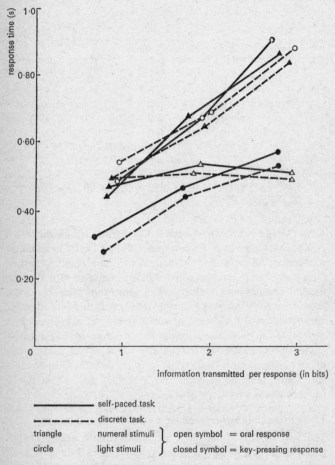

Figure 1 Reaction time as a function of information transmitted for four S–R codes and for self-paced versus discrete tasks

In the majority of cases the discrete reactions were made slightly slower and more accurately than the self-paced serial reactions; these changes tended to counteract each other, however, since average H_t/s was almost identical for the two conditions.

S–R compatibility effects

The most striking S–R compatibility effect is apparent from an examination of the slope constants for the linear equations of Table 1. In all cases the slopes of the functions relating RT and H_t for the less compatible tasks are greater than are those for the most compatible tasks. Thus, differences in RT attributable to the use of different S–R codes are present when only two alternatives are used, but increase markedly as the number of alternatives (and H_t per response) increases.

Discussion

The present results agree with those of previous investigations showing that RT is a linear function of H_t. They also agree with previous studies (cf. Alluisi, Muller and Fitts, 1957) in indicating that average information transmission rates increase, within limits, as the size of the coding alphabet is increased. These results, it should be noted, are for relatively naïve Ss whereas most previous studies have employed practiced Ss.

Various forms of linear equations were fitted to the data collected here, including the form proposed by Hick in 1952, $RT = b \log (n+1)$, where n is the antilogarithm of H_t. The best fit was obtained for the form used in Table 1, $RT = a+b (H_t)$. This mathematical model offers the additional advantage of providing estimates of RT as H_t approaches zero.[1]

1. Simple RTs of five Ss (one male and four women) who were members of the laboratory staff were measured with the same apparatus used in this study. Means of 0·316 and 0·440 s were obtained for the key pressing and vocal responses, respectively, to the numerals; means of 0·207 and 0·311 s were obtained for the same responses to the lights. The σ_ms of these means were 0·008, 0·022, 0·001 and 0·010 s, respectively. Each mean lies between the discrete and the self-paced serial-reaction intercepts of the appropriate equations of Table 1. The relatively high absolute values for the RTs to numerals may reflect the rise times and lower intensities of the projected numerals; vocal RTs include a slight lag time of the voice key.

Information transmission rate does not appear to be differentially affected by changes from discrete to self-paced serial reactions. There was a tendency for the discrete reactions to be made more accurately but more slowly than the serial; however, these differences in H_t and RT were small and compensating. Thus, the linear equations were essentially identical for each of the four comparisons. It appears, therefore, that the serial task, in which only the 0·15-s machine lag intervened between S's response and the appearance of the next stimulus, permitted as effective information processing as did a rest interval of 8 s followed by a 2-s warning signal.

Marked differences in the values of the intercept (a) and slope (b) constants were found as a function of the S–R coding combinations employed. In view of the number of previous studies that have obtained similar S–R compatibility effects, including studies comparing vocal and motor responses (Alluisi *et al.*, 1957; Muller, 1955), it is clear that human information processing time is highly dependent on the manner in which stimuli and responses are coded as well as upon the degree of stimulus and response uncertainty. The importance of such compatibility effects is further indicated by results that show these effects to persist even after considerable training (e.g. Fitts and Seeger, 1953) and to become increasingly important as the size of the coding alphabet is increased (as shown here). There is also some evidence that the importance of compatibility effects may increase with age (Suci, Davidoff and Surwillo, 1960; Welford, 1958), and several writers have proposed that the magnitude of these effects increases as the level of task stress increases.

The results obtained in the vocal-response-to-numerals task are basically different from the other findings. In both the discrete and the self-paced serial task, average RT was only slightly affected by the amount of information transmitted (H_t) per S–R event. As a matter of fact, RTs remained approximately constant for the 2- and the 3-bits/stimulus levels of stimulus uncertainty.

The failure of RT to decrease significantly as the number of alternative stimuli was reduced has been found (a) in studies that required S to read words with the number of possible stimulus words varying over a range from 2 to 256 (Pierce and Karlin,

1957; Sumby and Pollack, 1954), (b) in a study wherein S was trained for 45,000 trials on a task requiring finger responses to lights (Mowbray and Rhoades, 1959) and (c) in a study in which Ss made finger responses to vibratory stimuli applied to the finger tips (Leonard, 1959). From a consideration of the tasks used in these studies, the common finding may be given a plausible explanation in terms of the extended learning involved. It seems reasonable to expect that the stronger the habit strength of the S–R combinations required in a specific task, the less steep should be the function relating RT to H_t.

However, in the present study, there is little *a priori* basis for assuming stronger habit strength for numeral-vocal responses than for light-finger responses, i.e. for predicting less effect of H_t per response for the former type of coding. It appears possible, as an alternative, that the effects of learning may be reflected in the ability to deal effectively with particular sets of stimuli in combination. In the present case the 4–7 and 3–4–7–8 combinations of numerals may have been so incongruent with S's previous experience in dealing with subsets of numerals that he responded as though the entire alphabet of ten arabic numerals was being presented. Such a cognitive set presumably would not operate in the case of the lights, since there is no *a priori* reason to expect a set of any particular size.

Summary

This study investigated the effects on information processing of (a) the use of self-paced serial reactions *v.* discrete reactions, and (b) the use of different stimulus and response codes (both numerals and lights were used as stimuli, and both vocalizations and finger movements were used as responses), and (c) the use of three levels of stimulus uncertainty (ranging from 1 to 3 bits/stimulus in unit steps). These several conditions, and the use of naïve Ss, provided further tests of the generality of the function, $RT = a + b\,(H_t)$.

The results were: (a) Reaction time (RT) was an increasing linear function of the average amount of information transmitted (H_t) per stimulus–response event for three of the four S–R pairings employed. The RTs obtained for vocal responses to arabic numerals, however, were affected only slightly by number of alternatives in the range from 2 to 8. (b) The self-paced and discrete tasks gave very similar results. There was a slight tendency for the discrete reactions to be made more accurately but more slowly than the self-paced serial reactions, but the differences both in RT and H_t were small and compensating. The linear functions relating RT with H_t were essentially identical for the two modes of stimulus presentation.

These findings are interpreted as indicating the importance of overlearning in determining S–R compatibility effects. The findings also suggest that S's familiarity in dealing with specific subsets drawn from familiar alphabets may also affect his information-handling rates, when restricted subsets of stimuli and responses are used.

References

ALLUISI, E. A., MULLER, P. F., JR, and FITTS, P. M. (1957), 'An information analysis of verbal and motor responses in a forced-paced serial task', *J. exp. Psychol.*, vol. 53, pp. 153–8.

ARCHER, E. J. (1954), 'Identification of visual patterns as a function of information load', *J. exp. Psychol.*, vol. 48, pp. 313–17.

CROSSMAN, E. R. F. W. (1953), 'Entropy and choice time: the effect of frequency unbalance on choice-response', *Quart. J. exp. Psychol.*, vol. 5, pp. 41–51.

FITTS, P. M., and SEEGER, C. M. (1953), 'S–R compatibility: spatial characteristics of stimulus and response codes', *J. exp. Psychol.*, vol. 46. pp. 199–210.

GREGG, L. W. (1954), 'The effect of stimulus complexity on discrimination responses', *J. exp. Psychol.*, vol. 48, pp. 289–97.

HICK, W. E. (1952), 'On the rate of gain of information', *Quart. J. exp. Psychol.*, vol. 4, pp. 11–26.

HYMAN, R. (1953), 'Stimulus information as a determinant of reaction time', *J. exp. Psychol.*, vol. 45, pp. 188–96.

LEONARD, J. A. (1959), 'Tactual choice reactions: I', *Quart. J. exp. Psychol.*, vol. 11, pp. 76–83.

MOWBRAY, G. H., and RHOADES, M. V. (1959), 'On the reduction of choice reaction times with practice', *Quart. J. exp. Psychol.*, vol. 11, pp. 16–23.

MULLER, P. F., JR (1955), Verbalization as a factor in verbal versus motor responses to visual stimuli, *Unpublished Doctoral Dissertation, Ohio State University*.

PIERCE, J. R., and KARLIN, J. E. (1957), 'Reading rates and the information rate of a human channel', *Bell Sys. tech. J.*, vol. 36, pp. 497–516.

SHANNON, C., and WEAVER, W. (1949), *The Mathematical Theory of Communication*, University of Illinois Press.

SUCI, G. J., DAVIDOFF, M. D., and SURWILLO, W. W. (1960), 'Reaction time as a function of stimulus information and age', *J. exp. Psychol.*, vol. 60, pp. 242–4.

SUMBY, W. H., and POLLACK, I. (1954), Short-time processing of information, *USAF HFORL tech. Rep.*, no. 54–6.

WELFORD, A. T. (1958), *Ageing and Human Skill*, Oxford University Press.

7 E. C. Poulton

On Prediction in Skilled Movements

E. C. Poulton, 'On prediction in skilled movements', *Psychological Bulletin*, vol. 54, 1957, pp. 467–78.

No attempt will be made to give a detailed account of the role of prediction in a large number of specialized manual skills. Instead there will be a discussion of prediction in a single activity, pursuit or two-pointer tracking in one dimension. Then it will be shown how similar principles are involved in many everyday skills.

Pursuit Tracking

Pursuit tracking has two aspects which are common to a number of skills. First, it involves the acquisition of a moving target, as when an operative picks an object off a moving conveyor belt. Reaching for a stationary object can be regarded as a special case of this more general form of acquisition. And, second, pursuit tracking involves matching a function relating position and time, as in following a moving object with binoculars. Most of the other common examples of this kind of matching differ in two ways from conventional tracking: the task is self-paced, instead of paced by the movement of the target; and the path of the target can be seen ahead. In some cases it is the target path whose movement has to be controlled, as in following a contour with a sewing machine or power-operated fretsaw. In other cases the operative moves along a stationary target path, as in steering a car in traffic or along a winding road, following the contour of a window pane with a paint brush, and tracing the contours of a picture with a pencil.

Pursuit tracking in one dimension can be recommended as a task for study in the laboratory on two counts. First, the target movement or input can be varied along a psychological dimension from simple and repetitive to more complex and irregular. Two other dimensions of target movement, frequency and amplitude, can also be varied independently. And, second, both the input and the response can be recorded as wavy lines on the same moving paper tape, since they are restricted to a single spatial dimension. This record can then be analysed in a number of different ways, and, as Craik has shown (5, 6), the nature of the match or mismatch between the response and the input enables us to specify some of the psychological processes which are involved in the performance.

We shall not discuss rotary-pursuit tracking, for it has neither of these advantages. The input is fixed; and the only measure which is normally taken of the performance is whether S's stylus is touching the target area or not. Ammons (1) has described in detail the techniques of the different experimenters in this field. We shall also not consider compensatory or one-pointer tracking, for it demands more complex computations than are required in most other manual skills. A compensatory display shows S only an error function, which is the resultant of the input and his response movements. He receives no direct indication of the input, and the only direct indication of his response movements comes from the kinesthetic and other bodily sensations which they produce (31).

The rapid acquisition of a stationary target

A rapid aiming movement which is completed in about 0·5 s cannot contain a voluntary correction, for a voluntary movement has a reaction time (RT). Under the optimal condition where S is ready and waiting for the signal for the movement, this RT is about 0·2 s. Similarly, the voluntary correction of a movement also has a RT. Vince's results on the reactions to pairs of successive signals suggest that the sooner the voluntary correction is made after the initial movement, the longer this RT will be (40, table 1). Hick has shown that when S is half expecting to have to make a voluntary correction, and the signal which indicates that a correction must be made occurs as he starts his initial movement, the correction has a RT of about 0·3 s (21). If we add the 0·2-s latency of the original aiming movement to the 0·3-s latency of the voluntary correction, we obtain a total delay of 0·5 s.

This is the minimal time after the signal for an aiming movement, at which a voluntary correction of that movement could start to become effective. The commencement of a voluntary correction even as soon as this, assumes that S was more or less prepared for it, and took the decision at the time that the original aiming movement began, before the movement got under way.

It follows that a rapid aiming movement should be unaffected by visual monitoring, for there is no time to use this visual information. This hypothesis has been tested by Taylor and Birmingham (see 3, pp. 1–2) who used an oscilloscope display and a single practised acquisition movement. They compared three conditions: (a) visual monitoring of the response on the oscilloscope; (b) an unexpected failure of visual monitoring – the position of the spot on the oscilloscope was unaffected by the response; and (c) an unexpected reversal of the normal control–display relationship, such that the usual response made the spot move in the opposite direction. They found that in all three conditions the characteristics of the movement of the first attempt at acquisition were the same, although in condition (c) this movement was followed in due course by a response in the correct direction.

The decision to make a rapid aiming movement thus involves a prediction. As it were, S says to himself: 'if I contract such and such muscles to such and such an extent, I will end close to the target.' This appears to be the most elementary form of prediction shown in skilled movements. It will be called *effector anticipation*, and is listed in the top row of Table 1. The more obvious forms of prediction discussed later can be looked upon as extensions of this elementary form. To many psychologists this may not appear to involve prediction at all, only simple learning. But the point is that the use of any learning involves prediction of a kind. In a familiar situation S makes a particular response because in some sense he 'knows' from his past experience that it should turn out to be correct.

In the rapid acquisition of a stationary target some over-all time for the muscular contractions has also to be specified. But this time is not critical unless S has been told that he must acquire the target as rapidly as possible, or at some particular instant. For the sake of brevity and simplicity of exposition,

Table 1

Predictions Required in Pursuit Tracking

Task	Predictions	Name
Acquisition		
Rapid acquisition of a stationary target	(*a*) Prediction of nature and size of muscular contractions required	Effector anticipation
Rapid acquisition of a moving target whose future track is displayed ahead	(*a*)+(*b*) Prediction of duration of response movement	Receptor anticipation
Rapid acquisition of a moving target whose track is controlled by known constants or statistical properties	(*a*)+(*b*)+(*c*) Prediction of future position of target at time of completion of response movement	Perceptual anticipation
Matching		
Matching the movement of a target whose future track is displayed ahead	(*1*) Prediction of nature and size of response adjustment required +(*2*) Prediction of duration of response adjustment	Receptor anticipation
Matching the movement of a target whose track is controlled by known constants or statistical properties	(*1*)+(*2*)+(*3*) Prediction of future movement of target at time of completion of response adjustment	Perceptual anticipation

we shall not consider these special cases. We may simply note that by suitable experimental procedures it would no doubt be possible to produce situations which would require subdivisions of the relatively simple broad classifications which we are going to present.

A rapid aiming movement may be followed by one or more voluntary corrections, as it becomes clear that the present movement will not hit the target exactly. These voluntary corrections are often beautifully illustrated by records from step-tracking experiments, such as those of Vince (40, fig. 3), Searle and Taylor (37, fig. 3), Ellson and Wheeler (14, fig. 2), Craig (4, fig. 2), and Slack (39, fig. 2). In addition, a rapid aiming movement may involve several corrections at the level of the spinal reflex. For as Woodworth has pointed out (42, p. 116), the knee jerk, which is one of the classical instances of a reflex correction, has a latency as short as 0·03 to 0·04 s. It is only voluntary movements with which this paper is concerned.

The lengthening of the RT to the second of a pair of signals has been called 'psychological refractoriness'. Welford (41) has cited the evidence for this phenomenon up to 1950, and since then there have been papers by Elithorn and Lawrence (10) and Davis (7, 9), and also some comments on the Elithorn and Lawrence paper (8, 22). Refractoriness can be demonstrated under two distinct conditions, which are often confounded (28): (a) The S may not expect the second signal; (b) the second signal may follow the first so closely that he has no time to prepare for it, whether he expects it or not. Aiming responses made without adequate preparation also tend to be less accurate than well-prepared aiming responses (28, p. 104; 33, table 1).

The rapid acquisition of a moving target

As has been pointed out by Young (43), this is a more complex process than acquiring a stationary target, because the target will have moved before S has completed his response movement. For acquisition to be accurate, he has therefore to know in advance the position which the target will occupy at the time his response movement finishes. In addition, as with a stationary target, he has to make a prediction about the nature and size of the muscular contractions required to reach this point. There are two possible sources of information which can be used to determine the future position of the target.

First, the future track of the target may be displayed ahead. Examples are certain laboratory tasks which simulate a simplified form of driving. Thus in one experiment (32, harmonic tracking task), S was given a ball-point pen which could be moved against a transparent bar. He had to keep the point on a curved line drawn on a paper tape. The tape moved at a constant speed at right angles to the bar, and the curved line on it could be seen for varying distances ahead of the bar. Accurate acquisition is possible in these circumstances, provided S can predict how long his response movement will take. For he can then aim at the point ahead which the target will have reached as his response movement is completed. This whole procedure has been called *receptor anticipation* (30, p. 222), because the receptor mechanism has to function ahead of the response mechanism. It is listed in the second row of Table 1. Receptor anticipation may be looked upon as a special case of the more general receptor–effector span, such as the eye–hand span in touch-typing from copy. It is a special case because it involves more accurate judgements of timing than are usually required.

Second, the future track of the target may not be displayed ahead, but the track may contain constants or statistical properties which are known to S from past experience (31, 35). Thus the target may be traveling in a predictable direction at a predictable rate. Examples are aiming just ahead of an object which is traveling at a familiar speed, in order to pick it off a moving belt or rotating table, when the object can be seen but the belt or table is screened from view. For acquisition to be accurate under these conditions, S has to make the two predictions mentioned previously, and one additional prediction. He must now predict the position which the target will occupy as his response movement is completed. The whole procedure has been called *perceptual anticipation*, to distinguish it from the rather simpler receptor anticipation (30, pp. 222–3). It is listed in the third row of Table 1.

Matching the movement of a target

Matching the movement of a target without a response lag can be looked upon as the continuous acquisition of a moving target. It is the more general case, of which a discrete acquisition is a special instance. The predictions required are similar to those discussed above, and are listed in the bottom half of Table 1.

If matching were carried out by a series of rapid acquisition movements, S would be in alignment approximately every 0.5 s, but between these times he might be ahead of or behind the target. In practice, when receptor or perceptual anticipation is possible in pursuit tracking, the experienced S tends to match the rate of movement of the target, or even its acceleration. If he matches the target rate, he adjusts the rate of his movement to match the known or predicted rate of the target at the predicted time at which his decision will have been carried out. He may at the same time attempt to correct a small mismatch in position, by selecting a rate slightly greater or less than the known or predicted rate of the target. But if the target has a constant rate, Ellson, Hill and Gray have found that small misalignments may continue for several seconds at a time, although there is virtually no mismatch in rate (13). This is one line of evidence that the practised S can match the rate of the target.

Another line of evidence comes from Elkind (11, p. 43), who used noise inputs with various spectral shapes and cut-offs. With most inputs he found that the magnitude of the closed-loop transfer function increased at high frequencies. This, he stated (11, p. 41), 'is characteristic of systems that respond to input derivatives'. Additional evidence is supplied by Senders (38), who appears to have used inputs composed of two sinusoids. He found that display conditions which supplied the greatest amount of information about the target rate tended to give the best time-on-target scores.

In pursuit tracking with a simple harmonic input of 60 c.p.m., a difference in phase or amplitude, or a constant error in position, between the target and response pointers was sometimes found to have arisen gradually (34). When the difference became large enough, it was corrected. Somewhat similar results have been reported by Noble, Fitts and Warren (27). These errors can be looked upon as due to more or less constant mismatches in various rate functions. They suggest that S was predominantly matching the acceleration of the target, and was neglecting small differences in rate until they resulted in appreciable errors in position.

The nature of the tracking performance immediately following a blink (which completely obscures vision for about 0·25 s [23]) also suggests that S can respond to the acceleration of the target (36, p. 65). For theoretical errors calculated on the following two assumptions – (a) that S stopped initiating any movement while blinking, and (b) that he stopped initiating any change in rate of movement while blinking – were in both cases much greater than the observed errors.

However, when Gottsdanker (16, 17, 18) instructed his Ss to extrapolate accelerating and decelerating target movements, he found that they extrapolated the rate at which the target moved a little before it disappeared, but not its acceleration or deceleration. This was presumably due to lack of adequate practice with knowledge of results (KORs). For after only two practice runs with each course under a condition which could have afforded KORs if S had been aware of it (16, tracking a completed course), some response to acceleration was found. In a more recent review (19) Gottsdanker wrote as if he might be aware of this criticism, although he did not mention it. For he outlined a program of research on the perception of acceleration.

Where it is possible to match the acceleration of the target reasonably accurately, the mean tracking error is likely to be reduced. For a small error in acceleration produces initially only a small difference in rate between the two pointers. This difference in rate has to be left uncorrected for a time before it results in an appreciable error in position.

When the acquisition of a target is to be followed by matching, the two processes may be blended together. Instead of acquiring the target as quickly as possible, S can acquire the target more gradually. He may move at a rate which is intermediate between the fastest possible rate of acquisition, and the present rate of the target. Such a compromise reduces the acceleration component in the response. As we say, it makes the performance smoother. But smoothness is achieved at the price of a slightly greater error averaged over time. The use of these compromise responses in pursuit tracking is shown clearly when the two-pointer display is made invisible for a period of time. For on the reappearance of the display S is often confronted with a quite considerable discrepancy between the positions of the two pointers. In these circumstances it has been found that the practised S generally makes a compromise response (34, p. 191).

Matching with an average lag of practically zero has been reported in pursuit tracking when the future track of the target was visible ahead (32, table 3). A view of the track for 0·4 s ahead was found to be about as effective as a view for 8·0 s ahead. But a view for only 0·3 s ahead resulted in a significant increase in mean lag. Ellson and Gray (12, figs. 2 and 3) found a mean lag (or negative phase shift) of practically zero in pursuit tracking with predictable simple-harmonic inputs of either 30 or 60 c.p.m. In this case there was no preview of the target track. A certain amount of practice is required before the mean lag is reduced to practically zero under these conditions (30, fig. 4).

If the track of the target is neither displayed ahead nor predictable, S's responses will tend to be at least one RT behind the target. In these circumstances he has two extreme courses of action open to him. Either he can attempt to follow the track of the target more or less exactly, but with a relatively large and consistent lag. Or he can attempt to reduce the mean lag to his RT, by reacting as quickly as possible to each obvious discrepancy between the positions of the two pointers. This latter course of action reduces the mean error, but also reduces the smoothness of the response record. In practice, the mean performance of a group of Ss lies somewhere between these two extreme courses of action (32, table 3).

Everyday Skilled Movements

Smooth complex movements

Prediction plays an important role in smooth complex movements. We will consider first a complex movement which does not have to fit the environment at all, e.g. drawing the letter 'S' in space. The S does not have to wait until he has completed the first component of such a movement (whatever a component is taken to be), before he initiates the next component. For he knows from previous experience the approximate position he will have reached at the end of the first component, and the approximate time it will have taken him. He therefore initiates the next component, which will carry him on from this point, before he has ever reached it. He can thus make a single smooth movement, instead of a succession of simpler movements separated by short pauses.

Two predictions are involved for each component of such a smooth complex movement. First, a prediction has to be made as to where the component will end. If the movement is regarded as aiming at a series of imaginary targets, this prediction can be put the other way around: *S* has to predict the nature and size of the muscular contractions required to reach the imaginary target which is the endpoint of the component. And, second, he has to predict the time at which the endpoint will be reached. These predictions are listed in the fourth row of Table 2. A good deal

Table 2

Predictions Required in Everyday Skills

Movement	Prediction	Name	Analogous Verbal Task
Discrete aiming	(a) Prediction of nature and size of muscular contractions required	Open skill without advance information	Reading aloud a word on a memory drum
Variable smooth complex	(a)+(b) Prediction of duration of each component	Open skill with advance information	Reading aloud from manuscript
Relatively invariant smooth complex	(a)+(b)+(c) Prediction of future requirements	Closed skill with predictable requirements	Reciting aloud
Relatively invariant smooth complex	(a)+(b) only	Closed skill without external requirements	Rehearsing silently
Aiming with amendment	(1) Prediction of unsuccessful outcome of present response (2) Prediction of future position and movement of responding member in one RT (3) Prediction of nature and size of response adjustment required at this point	Open skill with exacting positional requirements	Amending the pronunciation of a difficult foreign word

of practice is needed, both in order to ensure that each component movement is made with sufficient precision to have a suitable and reasonably predictable endpoint in space and time, and so that *S* can learn the range within which this endpoint will fall. In our example of drawing an S, most of this practice presumably occurred on first going to school.

A smooth complex movement of this kind can be called a *closed skill without external requirements*. The term 'closed' was selected (29, p. 4) because the performance can be carried out successfully without reference to the environment. A somewhat analogous verbal task is rehearsing to oneself an overlearned sequence of words or nonsense syllables. (A closed skill does not need to be a single smooth complex movement. Thus a succession of taps, each separated by periods of inactivity, may also be a closed skill without external requirements. But in this paper we are concerned with periods of more or less continuous movement, not with periods of inactivity.)

A closed skill can be made to fit the environment, provided the requirements are not too exacting, and can be predicted in advance. An example is dealing a pack of playing cards into four piles. This can be done by almost any experienced player with his eyes closed. For he has only to ensure that the cards land face downwards, that each pile receives a card in turn, that the piles are located on the table, and that they do not run together. Except for these restrictions, the exact position of each card does not matter, and the task is unpaced.

A closed skill of this kind can be looked upon as the more general case, of which a closed skill without external requirements is a special instance. The same two predictions have to be made about each component as in a closed skill without external requirements. And, in addition, a prediction has to be made about the requirements of the environment. These predictions are listed in the third row of Table 2, under the title 'Closed skill with predictable requirements'. Certain of the imaginary targets of the closed skill without external requirements have simply become real. Practice is again necessary. Reciting aloud an overlearned sequence is a somewhat analogous verbal task.

Lincoln (26) has published a study in which one condition involved the learning of a closed skill with predictable requirements. This study differed from our example of dealing a pack of cards, in that it was the rate of a movement which had to be learned; the nature of the movement can be looked upon as either predetermined or irrelevant. A handwheel had to be turned for periods of 15 s at a rate of 100 r.p.m. In the relevant condition the only knowledge of results was given at the end of each period, when S was told his average error. Lincoln found that, after the first few trials, Ss trained in this way performed as accurately as Ss who had the additional advantage of seeing all the time how their rate of turning deviated from the required rate. Another study used pursuit tracking with a simple-harmonic input of 60 c.p.m. (34). In this case both the nature and the rate of the movement had to be learned. It was found that, after a relatively short learning period, S could sometimes respond for 5·0 s with his eyes shut without any appreciable effect upon his performance.

A closed skill with predictable requirements needs to be checked intermittently against the environment. This is because with the passage of time the performance tends gradually to drift in its positioning and/or timing from the optimal requirements. The less exacting the requirements are, and the more practiced the S is, the longer will be the time for which the skill can proceed without a check. In the two examples we have just considered, the performance only proceeded for 15·0 and 5·0 s respectively before a check was made. In the case of tracking with the eyes shut, an error in phase had generally developed by the end of the 5·0 s, as a result of a small error in wave length (34, p. 192).

Closed skills may be contrasted with *open skills*. An open skill is a skill which has to fit either an unpredictable series of environmental requirements, or a very exacting series, whether predictable or unpredictable. Provided (a) that the unpredictable series of requirements is not too exacting, (b) that each requirement is presented either before S is ready for it, or before it needs to be considered, and (c) that the requirements are not separated by spells of inactivity, a smooth complex movement can still be made to fit the series after practice. For once S has apprehended the next one or more requirements, he can proceed in the same fashion as in a closed skill with predictable requirements. The two predictions involved are listed in the second row of Table 2, under the title 'Open skill with advance information'. Reading aloud from a manuscript is a somewhat analogous task.

There are certain characteristic differences between a closed skill with predictable requirements and an open skill with advance information. Leonard found that with a four-choice self-paced task, an open skill with advance information could not be performed as rapidly as the comparable closed skill (25). He attributed this to the need to take in the advance information in the open skill. On the other hand, when the relative timing of the responses (or changes in response) was all important, a condition which allowed S to see the future requirements all the time resulted in greater speed and accuracy than conditions in which the future requirements had to be remembered, or deduced from previous requirements (35).

Serial aiming movements

The requirements of the environment may be relatively unexacting, but the next requirement may not be presented until S is ready for it, and it needs to be considered immediately. In this case the aiming movement which corresponds to each requirement must be separated from the aiming movement which corresponds to the next requirement by a pause at least as long as an RT. Each aiming movement is similar to the rapid acquisition of a stationary target in tracking. The only prediction involved is thus of the nature and size of the muscular contractions needed to hit each target. This type of movement is listed in the first row of Table 2, under the title 'Open skill without advance information'. An analogous verbal task is reading single words presented one at a time on a memory drum. (If S has been instructed to respond as quickly as possible after the presentation of the signal, the over-all time for the muscular contractions has also to be included in the prediction. For simplicity of exposition this special case is not covered by Table 2.)

Leonard (24) has compared open skills with and without advance information. He used both a two-choice task in which movements were constrained to a triangular path, and a four-choice task with a free-moving stylus. In both tasks S was instructed to work as fast as he could, while making as few errors as possible. Leonard found that with advance information the component movements tended to merge into each other; more time was spent on moving and less time on pausing. Whereas without advance information the component movements tended to be separated by pauses; less time was spent on moving and more time on pausing. Thus greater smoothness was possible with advance information. Leonard noted (24, p. 148) that to appreciate this difference fully it had to be observed, or, better still, experienced. The changes in movement time were smaller than the changes in the time spent on pausing, and hence the tasks were also performed rather more quickly with advance information.

When the positional requirements of the environment are more exacting, two or more aiming movements may be needed for each target, owing to the residual noise in the response system. With a relatively unpractised S, these successive movements may be separated by RTs. They are thus similar to the discrete aiming movements which we have just discussed. But with practice the successive aiming movements tend to merge into each other, so that it is often difficult to tell exactly where a movement would have ended if it had not been amended (33, p. 99).

The amendment of a movement to make it hit a target involves a number of predictions. First, S had to predict that the movement will not hit the target without amendment. Secondly, when he is about to amend the movement, he has to predict approximately where his responding member will be in one RT, and what it will then be doing. And finally, he has to predict the nature and size of the change in movement which is required at this point in order to hit the target. These predictions are listed in the bottom row of Table 2, under the title 'Open skill with exacting positional requirements'. Amending the pronunciation of a difficult word in a foreign language is an analogous verbal task. (A prediction related to the duration of the amending response has also to be included if S is working as quickly as possible.)

An open skill with exacting positional requirements employs a relatively variable sequence of components in order to achieve a highly precise endpoint. It can be contrasted with a closed skill, which employs a relatively invariant sequence of components, but achieves only a less precise endpoint. This is because the closed skill does vary to some extent, and this variation is not corrected as is the case in the open skill.

Mixed movements

Different parts of a cycle of operations may demand different degrees of precision. Where great precision is not necessary, the successive parts which are related to known requirements can be welded into a single, smooth, complex movement. But a part which demands great precision will always tend to need some additional aiming. Thus a cycle of operations may involve both smooth complex movements and serial aiming movements.

An example of a mixed movement is given by Golby, Annett and Kay (15). They recorded the performance of practised Ss carrying a peg 8·0 in and putting it into a hole, by means of high-speed cinematography. The Ss had to work as quickly as they could. As the size of the hole was reduced, the time taken by the first 7·5 in of the carrying movement was found to remain practically constant. It was only the time taken by the last 0·5 in of the movement which increased appreciably (15, fig. 1). In our terminology, the first 7·5 in of the movement was an open skill with advance information, or even a closed skill with predictable requirements, while the last 0·5 in was an open skill with exacting positional requirements.

Golby, Annett and Kay also employed the contact method of recording movements, which has been used extensively by Smith and his collaborators (20). As the size of the hole was reduced, this method showed an increase in both the movement-loaded and the positioning components of the task (15, fig. 1). Clearly this method of recording confounded the low-precision carrying stage with part of the final high-precision aiming. In view of these findings, the authors claim that the cinematograph method of recording movements can give the greater insight into their nature, even though it does involve a good deal more work in analysing records.

Most of the sensorimotor skills of industry must start at the beginning of training as a series of aiming movements. Where an operation needs great precision, or where a requirement cannot either be learned or apprehended in advance, there is a limit to the amount of smoothing which is possible. But where less precision is necessary, and the requirements can be learned or apprehended in advance, each series of aiming movements may become in time a single, smooth, complex movement.

Closed and open have been used in a different sense from the closed and open loops of the electrical engineer. In the engineer's terminology, both closed and open skills involve closed loops within the effector mechanism, i.e. kinesthetic feedback, at least at the level of the spinal reflex. If we consider the over-all input–output relationship, only the open skill with exacting positional requirements necessarily works closed loop on the input, and here there is a delay in the feedback loop corresponding to S's RT. All the other skills listed in Table 2 with external requirements may work open loop on the input for longer or shorter periods of time. Our distinction between closed and open skills corresponds to Campbell's distinction between 'body-consistent' and 'object-consistent' responses respectively (2, p. 334). In his paper, Campbell has discussed the relationship of this distinction to other theoretical viewpoints.

Summary

Table 1 shows three kinds of acquisition which have been studied in the field of pursuit or two-pointer tracking. It also lists the predictions which have to be made in order to carry out each task successfully, and suggests names. Matching a moving target is a more general case of the acquisition of a moving target. Instead of simply matching positions, the practised S tends to match rates or even accelerations.

Table 2 presents a classification for everyday skills. It also shows the predictions which are needed in each case, and suggests a terminology. Many manual operations probably contain as components two or more of the kinds of skill listed.

References
1. R. B. AMMONS, 'Rotary pursuit apparatus: 1. Survey of variables', *Psychol. Bull.*, vol. 52 (1955), pp. 69–76.
2. D. T. CAMPBELL, 'Perception as substitute trial and error', *Psychol. Rev.*, vol. 63 (1956), pp. 330–42.
3. R. CHERNIKOFF and F. V. TAYLOR, 'Reaction time to kinesthetic stimulation resulting from sudden arm displacement', *J. exp. Psychol.*, vol. 43 (1952), pp. 1–8.
4. D. R. CRAIG, Effect of amplitude range on duration of responses to step function displacements, *U.S.A.F., Air Material Command, Tech. Rep.*, no. 5913, 1949.
5. K. J. W. CRAIK, 'Theory of the human operator in control systems. 1. The operator as an engineering system', *Brit. J. Psychol.*, vol. 38 (1947), pp. 56–61.

6. K. J. W. CRAIK, 'Theory of the human operator in control systems. 2. Man as an element in a control system', *Brit. J. Psychol.*, vol. 38 (1948), pp. 142–8.

7. R. DAVIS, 'The limits of the "psychological refractory period"', *Quart. J. exp. Psychol.*, vol. 8 (1956), pp. 24–38.

8. R. DAVIS, 'Comments on "Central inhibition: some refractory observations" by A. Elithorn and C. Lawrence', *Quart. J. exp. Psychol.*, vol. 8 (1956), p. 39.

9. R. DAVIS, 'The human operator as a single channel information system', *Quart. J. exp. Psychol.*, vol. 9 (1957), pp. 119–29.

10. A. ELITHORN and C. LAWRENCE, 'Central inhibition: some refractory observations', *Quart. J. exp. Psychol.*, vol. 7 (1955), pp. 116–27.

11. J. I. ELKIND, Characteristics of simple manual control systems, *M.I.T., Lincoln Lab., Tech. Rep.*, no. 111, 1956.

12. D. G. ELLSON and F. E. GRAY, Frequency responses of human operators following a sine wave input, *U.S.A.F., Air Material Command, Memo. Rep.*, no. MCREXD-694-2N, 1948.

13. D. G. ELLSON, H. HILL and F. GRAY, Wave length and amplitude characteristics of tracking error curves, *U.S.A.F., Air Material Command, Memo. Rep.*, no. TSEAA-694-2D, 1947.

14. D. G. ELLSON and L. WHEELER, JR. The range effect, *U.S.A.F., Air Material Command, Tech. Rep.*, no. 5813, 1949.

15. C. W. GOLBY, J. ANNETT and H. KAY, Measurement of elements in an assembly task – the information output of the human motor system, *Inst. Exp. Psychol., Oxford. Final Rep. to Joint Committee on Individual Efficiency*, 1956, appx. C.

16. R. M. GOTTSDANKER, 'The accuracy of prediction motion', *J. exp. Psychol.*, vol. 43 (1952), pp. 36–46.

17. R. M. GOTTSDANKER, 'Prediction motion with and without vision', *Amer. J. Psychol.*, vol. 65 (1952), pp. 533–43.

18. R. M. GOTTSDANKER, 'A further study of prediction motion', *Amer. J. Psychol.*, vol. 68 (1955), pp. 432–7.

19. R. M. GOTTSDANKER, 'The ability of human operators to detect acceleration of target motion', *Psychol. Bull.*, vol. 53 (1965), pp. 477–87.

20. D. HECKER, D. GREEN and K. U. SMITH, 'Dimensional analysis of motion. 10: Experimental evaluation of a time-study problem', *J. appl. Psychol.*, vol. 40 (1956), pp. 220–27.

21. W. E. HICK, 'Reaction time for the amendment of a response', *Quart. J. exp. Psychol.*, vol. 1 (1949), pp. 175–9.

22. W. E. HICK and A. T. WELFORD, 'Comments on "Central inhibition: some refractory observations" by A. Elithorn and C. Lawrence', *Quart. J. exp. Psychol.*, vol. 8 (1956), pp. 39–41.

23. R. W. LAWSON, 'Blinking: its role in physical measurement', *Nature*, vol. 161 (1948), pp. 154–7.

24. J. A. LEONARD, 'Advance information in sensori-motor skills', *Quart. J. exp. Psychol.*, vol. 5 (1953), pp. 141–9.

25. J. A. LEONARD, Personal communication.

26. R. S. LINCOLN, 'Learning a rate of movement', *J. exp. Psychol.*, vol. 47 (1954), pp. 465–70.

27. M. NOBLE, P. M. FITTS and C. E. WARREN, 'The frequency response of skilled subjects in a pursuit tracking task', *J. exp. Psychol.*, vol. 49 (1955), pp. 249–56.

28. E. C. POULTON, 'Perceptual anticipation and reaction time', *Quart. J. exp. Psychol.*, vol. 2 (1950), pp. 99–112.

29. E. C. POULTON, Anticipation in open and closed sensorimotor skills, *Cambridge, England: Appl. Psychol. Unit Rep.*, no. 138, 1950.

30. E. C. POULTON, 'Perceptual anticipation in tracking with two-pointer and one-pointer displays', *Brit. J. Psychol.*, vol. 43 (1952), pp. 222–9.

31. E. C. POULTON, 'The basis of perceptual anticipation in tracking', *Brit. J. Psychol.*, vol. 43 (1952), pp. 295–302.

32. E. C. POULTON, 'Eye-hand span in simple serial tasks', *J. exp. Psychol.*, vol. 47 (1954), pp. 403–10.

33. E. C. POULTON, 'The precision of choice reactions', *J. exp. Psychol.*, vol. 51 (1956), pp. 98–102.

34. E. C. POULTON, 'On the stimulus and response in pursuit tracking', *J. exp. Psychol.*, vol. 53 (1957), pp. 189–94.

35. E. C. POULTON, 'Learning the statistical properties of the input in pursuit tracking', *J. exp. Psychol.*, vol. 54 (1957), pp. 28–32.

36. E. C. POULTON and R. L. GREGORY, 'Blinking during visual tracking', *Quart. J. exp. Psychol.*, vol. 4 (1952), pp. 57–65.

37. L. V. SEARLE and F. V. TAYLOR, 'Studies of tracking behavior. 1. Rate and time characteristics of simple corrective movements', *J. exp. Psychol.*, vol. 38 (1948), pp. 615–31.

38. J. W. SENDERS, The influence of surround on tracking performance. Part 1. Tracking on combined pursuit and compensatory one-dimensional tasks with and without a structured surround, *U.S.A.F., Wright Air Development Center, Tech. Rep.*, no. 52–229, part 1, 1953.

39. C. W. SLACK, 'Learning in simple one-dimensional tracking', *Amer. J. Psychol.*, vol. 66 (1953), pp. 33–44.

40. M. A. VINCE, 'The intermittency of control movements and the psychological refractory period', *Brit. J. Psychol.*, vol. 38 (1948), pp. 149–57.

41. A. T. WELFORD, 'The "Psychological refractory period" and the timing of high-speed performance – a review and a theory', *Brit. J. Psychol.*, vol. 43 (1952), pp. 2–19.

42. R. S. WOODWORTH, *Experimental Psychology*, Holt, 1938.

43. M. L. YOUNG, Psychological studies of tracking behavior, Part 3. The characteristics of quick manual corrective movements made in response to step-function velocity inputs, *U.S. Naval Res. Lab. Rep.*, no. 3850, 1951.

8 E. R. F. W. Crossman

The Information Capacity of the Human Motor System in Pursuit Tracking

Excerpts from E. R. F. W. Crossman, 'The information capacity of the human motor system in pursuit tracking', *Quarterly Journal of Experimental Psychology*, vol. 12, 1960, pp. 1–16.

Introduction

The usual experimental pursuit-tracking task consists of a display with a pointer which moves from side to side providing a course or input, $i(t)$. The subject has a control connected to a controlled member, a pointer or pen, which produces a track or output, $o(t)$, and his task is to keep the controlled member aligned with the course pointer so that the error, $e(t)$, is a minimum where

$$e(t) = o(t) - i(t). \qquad 1$$

In engineering terms the subject is then part of a closed-loop control system or servo-mechanism whose function is to 'follow-up' the course-pointer. There is a well-developed mathematical theory of linear servo-mechanisms and one of its central concepts is the *transfer function*, which gives $o(t)$ as a function of $e(t)$ and its differential coefficients; hence several workers have attempted to specify the human transfer function and they have had some success (Hick and Bates, 1951; North, 1950). Others (e.g. Fitts, Noble and Warren, 1955) thinking along similar lines have measured subjects' 'frequency response' and 'phase lag' when following sinusoidal inputs. However, this approach does not take account of the fact that the human subject has the ability, not shared by engineering control devices, to learn the pattern of the course and hence predict ahead, a fact which has been demonstrated by Poulton (1952, 1957) and called by him 'perceptual anticipation'. Nor does it allow for his ability to behave at will as an open-chain controller, by attending to the course itself rather than to the error, or to select certain parts of the course for special attention.

The latter aspects of performance can only be taken into account by considering the *statistical* rather than the functional properties of input, output and error, a step suggested by North (1950) but not followed up experimentally. Information theory is the natural tool to choose for this purpose, and one is led to ask, not what is the output as a function of the error, but at what rate is information transmitted from input to output, as a function of the input entropy. The important quantities to study are not then the actual functions $i(t)$, $o(t)$ and $e(t)$, but the time-averaged distributions of their values, $p(i)$, $p(o)$ and $p(i, o)$, and the entropies $H(i)$, $H(o)$ and $H(i, o)$ which measure their predictability. The subject's performance is measured by the rate R at which he can accept information from the course and reproduce it as track where

$$R = H(i) + H(o) - H(i, o). \qquad 2$$

The quantities in equation **2**, being parameters of a continuous signal or ensemble of signals, must be handled according to the theory of continuous information, which differs in important respects from the discrete theory hitherto chiefly used in psychology.

The Theory of Continuous Information

(a) The dependence of information rate on the choice of units

In a discrete information system the entropy of a signal depends only on the relative frequencies with which its different states occur, but in a continuous system it depends also on the size of the step, unit, grouping interval, or quantum used to measure it, increasing with the smallness of this unit (see Shannon and Weaver, 1949, chap. III). However, provided that all the entropies are computed in the same terms and that the unit is small compared to the finest detail in the probability distribution of the variable being considered, the rate is independent of it.

If the unit or grouping interval is too large, genuine fine structure may be blurred out and the rate will be underestimated. But if it is too small, a large sample of performance is needed to give a good estimate of the probability distribution. If the distribution is estimated from a small sample, chance differences of frequency due to sampling error appear as spurious fine detail and the rate is overestimated. The size of this bias has been calculated (Draper, 1954) and a correction can be applied, but the choice of unit must still be a compromise between the two conflicting requirements. For a given size of unit the rate has a definite maximum, equal to the input entropy.

(b) Time sampling

The theory of continuous information sets a limit to the fineness with which the time-scale need be divided up. Since variables in the physical world cannot change instantaneously, their successive values at short time intervals are highly correlated, which reduces the average information per value; and it has been shown (Shannon and Weaver, 1949, p. 53) that all the information contained in a given variable can be extracted by sampling it at least twice per period of the highest frequency W it can contain (i.e. its bandwidth), that is at intervals Δ, where

$$\Delta = \frac{1}{2W}. \qquad\qquad 3$$

(c) Distortion and noise

A distinction is drawn in the theory between two possible sources of discrepancy between the input and output signals in a channel, namely *distortion* and *noise*, and only the latter is considered as a loss of information. Distortion is any discrepancy due to a known systematic effect, and it can in principle be corrected at the receiving end without loss of information; the remainder, due to unpredictable effects, is noise which does cause loss of information. Distortion arose in the present experiments from delay in the subject's response and from a loss of amplitude at high speeds, and both were corrected before calculating the rate.

These and other theoretical considerations indicate that a tracking experiment must fulfil certain conditions if the calculated information rate is to be meaningful. First, the course and the subject's performance must both be statistically 'stationary' during a trial, so that the averaging processes shall be valid. Second, the successive samples of the course must be, or appear to the subject to be, uncorrelated, so that the calculated input entropy shall fairly represent what he experiences. Third, the bandwiths of course and track must be known and similar, so that the proper sampling interval for both can be calculated from equation 3. Having obtained a record of the subject's performance the following steps must then be taken to obtain his information rate:

1. Measure the values of corresponding sample points of course and track at time intervals Δ chosen according to the bandwidth.

2. Compute the frequency distributions of the sample values of course and track and their joint distribution, with a properly chosen grouping interval, allowing if necessary for distortion.

3. Compute the input, output and joint entropies per sample point.

4. Compute the rate per sample from equation 2, and hence the rate per sec.

Experimental Method

The apparatus used for the present experiments is illustrated in Figure 1. The main unit consisted of a paper drive and course generator driven by a variable speed velodyne motor, and the control was an 18-in vertical hand-wheel geared directly to a laterally moving pen, the controlled member. The subject stood facing a window within which he could see the course drawn by a hidden pen in black ink on a band of paper 8·5 cm wide and his own pen made a red line. The amount of the course visible above his pen, the *preview*, could be reduced by a sliding blind; both course and track were visible for a short distance below the subject's pen. The hand-wheel had to be moved through about 40° to cover the full width of the track and the subject's hand movements thus extended about 6 in up or down in a slight curve; the wheel offered little resistance. For a trial the motor was started by a switch after a verbal warning, and the paper then ran at set speed until one cycle of the course generator had been completed, when it stopped automatically. Eight speeds were used; they are given in Table 3.

The subjects were instructed to do their best to keep the pen-point on the course, but that if unable to follow all its variations they were to attempt to reproduce it even if late. Four subjects were tested in the main experiment; each was given two practice runs, then one experimental run at each of the eight speeds with short ($\frac{1}{2}$ cm) and long (8 cm) preview, making sixteen runs in all, the conditions being taken in random order. For the first

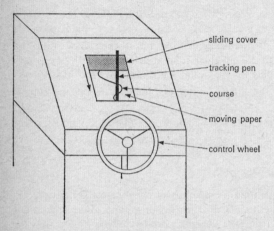

Figure 1 The apparatus used in the tracking experiment

two subjects the course was a pair of black lines 1 cm apart, and for the second two a single line. The time variation of the course was generated by a pair of epicyclic gears driven from the same shaft as the paper drive, so that the course had the same shape on the paper at any speed. The gears had ratios of 5/3 and 3/4 and slightly different radii, the course function being:

$$i(x) = 1 \cdot 25 \sin x + 1 \cdot 10 \sin \frac{8}{3} x + 1 \cdot 27 \sin \frac{17}{12} x$$

where x = distance along the paper in units of 3·8 cm.

The h.c.f. of the three frequency components in the course is $\frac{1}{12}$ and it therefore repeated after respectively twelve, thirty-two and seventeen cycles. The apparatus automatically stopped after one such repetition, which constituted a run. There were ninety-four peaks (reversals of direction) during one run.

The course was intended to be an approximation to a band-limited random signal, in that the subjects were not supposed to be able to predict ahead by learning the pattern. Its autocorrelation function, which is very similar to a part of the course itself, is given in Figure 2, and it can be seen that the maximum correla-

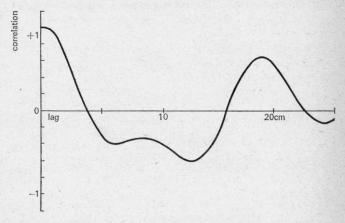

Figure 2 The autocorrelation function for the course used

tion in the first 25 cm is $r = +0.64$; r does not reach unity until at the end of one complete cycle, so that subjects cannot in principle improve their performance greatly except by learning the course as a whole, which did not appear to happen. It was therefore considered reasonable to regard the course as unpredictable over any range greater than 2 cm.

Analysis of Performance

The bandwidth of the course was taken to equal the highest frequency present in it, whose wave-length was 8.8 cm on the paper; by the sampling theorem, equation 3, it would therefore be sufficient to sample its value every 4.4 cm. Since the subject's finite response time always caused the track to lag behind the course, and it was desired to correct this distortion by comparing them at equivalent rather than simultaneous points, it was necessary to have readily recognizable sample points. The

successive peaks on the course were spaced 2·5 to 4 cm apart
and they were therefore chosen as sample points, being both
recognizable and slightly less far apart than the maximum
permissible according to theory; thus there were ninety-four
sample points per run.

It can be seen from the autocorrelation diagram (Figure 2)
that the positions of successive course samples are correlated at
about $r = -0·4$. While the subject could in principle derive
some help from this correlation, the calculation of input entropy
has been based on the assumption that they were independent,
i.e. that the entropy depended only on the probability distribution of sample values of the course. This distribution (Figure 3)

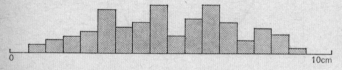

Figure 3 The amplitude distribution of course samples (94 samples;
group interval $\frac{1}{2}$ cm)

was roughly rectangular; with a grouping interval of $\frac{1}{2}$ cm there
were sixteen groups in the maximum excursion of 7 cm. The
input entropy was therefore approximately $\log_2 16$ or 4·00 bits
per sample, though the value calculated from the actual distribution is 3·91 bits. The choice of $\frac{1}{2}$ cm as grouping interval is
equivalent to a choice of $\pm \frac{1}{4}$ cm as the criterion of fidelity in
performance, so that a maximum of 3·91 bits could be transmitted per sample if the subject were to keep his error to less
than $\frac{1}{4}$ cm at each sample point. For a less stringent criterion, the
information per sample would decrease; for example, a unit of
1 cm ($\pm \frac{1}{2}$ cm) decreases the input entropy and the maximum
rate to 2·91 bits per sample.

The track was found to lag behind the course by a fairly
definite amount on any one run (see later discussion and Figure 4).
In principle, this lag represents a distortion which should be corrected by computing the correlation between course and track for
various lags, and then adjusting the track by the one giving
maximum correlation. (In so far as the lag fluctuates, it repre-

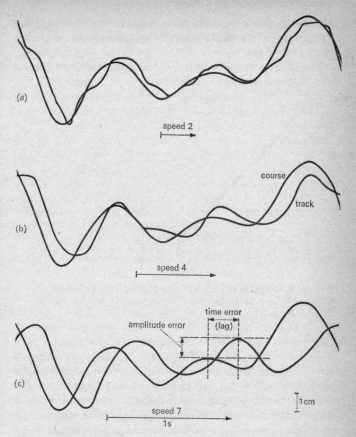

Figure 4 Examples of tracking performance and the indentification of amplitude and time errors: (a) speed 2, no preview; (b) speed 4, no preview; (c) speed 7, no preview

sents a calculable loss of information.) However, for each course peak the corresponding track peak was simply identified by visual inspection (see Figure 4) and for each of the ninety-four pairs the course and track amplitudes i and o relative to the left-hand edge of the paper were recorded, the amplitude error e being obtained by subtraction. Very occasionally (once in a thousand peaks) it was impossible to find a proper sample point on the track and then the error was measured from the average value of the track.

The ninety-four pairs obtained from a run were now entered in a scatter diagram or input–output matrix (Figure 5). A per-

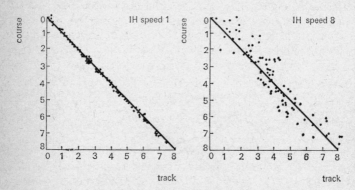

Figure 5 Scattergrams of course and track samples for subject IH. (94 samples are plotted; for perfect performance all points would lie on the diagonal)

fect performance would be represented on the diagram by a diagonal straight line, and complete failure either by a vertical straight line or by a random distribution of dots. The examples given illustrate the fact that performance was found to deteriorate in three ways with increasing speed. First, there was always more scatter about the mean regression line (more random error or 'noise'); second, the mean regression line sometimes had a steeper slope; third, and more rarely, the track was sometimes distributed bimodally, the regression line being then in two parts each parallel to the axis, suggesting that the subject could do no more than get his pointer on to the correct side of the midline. The first and third of these represent loss of information, but the second is a distortion, which was automatically allowed for in the later computations.

There are several alternative formulae from which the input, output and joint distributions in the scattergram could be used to compute the entropies and the information rate (see Shannon and Weaver, 1949, chap. IV); that of equation **2** was used here. If a very large number of sample points had been available on each run, the input–output matrix would have yielded functional probability distributions, and the entropies could then have been evaluated with small error. But there were only 94 samples in each run and since the input sample points were predetermined, not much improvement could be obtained by repeating runs. With a grouping interval of $\frac{1}{2}$ cm there were fifteen possible sample values of the course and track and so 15^2 cells in the input–output matrix. If all of them were occupied, the average cell frequency would be about $0\cdot5$; but only 15 to 40 were actually occupied, giving an average frequency of 2 to 5. The estimated joint entropy $H'(i, o)$ was calculated from the cell frequencies by the formula

$$H'(i, o) = -\sum f(i, o) \log_2 \times f(i, o) \qquad 4$$

where $f(i, o) =$ relative frequency of entries in cell (i, o).

(To simplify the computation a table was drawn up to give the contribution of each cell frequency to the total entropy, and the contributions were then added up directly.) The estimated entropies are perturbed both by sampling error and by systematic bias which are greater for smaller average cell frequency. Draper (1954) and Hick (1956) have given expressions for them but it was not entirely clear how their formulae should apply in the present case; after trying different formulae the following correction for bias was chosen:

$$H(i, o) = H'(i, o) - \frac{k-1}{2N} \qquad 5$$

where $k =$ number of cells in the occupied region of the matrix
$N =$ number of sample-points.

The correction term never exceeded 10 per cent and was usually much less. Table 1 shows the result of applying a different grouping interval to the same data, with and without correction, from which it can be seen that the bias is partly but not completely offset by the correction. As the same interval ($\frac{1}{2}$ cm) has been used throughout, comparisons between speeds and subjects should, however, be little affected by the residual bias in the present experiments.

Table 1

The Effect of Grouping Interval on the Estimated Information Rate

(100 sample points: subject PW, speed 4 with preview)

	Grouping Interval (cm)		
	0·25	0·50	1·00
Input entropy	4·74	3·82	2·88
Cells occupied (*k*)	30	16	9
Corrected value	4·89	3·90	2·92
Output entropy	4·72	3·83	2·91
Cells occupied	29	16	9
Corrected value	4·86	3·91	2·99
Joint entropy	4·84	4·88	3·45
Cells occupied	150	54	9
Corrected value	6·59	5·14	3·50
Rate per sample	3·62	2·77	2·35
Corrected value	3·16	2·67	2·41
Rate per sec	5·25	4·02	3·41
Corrected value	4·58	3·87	3·49

Results

At low speeds (Figure 4a) subjects track accurately. They do not produce smooth tracks with the same bandwith as the course, as they would were they acting as linear servo-mechanisms. Instead there are many small 'ripples' which cross the course several times between sample points, and are presumably due (Hick, 1948) to the discontinuous functioning occasioned by the subject's finite reaction time. The bandwith of the track being greater than that of the course, the track had to be 'smoothed' before computing the rate, and this was done by inspection. At moderate speeds (Figure 4b) the track is very similar to the course in general shape and follows it closely, usually with a small time lag, and some amplitude error; no discrete corrections can now be seen. At high speeds without preview (Figure 4c) the track maintains the general shape and form of the course, but the lag becomes large and substantial errors of amplitude appear. One subject reported 'I am doing no good at all; the thing is

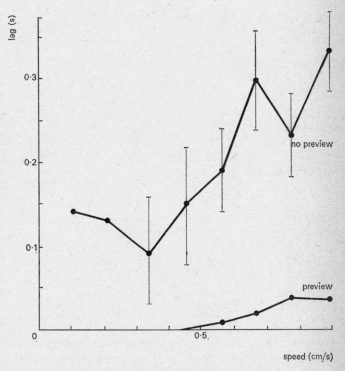

Figure 6 The average lag in tracking. Each point is the average lag over one run for one subject

simply flashing by and I can do no more than make frantic attempts to catch up with it.' In spite of this comment, the performance was considerably better than random, to the subject's later surprise. It was clear from the subjects' remarks that at speeds above 2 or 3 without preview, they aim at each successive peak as it comes up, and make no attempt to follow in between.

Nevertheless, the track is a good copy of the course, which tends to confirm the rightness of the time-sampling procedure. With preview the deterioration is much less marked. Without preview the time lag increased with speed up to a certain point (Figure 6); with it there was a much smaller increase. [. . .]

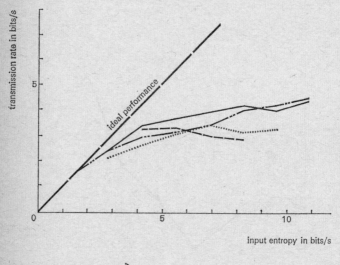

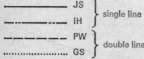

———————— JS	}	single line
—·—·—·—·— IH		
— — — — — PW	}	double line
·················· GS		

Figure 7 Course speed and information – tracking without preview. Information rate per s is shown as a function of course speed for pursuit tracking with minimal preview. Each point represents one run by one subject

The theoretical maximum information rate per s is equal to the input entropy, and hence the curve of ideal performance is a line with unit slope. All subjects achieved this at low speeds, beginning to depart from it at about 2 bits per s without preview and thereafter performance tended to level off at 3 to 5 bits per s (Figure 7). The flat-topped curve suggests that the subjects had an informational 'ceiling' or *channel capacity* of about 4 bits per s.

With preview the curve of performance began to depart from the ideal one at about 3 bits per s (see Figure 8), and thereafter increased linearly. The average slope for all four subjects was about half (0·512 times) the ideal slope. At the highest input

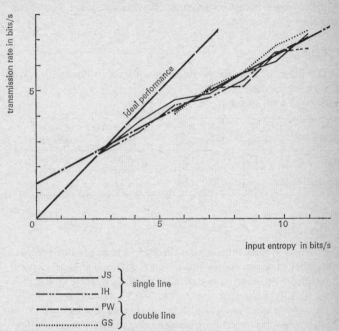

Figure 8 Course speed and information – tracking without preview. Information rate per s is shown as a speed course for pursuit tracking with ample preview. Each point represents one run by one subject. The dotted line has been fitted by the method of least squares; its equation is

$$R = 0.51H(i) + 1.36 \text{ bits}$$

entropy possible with the apparatus, there was no sign of the levelling off which would indicate the presence of a definite channel capacity.

Practice might be expected to have some effect on the rate attainable for any given input speed, and so indeed it did. Table 2 shows the rates for three successive runs for one subject on the same condition. There was a positive but relatively not large increase in information rate. This is in line with the results of earlier studies of pursuit tracking. No attempt was made to measure fatigue effects, but within single runs at high speed there were indications from subjects' reports that fatigue was beginning to be felt.

Table 2

The Effect of Practice on Information Rate in Pursuit Tracking without Preview
(subject PW; speed 4)

Run	H(i) bits	H(o) bits	H(i, o) bits	Rate, bits per s
1	3·91	3·63	6·20	3·04
2	3·91	3·74	6·20	3·16
3	3·91	3·93	6·22	3·32

Discussion

In recent studies information theory has been used to analyse a number of sensorimotor tasks, and the human channel capacity has been measured in two distinct ways. In discrete choice tasks such as light-key reactions (Hick, 1952) and card sorting when the subject does not know exactly what he will have to do on each trial – his uncertainty being measured by the *input entropy* – the average capacity seems to be about 5 bits per s, though with very long practice, as in typewriting or piano playing (Quastler, 1956) or with high 'compatibility' as in target aiming (Crossman, 1956), he may reach 15 to 20 bits per s. In these studies information rate may be measured by the total time taken to make a response of given information, or by the increment of time needed to deal with an increment of information, and the two approaches yield rather different results (Crossman and Szafran, 1956). In particular the time taken to complete the response, which is strictly irrelevant since it does not depend on information, has to be small and constant if the two methods of calculating are to give similar results.

The second type of channel capacity, however, appears in the response itself, as a relation between speed and accuracy. Hand movements only have so far been subjected to study, and the pioneer work is that of Fitts (1954) confirmed by Crossman (1956) and Annett, Golby and Kay (1958). In Fitts' experiment the subject had to tap in turn two metal plates of width w set a distance a apart as fast as he could. The time per tap, t, was found to obey the relation

$$t = -k \log \left(\frac{w}{a} \right) = -k(\log w - \log a) \qquad 6$$

where k is a constant for one subject, a result which will be referred to as Fitts' Law. The right-hand side of the equation can be interpreted informationally (Crossman, 1956) as the difference between an initial entropy $\log a$, and a final one $\log w$, and hence it represents the reduction of uncertainty of the endpoint of movement achieved on a single tap. The information-capacity (the reciprocal of k) was found to lie between 8 and 15 bits per s in all the studies mentioned. In this task the subject knows exactly what to do on each trial, so the input entropy is zero. Therefore the time cannot, as in the previous case, be occupied in transmitting the information in the input, and Fitts suggests that it is taken up in overcoming the 'internal random noise' which prevents a subject repeating a movement precisely.

On the evidence of these studies it seems reasonable to postulate that the human sensorimotor apparatus comprises at least two functionally distinct parts (Figure 9). The first, which may be called the decision or D-mechanism, is concerned with translating visual or other signals into orders which the second, the effector or E-mechanism, carries out. The D-mechanism has a capacity of 5 bits per s in most cases, and up to 15 or 20 bits per s in highly practised or 'compatible' tasks; the E-mechanism achieves about 10 bits per s for hand movements. According to this model a subject's performance at a task such as pursuit tracking will depend on exactly how the two mechanisms are loaded and on the time relations between their activities and the external situation.

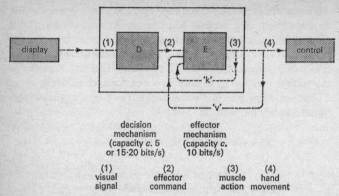

decision mechanism (capacity c. 5 or 15·20 bits/s)   effector mechanism (capacity c. 10 bits/s)

(1) visual signal   (2) effector command   (3) muscle action   (4) hand movement

'k' – kinaesthetic feedback path

'v' – visual feedback path

Figure 9 A schematic representation of information flow in the human perceptual–motor system. The decision (D) mechanism translates perceived signals into instructions for the effector system. The effector (E) mechanism controls the muscular activity needed to carry out the instructions. It may use visual feedback, 'v', and/or kinaesthetic feedback, 'k'

Tracking with preview

The tracking task certainly had high 'compatibility' and the D-mechanism would therefore be expected to work at 15 or 20 bits per s: though the control was by hand-wheel rather than direct movement, it seems reasonable to ascribe a capacity of about 10 bits per s to the E-mechanism. With preview the subject could look ahead as far as he liked and so offset the delays due to the working of the D- and E-mechanisms, by receptor antici- pation (Poulton, 1957). This being so, the smaller of the two capacities should be limiting and one might thus expect an over- all capacity of 10 bits per s. This level was never attained in the experiment (see Figure 8), though no definite ceiling appeared at a lower level.

The fact that the performance increased linearly with input load, yet at less than the ideal slope, suggests that another limita- tion, one allowing a constant fraction, rather than a constant absolute amount of information to be transmitted, must have been present and its locus may be sought in the division of visual attention between course and error. At high speeds, when looking ahead at the course, the subject was only able to see his own pen in peripheral vision, and actually to look at it would have entailed missing some of the course. Now the information capacity measured by Fitts was for a fully visual task, represented in Figure 9 by the E-mechanism with the visual feedback path 'v' in action. An equivalent task done without visual control has been studied by Vince (1948) who reports that hand movements of a few inches' extent made without vision were distributed normally with about $\pm$ 7 per cent error, and took 0·25 s or less. This much error is equivalent to $\log_2$ 100/14 or about 2·8 bits per movement. In the present task, it would imply that as soon as the subject's visual channel, attending to the course some distance ahead of his pen, were loaded sufficiently near to its full capacity of 15 or 20 bits per s to be confined there, the information transmitted per *sample* should settle at about 2·8 bits, and the rate per sec. would be given by 2·8 × (number of samples per s), until the E-mechanism's upper limit of 10 bits per s were reached. The observed performance curve agrees reasonably well with this view, and it may be noted in its support that the curve of transmitted information does appear to flatten out at about 2·5 bits per sample. Figure 10 shows how the performance curve for the preview condition might be expected to behave at loads greater

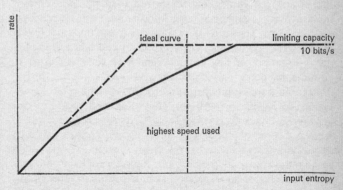

Figure 10 The expected behaviour of subjects tracking at higher speeds than those used. The upper limit represents a channel of 10 bits/s

than those used in the present experiment. It is also noteworthy that subjects reported that they had adequate time for movement at even the highest speeds in the preview condition. If this explanation is correct, then at high speeds with preview subjects made purely positional responses to successive peaks and ignored the velocity and acceleration of the track in between.

(b) Tracking without preview

Without preview the subject's attention must be centred on the narrow slit in which both course and controlled member appear. Bearing in mind that subjects were instructed to *reproduce* rather than strictly *track* the course, and that lag did not necessarily diminish their computed performance, the capacity expected according to the model would be just the same as in the preview condition, but in fact a capacity of only 4 bits per s was found. Again according to the model, the lag should be

$$\frac{3\cdot91}{20} + \frac{3\cdot91}{10}$$

or about 0·6 s, if the subject makes a positional response to each peak in turn; yet the observed lag (Figure 6, Table 3) was less than half this amount, which suggests that subjects may have been sacrificing information (i.e. accuracy of reproduction) to reduce their lag. Least lag is introduced by responding quickest, that is at low accuracy, but for correct tracking each response must on average contain as much information as the track does in the same time. Therefore if the subject is trying to reduce his lag at low track speeds, one would expect to find him making frequent responses of low accuracy and vice versa. In order to examine this point, one subject's records were examined closely; it was found that individual response movements could be distinguished sufficiently well to count them and measure their duration, with results given in Table 3. At low speeds (1, 2 and 3) the expected behaviour clearly occurs; it also appears that even when allowance is made for the residual receptor anticipation permitted by the small preview, this subject must have been predicting course positions (perceptual anticipation) to some extent, since response movements were consistently initiated before their targets came into view. At higher speeds (4 and above) the number of movements fell to one per sample point as had been expected, but the lag was still less than the movement time at all speeds except possibly the highest, and the subject must therefore always have been anticipating course positions.

Table 3

	Speed							
	1	2	3	4	5	6	7	8
(a) Characteristics of the tracking task								
Paper speed (cm per s)	1·09	2·22	3·40	4·53	5·62	6·75	7·80	8·93
Time per sample (s)	2·78	1·37	0·89	0·67	0·54	0·45	0·39	0·34
Input entropy (bits per s)	1·41	2·86	4·38	5·84	7·24	8·69	10·00	11·50
Preview time (8 cm) (s)	7·3	3·6	2·4	1·8	1·4	1·2	1·0	0·9
Preview time ($\frac{1}{2}$ cm) (s)	0·46	0·23	0·15	0·11	0·09	0·07	0·06	0·06
(b) Information rates (average of four subjects)								
Per sample – with preview (bits)	3·86	3·66	3·26	2·92	2·67	2·48	2·50	2·40
Per sample without preview (bits)	3·86	3·18	2·83	2·35	1·91	1·66	1·61	1·77
Per s – with preview (bits)	1·39	2·67	3·66	4·35	4·95	5·50	6·42	7·07
Per s – without preview (bits)	1·39	2·32	3·18	3·50	3·54	3·68	4·10	5·20
(c) Tracking without preview: an analysis of one subject's performance								
Average lag (s)	0·14	0·13	0·09	0·15	0·19	0·30	0·23	0·33
SD of lag (s)	—	—	0·07	0·07	0·05	0·06	0·06	0·05
Average duration of response movements (s)	0·45	0·32	0·30	0·33	0·45	0·44	0·38	0·33
No. of movements per sample-point	4–8	3–4	2–3	1–2	1–2	1	1	1
Information per movement (bits) for perfect performance)	$\frac{1}{2}$–1	1–1·3	1·3–2	2·0	2·0 or 3·9	3·9	3·9	3·9

According to Poulton (1952, 1957) and others, prediction of the future position of a course is based mainly on its speed at the time of observation. If the subject were capable of making such a prediction with the same accuracy and speed as he can observe position itself, the changeover would entail no loss in information rate, but this seems unlikely as the accuracy of prediction must inevitably diminish with its range, and prediction is also perceptually more complicated than direct observation of position. In terms of the model, then, one might suppose the prediction to be carried out by a third mechanism with a capacity of 4 bits per s approximately, whose output would pass to the D-mechanism for translation into motor instruction: but a more parsimonious explanation is suggested by the similarity between the rate found here and that observed in choice tasks of low compatibility (e.g. Hick, 1952), which leads one to suppose that the prediction task is an 'incompatible' one and that the capacity of 4 bits per s can simply be ascribed to the D-mechanism operating in its usual manner. This hypothesis could be tested by setting up a simple choice task involving prediction and measuring the capacity directly.

If it is indeed the use of prediction which lowers the rate, a change might be expected to occur when the course speed no longer allows time for it, that is, when peaks recur at less than about 0·3 s. The subject should then be forced into making pure positional responses lagging by just the spacing of one sample, and the rate should rise steadily with speed from 4 to 10 bits per s. Unfortunately the highest track speed available fell just short of the point where this would begin to happen.

It remains to consider why the subject should avoid lagging by the time (about 0·6 s) needed for pure positional responses. Four reasons can be suggested: (a) that subjects could have done so but were given insufficient practice to overcome their initial reluctance to 'get behindhand'; (b) that too great difference between the current motions of course and track would have produced intolerable visual confusion; (c) that course information might have been forgotten during such a comparatively long delay; (d) that too little feedback information about the response movements would then have been available. Further work will be needed to decide between these alternatives.

Conclusions

The informational analysis of pursuit-tracking performance appears to be feasible and to yield fresh understanding of the mechanisms involved. According to the relatively crude results of the present study the subject's performance seems capable of being fully explained in terms of a theoretical model derived from the results of previous work. In particular, the capacity in tracking with preview is just that of the effector system acting without visual feedback at about 2·5 bits per response or 10 bits per s, whichever is less. Without preview and when the lag is kept small the limit appears to be set at about 4 bits per s by the decision mechanism predicting future course positions.

It is hoped to carry out further work on these lines, with certain improvements. First, the present study was hindered by the need to use a predetermined course pattern, which had too much autocorrelation to be really satisfactory. It now appears technically feasible to provide a truly random course generator of limited bandwidth. Second, it is possible that the speed of eye movements may limit certain features of performance, such as the vision of attention between course and track in the preview condition; eye movements should therefore be recorded and compared with the current hand movements. Third, in the discussion free use has been made of information capacities drawn from earlier work. Since there is considerable variation between individuals, a much more accurate analysis would be possible if each subject's capacity were measured on subsidiary tasks at the time of his tracking performance. Fourth, the present approach could also be extended to study the effect of statistical structure in the course, that is, how far the subject can make use of observed patterns of course behaviour to facilitate his performance.

Finally it may be said that the statistical information theory approach to the study of tracking outlined in this paper is quite compatible with the analytic approach. It does, however, appear that the informational conditions of tracking should be closely specified before a definite transfer function can be identified by analytic means, and that its parameters may be expected to change with the statistical structure of the task.

References

ANNETT, J., GOLBY, C. W., and KAY, H. (1958), 'The measurement of elements in an assembly task – the information output of the human motor system', *Quart. J. exp. Psychol.*, vol. 10, pp. 1–11.

CROSSMAN, E. R. F. W. (1956), The measurement of perceptual load in manual operations, *Unpublished Ph.D. Thesis, Birmingham University*.

CROSSMAN, E. R. F. W., and SZAFRAN, J. (1956), 'Changes with age in the speed of information-intake and discrimination', *Experientia Supp. IV.*, pp. 128–35.

DRAPER, J. (1954), An introduction to information theory with reference to the human operator, *Paper presented to conference at the Military College of Science, Shrivenham.*

FITTS, P. M. (1954), 'The information-capacity of the human motor system in controlling the amplitude of hand-movements', *J. exp. Psychol.*, vol. 47, pp. 381–91.

FITTS, P. M., NOBLE, M., and WARREN, C. E. (1955), 'The frequency-response of skilled subjects in a pursuit-tracking task', *J. exp. Psychol.*, vol. 49, pp. 249–50.

HICK, W. E. (1948), 'The discontinuous functioning of the human operator in pursuit tasks', *Quart. J. exp. Psychol.*, vol. 1, p. 36.

HICK, W. E. (1952), 'On the rate of gain of information', *Quart. J. exp. Psychol.*, vol. 4, pp. 11–26.

HICK, W. E. (1956), Some miscellanea on information theory and the human operator, *Ministry of Supply Report WR/D/2/56.*

HICK, W. E., and BATES, J. A. V. (1951), The human operator of control mechanisms. *Ministry of Supply Monograph 17*, pp. 204.

NORTH, J. D. (1950), The human transfer-function in servo-systems, *Ministry of Supply Report WRD/6/50.*

POULTON, E. C. (1952), 'The basis of perceptual anticipation in tracking', *Brit. J. Psychol.*, vol. 43, pp. 295–302.

POULTON, E. C. (1957), 'On prediction in skilled movements', *Psychol. Bull.*, vol. 54, pp. 467–78.

QUASTLER, H. (1956), The force of habit, *University of Illinois Control Systems Laboratory Report R-70.*

SHANNON, C. E., and WEAVER, W. (1949), *The Mathematical Theory of Communication*, University of Illinois.

VINCE, M. A. (1948), Corrective movements in a pursuit task, *Medical Research Council A.P.U. Report No. 75.*

Part Three
The Nature of Movement and Response Modulation

In 1899 Woodworth (Reading 9) published a series of observations on the accuracy with which movements are made at different speeds. He distinguished two parts of movements, an initial impulse which is programmed in advance and secondary adjustments which are made to attain the required degree of accuracy. If successive repetitive movements are made at a rate of 120 per minute the secondary adjustments disappear and the accuracy of the movements reflects simply the accuracy of the initial impulses. These experiments effectively defined the conditions for observing 'ballistic' movements which are discussed more fully by Craik (Reading 10) and Begbie (1959).

Craik presents a model of the human operator in a system demanding continuous response modulation. Evidence suggests that continuous response modulation is an artifact of the experimental situation and that the underlying mechanisms function intermittently. He suggests that each intermittent modulation is a ballistic movement with a predetermined time-pattern.

The fundamental intermittency of operation of the underlying response control mechanisms has also been studied using reaction time tasks. If these mechanisms can only produce about two modulations per second, then the response to a second signal should be delayed as the interval between the first and second signals is reduced below half a second. Welford (Reading 11) describes five theories which have been advanced to account for the delays in responding to a second signal that have been widely reported. This field has been further developed recently with the observations by Way and

Gottsdanker (1968) and Brebner (1968) that though the second response is delayed the first response may be affected by a second signal. These results refute the simple idea that only one signal is processed at a time and that it is inviolate during its processing. Clearly, the way in which successively arriving signals are dealt with is far from being completely understood.

References

BEGBIE, G. H. (1959), 'Accuracy of aiming in linear hand-movements', *Quart. J. exp. Psychol.*, vol. 11, pp. 65–75.

BREBNER, J. (1968), 'Continuing and reversing the direction of responding movements: some exceptions to the so-called "psychological refractory period"', *J. exp. Psychol.*, vol. 78, pp. 120–27.

WAY, T. C., and GOTTSDANKER, R. (1968), 'Psychological refractoriness with varying differences between tasks', *J. exp. Psychol.*, vol. 78, pp. 38–45.

9 R. S. Woodworth

The Accuracy of Voluntary Movement

Excerpts from R. S. Woodworth, 'The accuracy of voluntary movement', *Psychological Review Monograph Supplement*, vol. 3, 1899, no. 2, pp. 54–9.

If the reader desires a demonstration of the existence of the 'later adjustments' which constitute the most evident part of the 'current control', let him watch the movements made in bringing the point of his pencil to rest on a certain dot. He will notice that after the bulk of the movement has brought the pencil point near its goal, little extra movements are added, serving to bring the point to its mark with any required degree of accuracy. Probably the bulk of the movement is made by the arm as a whole, and the little additions by the fingers. If now the reader will decrease the time allowed for the whole movement, he will find it more difficult, and finally impossible, to make the little additions. Rapid movements have to be made as wholes. If similar movements are made with eyes closed, it is soon found that the little additions are of no value. They may bring us further from the goal as likely as nearer. We have no exact knowledge of where the goal is and so cannot use our finer adjustments.

Another demonstration can be had by drawing a free hand line joining two points. The line will record the changes in direction, and so give us an insight into the later adjustments as far as they are applied to the direction of the movement. Increasing the speed of shutting the eyes produces the same effects as before. There is, however, one new fact that appears and gives us an insight into the character of the first adjustment. If lines of considerable length, say a foot or two, are made at a rapid rate, the changes in direction will probably be found to be about the same in them all. They all start out at nearly the same angle from the true direction and make about the same sweeping curve around to the goal. This curve is not a simple arc but bends back on itself. As this curve appears, moreover, when the eyes are closed, the changes in its direction cannot be due to later adjustments. The initial impulse takes the hand along a curve. We aim around a corner; not according to geometrical straight lines, but according to the make-up of our arm. From the geometrical point of view, the simplest movement that we can make – the movement as determined solely by its first impulse, and not complicated with later adjustments – is still a complex affair. The initial adjustment is itself complex. It includes the innervation of different muscles one after another. The coordination adapted to produce a straight line is probably more complex than that to produce certain curves. The first impulse includes also a command to stop after a certain distance. These later effects of the first impulse are probably in some degree reflex. The proper continuation of a movement which has been started seems, from pathological cases, to be dependent on the preservation of the arm's sensibility. Yet the first impulse of a movement contains, in some way, the entire movement. The *intention* certainly applies to the movement as a whole. And the reflex mechanism acts differently according to the difference in intention. We must suppose that the initial adjustment is an adjustment of the movement as a whole.

A graphic demonstration of the later adjustments in the matter of extent of movement is not so easy as in the matter of direction. But by means of a rapidly rotating kymograph it can be accomplished. By this means a curve of the speed of the movement – similar to the curve of muscular contraction – is obtained, and any little additions to the movement can be detected.

As representing the standard curve of a movement governed entirely by its initial adjustment, we take the curve of 'automatic' movements. Since no attention was paid to the extent of these movements, there is no call for later adjustments. With this standard we may compare the curves obtained when each movement was required to imitate the preceding, or to terminate at a given line. We may compare movements also at different speeds, and of the right and left hands. The comparison will reveal the causes of the differences in accuracy between these several movements. See Figures 1 and 2.

The most striking difference between these tracings is that between the sharpness of their tops. At the slowest rate the automatic movement gives a sharper top than any other, and the studied movements with eyes open the bluntest. The order of sharpness is: automatic, left hand with eyes shut, right hand with eyes shut, left hand with eyes open, right hand with eyes open.

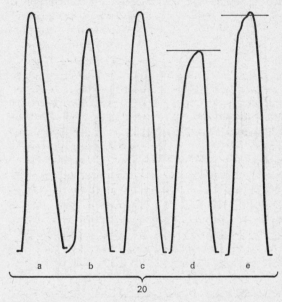

Figure 1 Tracings on a rapid kymograph of different sorts of movements: a, automatic; b, eyes shut, left hand; c, eyes shut, right hand; d, eyes open, left hand,; e, eyes open, right hand. Rate, 20 movements/min. The movements with eyes shut were required to be equal, each to the preceding. Those with eyes open were required to terminate on a line previously ruled on the paper. Selected records (not continuous). Reduced to ½ original size

The blunt top is an expression of extreme slowness of movement at the close. To make up for this, the beginning and middle of the movement, and also the return to the starting-point, are considerably hastened. This slowness at the end is useful because it allows for the fine adjustments. Evidences of these can be seen in the curves. They are visible as irregularities in direction or as marked differences from the run of the automatic movement.

145

Some of the fine adjustments consist in little *additions* to the movement, carrying it beyond where it would otherwise have gone; and others in a *subtraction* or inhibition of the movement, making it shorter than it would otherwise have been. The latter seem to give the best results; the former seem to be corrections of

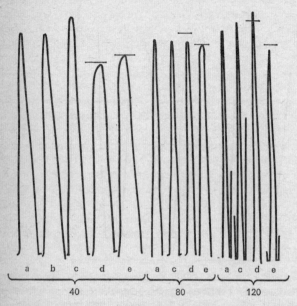

Figure 2 Same as Figure 1 but at rates of 40, 80 and 120. Letters have the same meaning as in Figure 1

mistakes. The best type of later adjustment is that which brings the movement so smoothly to a stop that no sharp change in direction is possible. This type is the best, since it is clearly the least awkward. The whole movement runs smoothly to its desired end, without any break or correction.

Turning now to the records of movements at more rapid rates, we see the differences between the different sorts gradually disappear. At 40 the differences are still present; the time allowed is still sufficient for nearly all the later adjustment that can be profitably used. At 80 only the right hand, eyes open, shows any perceptible broadening of the top; at 120 even this is almost gone. Above this the later adjustments are about *nil*, and all movements have to depend on their initial adjustment.

These tracings demonstrate the truth of our previous assumption that the loss of accuracy at high speeds was due to impossibility of later adjustments. Or, as it was expressed, the *bad effect of speed is exerted on the current control of the movement.* A rapid movement does not allow time enough for the later adjustments. The later adjustments are reactions to stimuli set up by the movement and a rapid movement does not allow for the reaction time. That this is a sufficient explanation of the bad effect of speed, at least up to 120, is seen on comparing the degree of loss of accuracy with the degree of failure of the later adjustments [. . .]

The presence of later adjustments can be detected in many common movements, as, for instance, in singing. Ordinary singers do not always strike the note accurately at one jump, but must feel around a little after reaching the neighborhood, guiding themselves by the sense of pitch. Probably the ordinary run of violinists, and certainly the beginner, find their notes in this groping way. The path to skill lies in increasing the accuracy of the initial adjustment, so that the later groping need be only within narrow limits; and through increasing the speed of the groping process, so that finally there seems to be no groping at all. The later adjustments are combined with the bulk of the movement in that smooth and graceful way which we picked out from our tracings as the most perfect type. Whether the great virtuosos do away entirely with the later adjustments and achieve their wonderful accuracy by means of the first impulse, would be an interesting thing to find out. The speed and *verve* of their performances make it difficult to suppose there is anything there of the nature of groping. Yet these artists have had to work up through the groping stage, and it is likely that some traces of the process by which they reached perfection should remain in the perfected result. The later adjustment is probably there, but it is made with perfect smoothness, and has by long and efficient practice attained the sureness and the speed of a reflex.

10 K. J. W. Craik

The Operator as an Engineering System

K. J. W. Craik, 'Theory of the human operator in control systems. I. The operator as an engineering system', *British Journal of Psychology*, vol. 38, 1947, pp. 56–61.

The Human Operator Behaves Basically as an Intermittent Correction Servo

The evidence for this is the periodic or wavy nature of the time record of tracking errors, showing a spectrum with a predominant frequency of about 0·5 s with a smaller cluster of frequencies from 0·25 to 1 s. This periodicity might be attributed to a sensory threshold or 'dead zone', such that misalignments smaller than a certain value evoke no corrective movement; but there is evidence against this. First, the display magnification is usually such that the misalignments occurring during steady tracking exceed the known threshold (i.e. visual acuity). Secondly, if the rate of the course, or the magnification of the display for a given course, is increased by a certain factor, the periodicity of the corrections is little, if at all, affected; whereas if their periodicity were determined by the time taken for the misalignments to reach a certain 'threshold' value this alteration should shorten the periodicity of the corrections in the same ratio.

Consistently with the above principle, we find that the mean error in tracking any given variable-direction course is nearly proportional to the rate of the course, over a wide range of speeds. We should account for this by saying that the faster the course the greater the misalignments that occur in each period between two corrections, in strict proportion.

The Intermittent Corrections Consist of 'Ballistic' Movements

For example, they have a predetermined time pattern and are 'triggered off' as a whole. This behaviour may be contrasted with that of an intermittent correction servo in which, for instance, a follow-up motor is intermittently switched into a circuit in which it runs until it has reduced the misalignment to zero, and this action reduces the input to it to zero so that the motor stops. In the human operator, on the other hand, at a particular instant (i.e. about 0·3 s after the end of the preceding corrective movement), a corrective movement having a predetermined time course (usually occupying about 0·2 s) is triggered off. The evidence for this is based on studies of reaction time, i.e. on the internal time lag of the operator, due to the time taken by the sense organ to respond, for the nerve impulses to traverse the central nervous system, for the appropriate response to be 'selected' and for the nerve impulses reaching it to traverse the motor nerves. This lag is about 0·2–0·3 s. Thus, if a human operator's limb movement amplitude, or velocity, or acceleration, were determined continuously by the misalignment, continued oscillations of approximately 0·5-s periods, and of whatever amplitude they commenced at, would inevitably result. This tendency could be overcome if a misalignment triggered off a ballistic movement of fairly correct amplitude (say ±10 per cent); the eye would then detect the residual misalignment, which may be composed of two parts – the error in the first ballistic movement, and any movement of the target which has occurred in the meantime. In the absence of the latter (e.g. in aiming at a stationary target) the second corrective movement may again be accurate to ±10 per cent of its own value so that the misalignment is reduced to 1 per cent of its original value.

Direct evidence bearing on this ballistic behaviour can be obtained in various ways. First it is easy to present a misalignment to an operator, and then screen his eyes just before he makes his corrective movement. A movement accurate to within about 10 per cent will result, if he has previously learned the 'feel' of the control. If he operated like a follower motor, intermittently switched in, such obscuration of the misalignment would be equivalent to cutting the input connexions, and the motor would not of course make any further corrective movement.

Physiologists might make a further hypothesis to avoid the 'ballistic' theory. They might say that the visual misalignment, once it has been detected by the eye, becomes translated into a 'limb-movement misalignment' (i.e. a kinaesthetic misalignment) which acts as the continuous input to the limb until our kinaesthetic (i.e. joint and muscle senses) register 'correct position', or no misalignment. We certainly do possess such a sense, but it is less easy to abolish it experimentally and to see what happens in its absence, than in the case of vision. Patients with *tabes dorsalis* have considerable loss of kinaesthetic sensation, but it is difficult to know how complete this loss is in any particular case.

In any case, the same general argument as before – that a continuous series of oscillations of the initial amplitude would occur if elimination of kinaesthetic misalignment were the sole determinant of movements, owing to the inevitable reaction time lag – seems to apply. Further, it is possible to show that considerable precision of movement is maintained even when the movements are made so rapidly that they are completed before the kinaesthetic stimulus corresponding to their first approximation to the right position could have 'gone the round' of the central nervous system and controlled the subsequent output movement; unless indeed reaction times to kinaesthetic stimuli were vastly shorter than to any other kind. It is, however, possible to show experimentally that kinaesthetic reaction times are very little shorter than auditory, for instance. Thus, we may ask the operator to move a lever against a stiff spring, so as to make a rapid movement to correct a misalignment, and then to return to his starting point. After he has learned the 'feel' of the control (i.e. its gear ratio and spring tension) and is making fairly accurate movements, we suddenly alter the spring tension, so that he over- or under-shoots. A record of this on a fast-moving drum shows that about 0·15 s elapses after he begins his movement, until he is able to begin a readjustment of it, to meet the modification of resistance.

Similarly, it is possible to show that in playing musical instruments, typewriting, sending morse, etc., complicated patterns of movement are executed at a rate which would be impossible if they were continuously governed by the value of the misalignment, with the inevitable reaction time lag. Apparently they must be individually performed, triggered off ballistically, and the sensory feedback must take the form of a delayed modification of the amplitude of subsequent movements. Sensory control, in other words, alters the 'internal gear ratio' or amplification of the operator with a time lag and determines whether subsequent corrective movements will be made; it does not govern the amplitude of each individual movement while it is being made. We could make a servo, using existing engineering principles, which would show the features of intermittent, ballistic correction. But this last point – the fact that the sensory misalignment alters not merely the amplitude of the response but the *relation* between the input, or misalignment and the output, or response – introduces a further complication, the nearest approach to which, in engineering, seems to be 'floating plus proportional control'. Even this involves a quantitative alteration of the amplification of the system by the residual misalignment, whereas something more complex still seems to be occurring – a very wide alteration in the functional relationship between input and output.

For instance, if the operator is using a positional control, his successive ballistic corrective movements should be linearly proportional to the misalignments; but if he is using a velocity control they would have to be linearly proportional to the *derivatives* of the misalignments. Roughly speaking, we might call this *qualitative* modification or output on a basis of some response to the difference between instantaneous input and output at the previous instant, or 'qualitative feedback'.

A further complication is introduced by the operator's ability to 'anticipate' movements of the target, or alterations in misalignment. For instance, with a positional control, the errors in tracking a moving target are usually less than we should predict on the above theory of intermittent ballistic corrections. The operator goes on turning the handle steadily, or even accelerating it; his record, after some practice, becomes much smoother than it was initially; and if he finds that he is still lagging behind the target (as if the above theory is correct he is bound to do) he can put in an extra forward movement. Here we have several processes.

There are some Counteracting Processes tending to make Controls seem Continuous

First, there is one akin to momentum, or inertia. If the operator has been turning the handle, in a series of discrete movements, for some seconds, he will tend to convert this into as steady a rotation as he is capable of, and to continue doing so although the misalignment may be zero, i.e. he has zero input to produce this output! (This can be shown experimentally by suddenly stopping the target, when the operator will overshoot for the period of one reaction time, until the serious misalignment which results stops his steady output from continuing.) It is for this reason that in the first section it was stated that the human operator is *basically* an intermittent correction servo; he has in addition this mechanism for going on doing whatever is giving a satisfactory result, or zero misalignment, rather like a heavy flywheel and having the same valuable smoothing effect.

What are the essential features of this process, and can we conceive any mechanisms which will accomplish it? When the operator continues to turn the handle at the same speed, independently of whether there is any input or not, he is, in humanistic terms, assuming that he is justified in doing so, in order to compensate for his reaction time lag. Since he is always subject to this lag, in attempting to keep up with the present he is always in fact being a prophet and extrapolating from past data! It is really no different from the further kind of anticipation which enables him to extrapolate into the physical future. Now all scientific prediction consists in discovering, in data of the distant past and of the immediate past which we incorrectly call the present, laws or formulae which apply also to the future, so that if we act in accordance with those laws our behaviour will be appropriate to that future when it becomes the present. Thus the essential feature of extrapolation and anticipation is, again in humanistic terms, that the operator should detect the *constants* in what he is doing. Thus, he may move a handwheel in a series of jerks, so that its *position* changes from moment to moment, but he may realize after a few seconds that he is turning it at a *steady rate*, i.e. its *angular velocity* is constant; and having discovered this he may try whether it will not pay him to go on doing so; usually it will. He may, however, find that its rate is changing – the target has angular acceleration. He may, in theory, at any rate, be able to feel this acceleration which he is having to put into the hand-wheel, and if he happens to find that it is constant, or nearly so, and is able to put out a constant acceleration of this value in turning the wheel, again he may achieve better following.

Now let us look at the same thing from a mechanical point of view. There are many devices – such as speedometers and accelerometers – which do the differentiations involved in record-ing velocities and accelerations; and the problem would be how, for instance, to couple a number of such devices to a telephone selector-switch operating motor, so that if the output of the motor over a few seconds of intermittent corrective action showed a constant reading on the speedometer, or even on the accelero-meter, the motor would be caused to go on putting out this speed or acceleration, irrespective of whether there was any input or not, unless or until such behaviour gave rise to a large misalign-ment. If that happened the extrapolating system would be over-ridden and intermittent corrections would begin again, until a new value for a constant was found. The solution would seem to be to provide the motor with positive feedback of such a kind that it continued to go on doing whatever it was doing at the moment – running steadily or accelerating uniformly. Such a system would need considerable smoothing and stabilization, otherwise any slight disturbance, such as a slight acceleration, would very rapidly be cumulative, and the machine would reach its maximum speed; but if the feedback were delayed and smoothed, the system could be sufficiently stable and would not 'wander' too badly. This system would of course be combined with negative feedback of the ordinary kind (viz. actuation by the difference between input and output quantities), so that if the positive feedback led to overestimation of the velocity, or if the target started to decelerate, the motor would overshoot and this would introduce a positional misalignment, which would reverse the direction of mechanical control. This would alter the average value, for the last time interval, to the positive feedback system, which would therefore cease from perpetuating this velocity but would, when it had time to steady down, start putting in a new one.

Electrical Models Could Fairly Exactly Simulate the Human Operator's Behaviour in Tracking

In general terms, the extraction of the inputs for the positive feedback network consists of successive differentiations, while the extrapolations on the basis of them consist of successive integrations. Let us consider in more detail some circuits by which this might be accomplished. Suppose the motor drives a generator across whose output terminals is a capacity in series with a high resistance, constituting a differentiating circuit with a time lag or averaging effect, owing to the time constant of the system. Then the generator voltage is proportional to the speed of the motor and the voltage across the resistance of the differentiating system is proportional to its acceleration; if necessary, higher derivatives can be obtained in the same way. The lag in the first differentiation can be obtained by putting a resistance and capacity in series across the generator output and taking the voltage off the capacity. The output voltage from this smoothing system is taken to the input of the amplifier supplying the motor fields and should cause the motor to continue running at the mean speed, at which it has been manually rotated, for a sufficient time to cause the voltage to be delayed and smoothed across the generator to reach a steady value. The speed of running will of course wander slowly in time if the system also has ordinary velodyne negative feedback for velocity control. If the manually applied speed was an accelerating one, the system will maintain a mean steady speed if it is supplied with one differentiating stage only (i.e. the generator with its delaying system). But if there is a second differentiating system, with a longer time constant, it will register a manually imposed change of velocity over several periods of operation of the first differentiating system, i.e. an acceleration, and if this is integrated by a resistance-capacity circuit and applied to the amplifier serving the fields, a uniform acceleration will occur.

Of course, it is not necessary for the original speeds to be put in manually; with a velodyne fitted up as a servo auto-following system in which the task of the velodyne is to make a slider keep on the centre of a potentiometer, for instance, which is moved by an external agency, the mechanical control will commence by ordinary positional following, being actuated by the misalignments. Further, though this alone would lead to a lag behind a uniformly moving target, once it has started to run at a constant velocity, the remaining misalignment will still be operative, if arranged to be in series with the positive feedback voltage, so as to cause the shaft to step on and make up for the lag. This system would have many of the same characteristics as a velodyne with phase advance produced by delayed negative feedback – i.e. a condenser across the generator output.

It should be possible to make a velodyne simulate the 'intermittent ballistic correction' process considered in the first and second principles. Thus, the error voltage representing the misalignment could be connected periodically by a rotating contact to a condenser which is charged. This condenser would then be switched on to the amplifier input and would result in a 'ballistic' rotation of the output shaft through an angle proportional to the charge on the condenser.

Little is known of possible physiological mechanisms for accomplishing this kind of thing. There is evidence (e.g. from sensory adaptation and accommodation of nerves) of differentiating systems, at least of the first order, which may serve to measure rates of change of stimulation, though our knowledge extends only to stimulus *intensity* and not to more complex stimuli such as misalignments in space. Even here, it is possible to suggest hypothetical spatial differentiating systems which are not physiologically inconceivable. The other aspect – the integration, resulting from positive feedback – would seem to require 'autorhythmic' nervous centres which continue to discharge once they have been forced to do so, and in a way which follows the original forcing stimulus. The beating of the isolated frog's heart and the spontaneous oscillatory potentials in the excised frog's brain and in the intact cortex of man (both Berger rhythms and the abnormal rhythms of epilepsy) are suggestive in this respect, for they are evidence of self-maintaining neural oscillators. Lorente de No's and Ransom's concept of the 'closed neurone circuit' would serve the same purpose. What has to be considered is clearly a form of positive feedback and the main difficulty in all the cases just mentioned would seem to be that what is required is continuous feedback of excitation in the form of nerve impulses following after the neurones have recovered from their refractory phase, whereas slow potential oscillations probably imply discharges of some other kind than trains of nerve impulses.

We should also consider long-lasting changes of stimulus–response relationship (i.e. learning) which, in an electrical model, would probably require to be imitated by some auto-selective switching device rather than regarded as time constants of a resistance-capacity system. Another type of control demands the establishing of complex response patterns which are 'triggered off' as a whole by the stimulus. Instances are the action of word habits in typewriting, or of blocks of stimuli in transmitting morse, or of associated movement groups in knitting. These seem to require some 'sequencing' switchgear, of the type used in the relay automatic telephone system, and make us think of the physiologists' 'chain reflexes' and of rhythmic reflexes such as walking and breathing.

11 A. T. Welford

Evidence of a Single-Channel Decision Mechanism Limiting Performance in a Serial Reaction Task

Excerpt from A. T. Welford, 'Evidence of a single-channel decision mechanism limiting performance in a serial reaction task', *Quarterly Journal of Experimental Psychology*, vol. 11, 1959, pp. 193–208.

The Present State of Theory

Looking back over the statements published in this field, we find five types of theory have been advanced to account for the delays in responding to a signal which closely follows a previous signal.

1. The first type, which was responsible for the term 'psychological refractory period' postulates that following some event in the chain of processes leading from signal to responding action there is a refractory state, analogous to that found in nerve fibres but of much longer duration – 100 to 500 ms in different formulations. The widely held suggestion, that there is a refractory period of about half a second following the making of a response seems to have come from Telford (1931). It has been clearly refuted by Vince's (1948) experiments and by all the evidence since. Fitts (1951, p. 1323) suggested that there might be a refractory period of the same kind but with a duration of only about 100 ms, and Davis (1957) has postulated a refractory period of about the same length following central activity rather than the actual making of a response.

2. Broadbent (1958, p. 280) has suggested that there may be a kind of quantizing of perception into samples about a third of a second long. He further suggests that the subject can begin a new sample when S_1 arrives and that delays to S_2 are due to the data having to wait until the next sample before they can be dealt with. This theory, although fundamentally different in conception from the previous type has some similar consequences.[1] It

1. S_1 = first signal; S_2 = second signal; TR_1 = reaction time to S_1; TR_2 = reaction time to S_2; M_1 = movement to S_1; M_2 = movement to S_2.

would, at first sight, account well for the data of the present experiment: the delays in the ungrouped cases when S_2 arrived during TR_1 were about what would be expected, and delays when S_2 came during M_1 would be due to S_2 'missing' the next sample and having to wait for a third. Broadbent's theory would further offer an attractive explanation of the variability of delay when S_2 arrived close to the beginning of M_1 as this would also be about the end of the first sample after S_2, so that in some cases S_2 would be in time for the second sample but in other cases would have to wait for the third. The theory would not, however, account for the tendency to lengthening of M_1 in cases in which I' was short. Further, one would expect that in cases in which S_2 came during M_1, TR_1 and TR_2 would have been positively correlated since short TR_2 would be secured if TR_1 ended and S_2 arrived before the end of the first sample. Plotting TR_2 against TR_1 it was clear that the correlation if any, was negligible.

Both these two types of theory postulate that delays are caused by some process occupying a fixed time interval which is, as the theories are stated, independent of the length of TR_1 and TM_1, and would presumably not change with the amount of information conveyed by S_1 or by the monitoring of M_1. Both theories thus have the severe disadvantage that they require an *ad hoc* quantity to be postulated for the refractory period or quantized interval. If all the existing evidence is to be accounted for, such a quantity would have to be assumed to vary with circumstances in some way not as yet understood. The theories can thus, at the present stage at least, have only *post hoc* descriptive value and are not yet reliably predictive. They cannot, however, be refuted on present evidence, they can only be shown to be unnecessary. The crucial experiments have not yet been done. It would be instructive, for example, to try experiments in which the average reaction times would be longer than those obtained so far – for example by requiring multichoice reactions. If under these conditions the delays were found to be no longer than those already observed, it would be evidence in favour of a theory such as that of Davis or Broadbent.

3. A different type of theory again states that the delays to S_2 are due to what we have called the 'Mowrer effect'. Mowrer

(1940) found that in a serial reaction time task signals arriving before (or after) a modal or mean interval were reacted to more slowly and he 'explained' the effect by saying that the subject's 'expectancy' of a signal was then lower. This type of theory was originally suggested as a possibility by Hick (1948), and was espoused by Poulton (1950) and by Elithorn and Lawrence (1955). If specification of the actual amount of delay is not attempted the theory can fit a great deal of the evidence very well. Preference for other theories depends upon their giving a better *quantitative* fit to the data. Its lack of quantitative precision is indeed its main disadvantage and makes it again non-predictive. If all the data already accumulated were to be accounted for, the delays would have to vary with circumstances according to principles as yet unknown. Further, there is no mechanism in terms of which the effect can, as yet, be confidently understood, so that the theory is at present purely descriptive: the effect of 'expectation' can only be observed *post hoc* from empirical data. Broadbent (1958, p. 272) refers to this theory as 'parsimonious'. It is so only if quantitative considerations are neglected. If they are taken into account, the additional postulates necessary to explain variations in the amount of the effect make the theory very much less parsimonious than it appears at first sight.

4. Elithorn and Lawrence (1955) seem to imply the suggestion that the results of experiments using pairs of responses made by different hands could be accounted for in terms of cortical or other central interaction. It is reasonable to suppose that this might be substantial between bilaterally symmetrical effectors. It is true that Fraisse (1957) has shown that a signal may cause delay even if no overt response to it is required, but inhibition of action might well have significant effects in this respect. The complementary experiment in which responses to different signals would be made by widely separated effectors, e.g. jaw and foot, has not, so far as the writer is aware, been done.

5. Lastly, we may consider the hypothesis that there is in the central mechanisms a single channel of limited capacity. This was implied in Craik's (1948) treatment, was made explicit by Hick (1948) and was developed by Hick and Bates (1950), the present author (Welford, 1952), Davis (1956, 1957), Fraisse

(1957) and Broadbent (1957, 1958). In its bare essentials this theory assumes, firstly, a number of sensory input mechanisms each capable of receiving data and storing it for a limited period so that, for example, a short *series* of signals can be received as a unit. Secondly, it assumes a number of effector mechanisms containing both central and peripheral elements and capable of carrying out a series of actions such as the pressing and release of a key or a series of taps (Vince, 1949) as a single unit. Thirdly, between these two it postulates a single-channel decision mechanism. This is regarded as being of limited capacity in the sense that it takes a finite time to process information and can thus only deal with a limited amount of information in a given time.

It is further implied that sensory input data can be accumulated while the decision channel is occupied by dealing with previous data, and can be passed together to the decision channel as soon as it is free. Similarly the decision channel can 'issue orders' to the effector side for a *series* of responses the execution of which can overlap with the decision channel's dealing with fresh input. Sensory feedback data from responding actions may, however, 'capture' the decision channel, i.e. responses may be monitored.

This theory does not have the disadvantages of the others although it is not without its own difficulties, of which the most pertinent are perhaps three:

(a) Some additional postulate is needed to account for 'grouping'. This, however, is a problem for any theory except, perhaps, that of Broadbent who might postulate that the subject would occasionally fail to begin a new sample with the arrival of S_1, and that S_2 would sometimes appear before he did so. A possible line of approach to the problem of grouping is to link it with the need to collect data over a period of time in order to distinguish a signal from 'neural noise' (see e.g. Gregory, 1955), or with the fact noted in several studies (e.g. Piéron, 1923, Cheatham, 1952) that perception of a stimulus can in certain circumstances be modified or prevented by another stimulus coming a short time after.

(b) The question arises of why movements are sometimes monitored and sometimes not. The present writer suggested (Welford,

1952) and Davis has reiterated (1956) that monitoring may be unnecessary when the accuracy required of the responding action is sufficiently low for it to be made ballistically without there being any appreciable likelihood that it will fail to be effective. If highly accurate movements are required, however, monitoring may be inevitable, and even when not strictly necessary it may give the subject confidence. It is understandable that monitoring for either of these reasons would tend to drop out with practice, and we may note in support of this view that Davis's original subjects (Davis, 1956) and Marill's (1957) subjects, who are the two groups failing to show delays when S_2 came after the end of TR_1, were substantially more practised than others. Experiments comparing delays at various stages of practice could settle whether this explanation is correct.

(c) The theory fits the evidence very reasonably well if we take the time for which the single channel is assumed to be occupied as equal to the total TR_1. Such a formulation neglects, as Davis (1957) has pointed out, the fact that appreciable times are required for data to reach the cortex from sense organs and for efferent nerve impulses and muscular action to make a response effective. The theory would certainly not work if these times were deducted from TR_1, as at first sight it would seem they should be, in order to arrive at the supposed time required for the decision mechanism to act in response to S_1. Any suggestion to overcome this difficulty must at present be speculative, but we may note that the difficulty would cease to exist if it could be shown that some minimum feedback from the responding action, indicating that it had begun, was necessary for the decision mechanism to be 'cleared'. If this were so the time taken to initiate a movement would automatically be included in the decision time, and there would be added a new time component of a few milliseconds for the feedback signals to get back from the responding member to the brain. If this time was approximately the same as that required for a stimulus to reach the brain from an exteroceptor it would mean that reaction time would be a reasonable measure of decision time although the equating of the two would be in a sense fortuitous. An indication in favour of such a scheme is contained in the finding by Fraisse (1957) that delays following an S_1 to which no response had to be made, and for which presumably the feedback did not occur, were shorter than when S_1 was followed by an overt responding movement.

Future Research

We may end by briefly urging two general points for future studies which emerge from what has been done so far. Firstly a wide variety of theories will fit substantial areas of the facts, and distinction between the various theories can often only be made following a detailed *quantitative* analysis of the data. Any new theory should be accompanied by a review in quantitative terms of *all* the rather formidable mass of data so far collected.

Secondly, there seems to be a danger that the study of reactions to discrete pairs of signals will become unduly preoccupied with minutiae. There is a fairly obvious series of experiments still to be done with this technique, and doubtless if they were done they would suggest others. The kind of question these could settle would, however, almost certainly be answered incidentally, and a great deal of valuable information obtained besides, if attention was returned to the original stimulus to such studies, namely the analysis of continuous performance.

References

BROADBENT, D. E. (1957), 'A mechanical model for human attention and immediate memory', *Psychol. Rev.*, vol. 64, pp. 205–15.

BROADBENT, D. E. (1958), *Perception and Communication*, Pergamon Press.

CHEATHAM, P. G. (1952), 'Visual perceptual latency as a function of stimulus brightness and contour shape', *J. exp. Psychol.*, vol. 43, pp. 369–80.

CRAIK, K. J. W. (1948), 'Theory of the human operator in control systems. II. Man as an element in a control system', *Brit. J. Psychol.*, vol. 38, pp. 142–8.

DAVIS, R. (1956), 'The limits of the "psychological refractory period"', *Quart. J. exp. Psychol.*, vol. 8, pp. 24–38.

DAVIS, R. (1957), 'The human operator as a single channel information system', *Quart. J. exp. Psychol.*, vol. 9, pp. 119–29.

ELITHORN, A., and LAWRENCE, C. (1955), 'Central inhibition – some refractory observations', *Quart. J. exp. Psychol.*, vol. 7, pp. 116–27.

FITTS, P. M. (1951), 'Engineering psychology and equipment design', in S. S. Stevens (ed.), *Handbook of Experimental Psychology*, Wiley, pp. 1287–340.

FRAISSE, P. (1957), 'La période refractoire psychologique', *Année Psychol.*, vol. 57, pp. 315–28.

GREGORY, R. L. (1955), 'A note on summation time of the eye indicated by signal/noise discrimination', *Quart. J. exp. Psychol.*, vol. 7, pp. 147–8.

HICK, W. E. (1948), 'The discontinuous functioning of the human operator in pursuit tasks', *Quart. J. exp. Psychol.*, vol. 1, pp. 36–51.

HICK, W. E., and BATES, J. A. V. (1950), 'The human operator of control mechanisms', *Min. Supply Res. & Develop. Monogr.*, no. 17, p. 204.

MARILL, T. (1957), 'The psychological refractory phase', *Brit. J. Psychol.*, vol. 48, pp. 93–7.

MOWRER, O. H. (1940), 'Preparatory set (expectancy) – some methods of measurement', *Psychol. Monogr.*, vol. 52. no. 233.

PIÉRON, H. (1923), 'De la variation des intervalles limites de masquage d'une excitation lumineuse par une excitation consécutive très intense en fonction de l'intensité de la première', *C.R. Soc. Biol. Paris*, vol. 88, pp. 736–89.

POULTON, E. C. (1950), 'Perceptual anticipation and reaction time', *Quart. J. exp. Psychol.*, vol. 2, pp. 99–112.

TELFORD, C. W. (1931), 'The refractory phase of voluntary and associative responses', *J. exp. Psychol.*, vol. 14, pp. 1–36.

VINCE, M. A. (1948), 'The intermittency of control movements and the psychological refractory period', *Brit. J. Psychol.*, vol. 38, pp. 149–57.

VINCE, M. A. (1949), 'Rapid response sequences and the psychological refractory period', *Brit. J. Psychol.*, vol. 40, pp. 23–40.

WELFORD, A. T. (1952), 'The "psychological refractory period" and the timing of high-speed performance – a review and a theory', *Brit. J. Psychol.*, vol. 43, pp. 2–19.

Part Four **The Role of Proprioception in Skill**

Any attempt to analyse the mechanisms which permit even so simple an action as placing a pencil on a desk immediately emphasizes the necessity for the brain to know where the pencil starts from and where it should be placed. Vision is the most accurate of man's senses and could be used to signal both locations. However, provided the brain knows the location of the hand which holds the pencil, the location of the pencil may be simply inferred. Proprioception, which signals the state of the muscles and joints, can take the place of vision and signal the starting point of the movement. With this information the brain can compute the movement required to carry the pencil to its required location. Proprioception may also provide similar background information even when the pencil is not at rest to begin with, and throughout the course of a movement proprioception maintains a monitoring function to check that the intended movement is indeed executed.

By altering the load against which a movement is made and the amplitude of its excursion the proprioceptive feedback from a movement may be experimentally manipulated. Bahrick (Reading 12) reviews several attempts to test a particular mathematical relationship between the physical characteristics of a manual control and the proprioceptive feedback it produces. A much more technical paper by Notterman and Page (1962) describes an intensive investigation into the relationship between performance and the physical characteristics of controls.

Gibbs (Reading 13) presents an experiment in which the time taken to amend errors introduced by reversing the usual effects of moving a control was recorded. It was predicted that as response monitoring was delegated from vision to proprioception, a systematic improvement in error-correction times would result. The predicted improvement occurred and Gibbs concludes that this provides further support for his thesis that movements are continuously monitored by proprioception.

The importance of proprioception in the control of movements has led some researchers to advance theories of motor dysfunction in terms of distorted or delayed proprioceptive feedback. Dinnerstein, Frigyesi and Lowenthal (Reading 14) present a theory that Parkinsonian disability may be due primarily to delayed proprioceptive feedback. There is some experimental support for their theory but there is also evidence that until further refined the theory is not yet satisfactory; it does not account for all clinical signs and some normal young subjects show patterns of perceptual behaviour characteristic of Parkinsonian patients.

Reference
NOTTERMAN, J. M., and PAGE, D. E. (1962), 'Evaluation of mathematically equivalent tracking systems', *Percept. mot. Skills*, vol. 15, pp. 683–716.

12 H. P. Bahrick

An Analysis of Stimulus Variables Influencing the Proprioceptive Control of Movements

H. P. Bahrick, 'An analysis of the stimulus variables influencing the proprioceptive control of movements', *Psychological Review*, vol. 64, 1957, pp. 324–8.

It is generally known that accurate execution of movements depends upon proprioceptive information reaching the central nervous system. Clinical evidence (7, p. 235) as well as experimental findings (8) indicates that control and perception of movements are very poor when this sensory channel is not functioning.

Little is known, however, about the specific characteristics of proprioceptive stimulation that permit the individual to control changes in position, rate or acceleration of his limbs. In other words, no detailed theories of proprioception comparable to the specific theories available for some other sense modalities have been developed (7, p. 234). Most of the available knowledge in this area is based upon anatomical investigations of the receptor system, its neural connexions and its central representations. Although several types of receptors have been identified (13, p. 1185; 14), differentiation of their function is as yet not clearly established. It is thought that forces internal to the body act as proprioceptive stimuli, but the processes by which these stimuli are encoded into messages which ultimately form the basis for perception and control of movements are not well understood (7, p. 234).

Behavioral data specifying the relations between stimulus and response characteristics have been difficult to obtain because of problems of controlling proprioceptive stimuli. Investigators have used drugs or faradic currents (8, 9) as means of reducing the effectiveness of proprioceptive stimuli. Recently, an indirect approach to this problem has been attempted. This approach consists of varying the type and degree of resistance to motion offered by a control which S uses in the execution of movements

The effect of this variation upon S's ability to perceive and control his movements is studied and an attempt is made to infer characteristics of the proprioceptive system. As a technique of investigating proprioception, this approach has obvious limitations. The forces which S applies to move a control are only indirectly related to the proprioceptive stimulation he receives during the execution of the movement. The cutaneous senses are also stimulated during movement, and unknown transformations are involved between the control force acting upon the limb and the proximal stimuli acting upon receptors in muscles, tendons or joints.

Despite these substantial limitations, the approach has some theoretical as well as practical advantages. The forces required to move a control and thus also the control forces acting upon the limb, can be specified as a function of four physical properties of the control, and these properties can all be regulated conveniently by E. They are mass, viscosity, elasticity and the degree of coulomb friction. In a control such as that used by Howland and Noble (11) these parameters combine according to the following time-varying system equation:

$$L_t = K\theta + B \, d\theta/dt + J \, d^2\theta/dt^2, \qquad 1$$

where the left-hand side of the equation is the force applied by the human arm, the right-hand side represents the component resistive forces offered by the external control, L_t is the torque required to move the control at any instant of time (t), K is the constant of elasticity of the control, B is the viscosity constant, J is the moment of inertia and θ is the angular displacement o the control with respect to its neutral, or spring-centered, position (6). Coulomb friction has been neglected in this equation, as have the internal resistive forces in the limb itself.

It has already been pointed out that the force which the control exerts upon the limb may not be equated to proprioceptive stimuli. However, one may assume that the forces which do act as proprioceptive stimuli during the movement of limbs are determined by physical properties of our limbs analogous to those specified in the above equation for the control. Previous investigation (4) has already established some of these physical properties of limbs and their significance in relation to the control of movements. These physical properties of limbs are difficult to control and the present approach attempts to infer their function in proprioception by studying the effects of analogous characteristics of controls where these properties can be manipulated conveniently.

From an applied viewpoint, this approach may be useful in that the data are relevant to the solution of human engineering problems related to the design of controls used in man–machine systems, or to the design of prosthetic devices.

In the present article some general hypotheses are developed about the effect of each of the physical control parameters specified in equation 1, and data are reported which test these hypotheses.

Inspection of equation 1 shows that the torque needed to move the control depends upon its position, rate and angular acceleration, the relative importance of these depending upon the respective values of the elasticity, damping and inertia constants. Thus, if the elasticity constant K is zero, the torque required to move the control will be independent of its position, but if K is relatively large, the torque will vary largely as a function of position. Analogous relations exist between the damping constant B and angular velocity, and between the moment of inertia and angular acceleration.

It is now hypothesized that a man can use the force cues obtained in moving the control to improve his perception of position, rate and acceleration of limb motion. Specifically, it is hypothesized that the elasticity constant of the control improves S's ability to perceive and control positions, the damping constant improves perception and control of rate, and the moment of inertia improves the perception and control of acceleration. Thus, an increase in each of these control constants should lead to improvement in the corresponding behavior. At the same time, it is hypothesized that an increase in any of the control constants will affect adversely performance which is aided by the other constants. Thus, increases in K are expected to interfere with the control and perception of rate and acceleration, while increases in B and J will affect adversely the control and perception of position. This hypothesis suggests itself, since the force required to move the control would not be expected to provide useful cues for the control of rate if it changes rapidly with position and, conversely, it should not offer useful cues for the detection of position if it varied greatly as a function of rate or acceleration.

Several experiments have been conducted in which the accuracy of movement was studied as a function of the physical characteristics of controls (1, 2, 3, 10, 11). A few of these (1, 2, 10) were designed specifically to test the above predictions. In one study (2) Ss performed simple circular and triangular control motions with a joystick control which was loaded with various degrees of spring stiffness, or damping, or mass. In each control-loading condition, the movements were first practiced with the help of a visual guide and paced by means of a metronome. The visual and auditory guides were then removed and Ss were instructed to reproduce the motions as accurately as possible. Photographic records of all motions were obtained and measured for accuracy of temporal and spatial reproduction. It was found that an increase of viscous damping or of inertia of the control resulted in greater uniformity of speed within individual motions, and also in greater uniformity of speed in successive reproductions of the same motion. In the case of the triangular motions, increased mass and increased damping led to greater uniformity of peak velocity on each side of the triangle on successive trials. Spring loading interfered with the control of rate and acceleration, but its effect upon spatial accuracy of the reproduced motion was, in general, not significant. It was suggested that extended practice is needed for effective utilization of cues provided by spring loading.

This hypothesis was checked in a second experiment (1) in which the accuracy of positioning a horizontal arm control was investigated as a function of changes in the torque-displacement relation of the control. Extended practice was given and knowledge of results was provided. It was found that positioning errors are smallest when the ratio of relative torque change to displacement is largest. Under optimum conditions of spring loading, average positioning errors were less than half the amount obtained for a control which was not spring loaded. It was concluded that force cues provided by a spring-loaded control can improve the accuracy of positioning a control, and that the amount of improvement is a function of the relative and absolute torque change per unit of amplitude change.

Further investigation of the usefulness of force cues in regulating the amplitude of motion has supported the above conclusions. It was shown that the transmission of amplitude information can be increased significantly by spring loading the control used by Ss. Optimum results were obtained with a control which provided geometric increments of force as a function of arithmetic changes of amplitude. This condition provides force cues which are equally discriminable over the range of amplitudes employed (12, 15), and yields the largest number of absolutely discriminable categories of amplitude response.

Although the above results support the general hypotheses regarding the effects of K, B and J constants upon the control of movements, many questions remain unanswered. In order to establish that the observed effects are due to changes in proprioceptive stimulation, it will be necessary to control cutaneous sensitivity. It is hypothesized here that the contribution of cutaneous receptors is most significant in relation to minute manipulatory responses, and least significant for larger movements of the type dealt with here.

Further problems arise because the control parameters under discussion have certain mechanical effects upon the nature of movements, and these must be separated from the effects upon proprioceptive stimulation. Large amounts of damping, for example, make rapid movements difficult and fatiguing, and greater uniformity of movement rate observed under these conditions may reflect mechanical effects rather than improved proprioceptive discrimination. The identification of these mechanical effects becomes more difficult when continuous movements are dealt with, as was shown in the study by Howland and Noble (11). Interactions among the physical parameters of controls may cause complex mechanical effects such as oscillation, and these may obscure or counteract the effects due to augmented proprioceptive stimulation. In general, the analysis of K, B and J effects is relatively simple for discrete, adjustive movements of the type primarily dealt with so far, but becomes increasingly complicated for complex or continuous motions.

Work now in progress attempts to establish relations between the forces exerted upon a control and intensity of stimulation at the receptors in the elbow. This analysis is based upon a simplified mechanical model of the arm (16) by means of which forces acting upon the hand are resolved at the elbow joint (5, p. 319). In this manner it may become possible to infer changing intensities of stimulation of receptors at the joint during the course of movements.

Ultimately, the development of proprioceptive theory described here must be supported by a more direct analysis of K, B and J factors within the body, and their effects upon the perception and control of movements. This, in turn, will require a better understanding of the biophysical principles by which forces internal to the body are brought to bear upon proprioceptive receptors.

References

1. H. P. BAHRICK, W. F. BENNETT and P. M. FITTS, 'Accuracy of positioning responses as a function of spring loading in a control', *J. exp. Psychol.*, vol. 49 (1955), pp. 437–46.

2. H. P. BAHRICK, P. M. FITTS and R. SCHNEIDER, 'The reproduction of simple movements as a function of proprioceptive feedback', *J. exp. Psychol.*, vol. 49 (1955), pp. 445–54.

3. A. DERWORT, 'Ueber die Formen unserer Bewegungen gegen verschiedenartige Widerstaende und ihre Bedeutung fuer die Wahrnehmung von Kraeften', *Z. f. Sinnesphysiol.*, vol. 70 (1943), pp. 135–83.

4. W. O. FENN, 'The mechanics of muscular contraction in man', *J. appl. Physics*, vol. 9 (1938), pp. 165–77.

5. R. FICK, *Handbuch der Anatomie und Mechanik der Gelenke*, Part II, Verlag von Gustav Fischer, Jena, 1910.

6. P. M. FITTS, 'Engineering psychology and equipment design', in S. S. Stevens (ed.), *Handbook of Experimental Psychology*, Wiley, 1951, pp. 1287–340.

7. F. A. GELDARD, *The Human Senses*, Wiley, 1953.

8. A. GOLDSCHEIDER, 'Untersuchungen ueber den Muskelsinn. I. Ueber die Bewegungsempfindung', in A. Goldscheider, *Gesammelte Abhandlungen*, Vol. II, Barth, Leipzig, 1898.

9. A. GOLDSCHEIDER, 'Untersuchungen ueber den Muskelsinn. II. Ueber die Empfindung der Schwere und des Widerstandes', in A. Goldscheider, *Gesammelte Abhandlungen*, Vol. II, Barth, Leipzig, 1898.

10. H. HELSON and W. H. HOWE, Inertia, friction, and diameter in handwheel tracking, *OSRD Rep. no. 3454, 1943*. (PB 406114.)

11. D. HOWLAND and M. E. NOBLE, 'The effect of physical constants of a control on tracking performance', *J. exp. Psychol.*, vol. 46 (1953), pp. 353–60.

12. W. L. JENKINS, 'The discrimination and reproduction of motor adjustment with various types of aircraft controls', *Amer. J. Psychol.*, vol. 60 (1947), pp. 397–406.
13. W. L. JENKINS, 'Somesthesis', in S. S. Stevens (ed.), *Handbook of Experimental Psychology*, Wiley, 1951, pp. 1172–90.
14. B. H. C. MATHEWS, 'Nerve endings in mammalian muscle', *J. Physiol.*, vol. 78 (1933), pp. 1–53.
15. M. E. NOBLE and H. P. BAHRICK, 'Response generalization as a function of intratask response similarity', *J. exp. Psychol.*, vol. 51 (1956), pp. 405–12.
16. H. E. WHITE, *Modern College Physics*, Van Nostrand, 1948.

13 C. B. Gibbs

Probability Learning in Step-Input Tracking

C. B. Gibbs, 'Probability learning in step-input tracking', *British Journal of Psychology*, vol. 56. 1965, pp. 233–42.

Introduction

There are lawful relations between the direction of movement and the discharge of specific groups of proprioceptors (Mountcastle, Poggio and Werner, 1963). The speed of movement is closely related to the rate of change of frequency in the discharge of primary nerve endings (Matthews, 1933). The speed and direction of movement could therefore be controlled directly by proprioceptive feedback, once the relevant relations were learned. The extent of movement could be determined by integrating the speed signals from proprioceptors over time, to provide integral error control (Gibbs, 1954). It is hypothesized that new movements are first controlled by exteroceptors, but that detailed duties of monitoring are delegated to proprioceptors for the longest possible period. The degree of dependence on vision depends on the probability and predictability of the outcome of specific responses. Delegation releases exteroceptors and the limited span of attention from detailed duties of monitoring.

A hypothetical function of proprioception is to provide negative feedback which ensures that a movement initiated by an error-stimulus reduces that error. Negative feedback depends on a definite directional relation between input data and the feedback data which define the output. A reversal of the normal learned relation between visual and proprioceptive data should therefore lead to positive feedback by which response to an error stimulus increases the error.

Two distinct types of learning underlie the effective control of movement. The learning of lawful relations between movements and sensory feedback (output–feedback relations) is to be distinguished from the learning of serial, S–R probability relations; they are exemplified by the tracking task that is described. A major purpose of the experiment is to demonstrate the existence, and some major effects of both types of learning.

The above hypotheses lead to unequivocal predictions and to consistent explanations of known phenomena. In a task of step-input tracking the direction of successive responses is not always equally probable; such tasks are convenient for the study of serial probability relations. It is easy to provide an incompatible directional relation between control and display, i.e. a control–display relation where the control joystick and the display cursor move in opposite directions. Such a relation is well adapted for the demonstration of positive feedback in early practice, which results in large directional errors and considerable delays before errors are amended. By hypothesis, the unfamiliar but constant control–display relation can be learned and negative feedback again develops with a consequent reduction of errors in responses of both high and low probability.

The delegation of monitoring from vision to proprioception, or from conscious to automatic level, reduces the time taken to amend directional errors. The approximate reduction should be from 0·25 to 0·10 s; the former time represents visual reaction time, and the latter corresponds to known latency in the motor-proprioceptor circle of nerves (cf. Ruch, 1951). Amendment times of 0·10 s would contrast with findings of psychological refractoriness, e.g. that in responses to two closely spaced stimuli, the reaction time to the second is longer than that to the first (e.g. Adams, 1961, 1962; Craik, 1948; Davis, 1956, 1957, 1959; Hick, 1948; Vince, 1948; Welford, 1952, 1959). Other predictions from the hypotheses are that the number of directional errors and the duration of visual reaction times depend on the relative probabilities of responses. The data reported here are compatible with these hypotheses.

Method

Six men and six women of ages ranging from 23 to 54 yr, used a joystick to position a cursor on an oscilloscope and track a target spot of light. Movement was limited to the horizontal plane. Three subjects of each sex used their preferred hand; the others used their non-preferred hand. In the main study the control–display relation was incompatible, but a control group of six subjects used a compatible relation in an otherwise identical procedure. Subjects were instructed to respond as rapidly and accurately as possible.

The target appeared for 1 s in any of five different positions, 1·125 in apart, disappeared for 1 s and reappeared in a new position. Each position and each possible pair of successive positions was used equally frequently in one complete 'run' of 100 steps. There was a three to one probability that a target at position 2 would move to the right rather than outward to position 1; a target at position 4 was more likely to move left than right. Steps are termed 'probable' when the movement actually demanded conformed to the higher probability; steps outward from 2 or 4 are termed 'improbable'. Responses beginning at position 3 are called 'equiprobable' because the two possible directions of movement were equally probable. Movements from positions 1 or 5 were 'unequivocal' with respect to direction.

Records of target and joystick movements were analysed for errors in the initial direction of movement, for response latencies and for amendment times. Response latency is the interval between the onset of a stimulus and the beginning of a response; the definition applies also to reaction time but a different term is needed for the delays which arise in tracking tasks. Amendment time is the interval between the beginning of an incorrect response and the commencement of an amended movement.

Results

The control group using a compatible control–display relation made eight errors in 600 responses as compared with the 272 errors made in the 1200 responses of the experimental group. There was a small but significant ($P < 0.01$) difference of 0·04 s in the mean response latencies of all types of responses, which also favoured the compatible control–display relation. Table 1 shows the proportion of experimental group errors in responses of different probability at the three stages of practice indicated in column 1. The first entry in column 2 under the heading E/R shows that between steps 1 and 33 the group made thirty-seven errors (E) in a total of forty-eight improbable responses (R). The adjacent entry expresses the fraction as a percentage (77 per cent). Other entries in the table show similar relations for other responses. The main findings are that the great majority of errors occurred on the relatively infrequent improbable and equi-probable responses. There was a monotonic decrease in all error percentages as practice continued, except for an increase on

Table 1

Total Number of Errors (E) in Responses (R) of Different Probability at Different Stages of Practice (Steps 1–33, 34–66 and 67–100)

		Improbable	Equiprobable	Probable	Unequivocal
	(1) Steps	(2) E/R %	(3) E/R %	(4) E/R %	(5) E/R %
	1–33	37/48 77	44/72 61	38/120 32	18/156 12
	34–66	25/36 69	27/96 28	13/120 11	4/144 3
	67–100	22/36 60	29/72 40	12/120 10	1/180 0·6
Totals	1–100	84/120 70	100/240 42	63/360 18	23/480 5

equiprobable steps in the last stage of practice. All twelve subjects made errors on step 1 which demanded an equiprobable response, but following step 33 a maximum of six subjects made errors on these steps. Nine subjects made errors on the first and on the last appearance of improbable steps (step 16 and step 89) percentage errors remained high (60 per cent) in the last stage of practice. In contrast, errors virtually disappeared in unequivocal responses.

Response latencies, like errors, were markedly reduced in early practice. The mean response latencies shown in Figure 1 relate to steps 15 to 100; the stage where response latencies became reasonably consistent. Figure 1 shows the striking and significant ($P < 0.01$) monotonic relation between serial probability and the mean response latencies of correct responses; a relation similar to that noted by Hyman (1953). The figure shows that on improbable steps the response latency for a correct movement

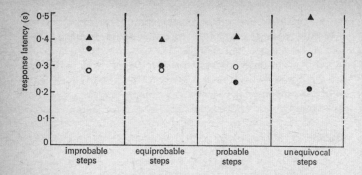

Figure 1 Relation between response latencies for correct and incorrect movements, and corrective response latencies, on steps of different probability (n = 12). ●, mean response latency for correct responses. O, mean response latency for incorrect responses. ▲, corrective response latency (response + amendment)

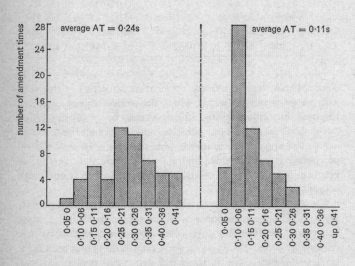

Figure 2 Histogram of amendment times in steps 1–10, and steps 71–100

was nearly 0·10 s longer than the response latency for an error. This is the expected relation between accuracy and speed. It was very surprising that the response latencies of correct and incorrect responses were virtually equal on equiprobable steps and that the latter response latency actually exceeded the former on probable and unequivocal steps, i.e. the larger latencies produced more errors.

The correlation between the response latencies and the errors of subjects was not significant, i.e. the subjects who responded most rapidly did not make most errors. Three male subjects had shorter response latencies and fewer errors than the group mean, and provided the three best combined scores. One male subject made the poorest combined score. The range of individual errors was 10–37.

A major prediction from hypotheses was that amendment times would be reduced from about 0·25 to 0·10 s. Figure 2 shows the actual distribution of amendment times in early and late practice (steps 1–10 and steps 71–100). There is a striking and significant change in mean amendment time from 0·24 to 0·11 s, as predicted.

The top half of Figure 3 shows the responses of a typical female subject on steps 15–20. The square form steps represent the various positions of the target from 1 to 5, denoted respectively by the squares of minimum and maximum height. The thick base lines between steps of different heights represent the 1-s periods of target absence. The continuous line above the steps is the subject's tracking response. A correct response was always in a direction that matched the changed height of a new step. The first step demanded an improbable response from position two to one; the tracking line should have moved downward in the figure. In fact, the subject made a small anticipatory movement in the probable and incorrect direction before light one appeared. Following its appearance, the subject made a large, all-or-none response of approximately correct extent in the wrong direction. Anticipatory movements were common in the subjects who made most errors. The response from position 2 to 4 was initially in the correct direction but was reversed, approximately 0·10 s after movement began. The reversal caused a large error in direction, which was amended after a delay that was compatible with visual reaction time. Responses that were initially correct, but rapidly reversed, accounted for 12 per cent of all the errors made in steps 1 to 33. Errors of less than 0·125 in at the display would not be detected in analysis because of size reduction in recording. The lower half of Figure 3 shows responses at a

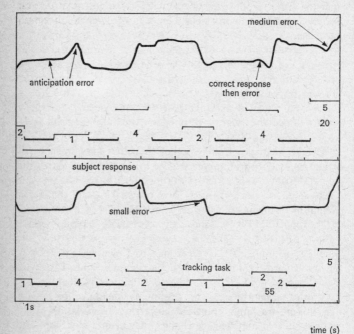

time (s)

Figure 3 Response of typical woman subject on steps 15–20 (upper) and steps 51–6 (lower)

later stage in practice (steps 51–6). Directional errors occurred in making a probable response from position 4 to 2 and an improbable response from position 2 to 1. In general, the size of errors was much reduced by practice.

In the 1200 responses made by the experimental group, 272 were initially in the wrong direction. The women made 168 and the men made 104 errors, a significant difference ($P < 0·01$). Five women and one man produced the six highest error scores. The errors made by both sexes were distributed in a similar manner between responses, of different probabilities, indicating similar estimates of response probability. Without regard to sex, 158 errors were made by the six subjects who used their non-preferred hand and 114 errors were made by the other six subjects who used their preferred hand. This difference also was significant ($P < 0.01$). As noted above, the control group using a compatible control–display relation made only eight errors in 600 responses.

Discussion

The small, rapidly amended errors observed in these tests have not been reported previously. Errors and response latencies provided highly sensitive measures that emphasized small but significant differences in performance due to hand, probability and sex.

It is not yet possible to explain why the majority of women subjects made more errors than most of the men. There was no reliable sex difference in probability matching; contrary to some established prejudices, the difference in errors did not stem from a feminine tendency to repose undue confidence in highly improbable events, e.g. that a target starting from the edge of the oscilloscope would move off the screen entirely.

Errors increased sharply when subjects were placed under minor stress, either by responding to stimuli of low probability or by using their non-preferred hand. These results indicate that these sensitive measures of performance may be particularly useful in studying stress. The method has now been applied successfully to a study of effects of alcohol and a report is in preparation.

The problem of control

Lawful relations must exist in any system to permit effective control of the speed, extent and direction of movement. In organisms, practice can improve performance only to the point where these relations are learned. There is a definite relation between the direction of movement and the discharge of specific groups of proprioceptors (Mountcastle *et al.*, 1963). High correlations exist between the rate of movement and the rate of change of frequency of the kinaesthetic discharge (Matthews, 1933). Proprioception could therefore monitor direction and speed directly; speed could be integrated over time in order to determine the extent of movement by integral error control.

Correlations also exist between movement and visual feedback but the typical errors of early practice show that vision does not continuously monitor rapid movements. Many movements were almost correct in extent but ran in the wrong direction for about 0·25 s. During that period visual feedback was not effective in amending error and it cannot therefore be credited with the continuous monitoring of direction, speed or extent. Many early responses were initially correct but were reversed after approximately 0·10 s to produce a large directional error. Had visual feedback been effective in that time, the correct initial adjustment would have continued.

Data reported by Helson and Steger (1962) suggest that visual feedback can produce a motor effect in 0·1 s. In the transition from visual to proprioceptive monitoring, some rapid amendments were possibly based on vision, but the purpose of delegation is to relieve visual attention of uneconomic duties of detailed monitoring.

Probability, latency and error

The delegation of monitoring from vision to proprioception, effects a change in the time for amending errors, from about 0·25 to 0·10 s. The former period represents visual reaction time, the latter is the known latency in the motor-proprioceptor circle of nerves (Ruch, 1951) and the minimum time to amend responses that are not monitored by vision, e.g. hand-tapping (Dresslar, 1892).

In early practice, the mean time to amend errors was 0·24 s (Figure 2). Subjects expected that a rapid, primary response could run for that period, under proprioceptive control, without developing serious error requiring a visual check. The expectation was invalidated by the reversal of normal directional relations, which permit control by negative, proprioceptive feedback. Subjects were presented with a choice between speed and accuracy until the new relation was learned. They could regress to slow, visual monitoring which would minimize errors, but increase the time needed to acquire the target, which appeared only briefly. Alternatively, they could respond rapidly using proprioceptive feedback, but the reversed relation would then produce frequent directional errors.

The mean amendment time was 0·11 s in late practice, indicating that subjects were probably using proprioceptive monitoring, despite a high percentage of errors on the less probable steps. The subjects were not aware of these rapid amendments. Delegation therefore largely relieved visual attention of the duties of detailed monitoring, although the incompatible relation was not fully learned. The over-all error percentage in the last stage of practice was about 16 per cent, and only 1·3 per cent of errors were made by the control group using a compatible relation.

A clear distinction exists between the lawful relations of movement and feedback, and the serial probability relations between input and output, that are exemplified by the different types of tracking steps. The latter permit tests of the hypothesis that the degree of visual attention depends on the input–output probability relation. Specifically, highly probable responses are initiated with a minimum of visual attention, which is indicated by short, visual response latency. Figure 1 indicates that the latency is related directly to response probability. Table 1 shows that the largest proportion of errors occurred on the less probable steps, so that a further disproportionate increase of visual attention would be needed on these steps, to minimize the errors.

The stimuli appeared at equal time intervals but there was always uncertainty of the extent of impending responses. The latency of a correct response was 0·'3 s on unequivocal steps, where the demand for direction was certain, but each of four different extents was equally probable. In steps starting from positions 2 or 4, the increase of directional uncertainty raised latency to 0·27 s for a correct response in the probable direction, but a similar mean latency of 0·28 s produced errors on directionally improbable steps. It was necessary to increase latency to 0·37 s to obtain correct responses on the latter steps. There were three times as many probable as improbable steps. Subjects therefore had a choice between short latency, producing about 25 per cent of errors, and a long latency on both probable and improbable steps, which would minimize errors. In late practice, errors could be amended in 0·10 s and this was near the difference between the short and long latency. Time loss would therefore be negligible even when errors were made and time was important owing to brief target presentation. A strategy that minimized the time to acquire the target, rather than error, would produce 25 per cent of errors on steps starting from positions 2 or 4. In late practice, the average group errors were 22 per cent.

It would be expected that increased care in identifying the direction demanded would increase response latency and diminish error. This relation obtained on improbable steps, but on equiprobable steps the latencies of correct and incorrect responses were virtually equal to 0·30 and 0·29 s respectively. On these steps, 50 per cent of responses would be correct by chance, even with the 'short' latency of about 0·30 s, and there would be little time loss in amending errors, as compared with using the 'long' latency of 0·37 s for all responses. Again, the group minimized target acquisition time rather than error, and accepted 40 per cent of error in late practice.

Figure 1 shows that on probable and unequivocal steps, errors were actually associated with the longer latencies, i.e. the opposite of the expected relation. However, most of the relevant, plotted data were obtained in early practice, when error and long latency were associated on all types of responses. After step 67, there were only thirteen errors on probable and unequivocal steps; these were probably due to temporary regressions in learning the incompatible, control–display relation. They are not significant exceptions to the normal, inverse relation between accuracy and speed.

The development of a short amendment time of 0·1 s was an alternative to accepting long response latency on all steps, and it produced an effective compromise between the opposed requirements for accuracy and speed. The relations that developed, between response probability, latency and error reflect surprisingly high predictive capacity. Subjects developed, in 1 min practice, a highly adaptive strategy based upon relations that are extremely complex and obscure at the conscious, intellectual level. The group as a whole, and the women in particular, adopted the strategy that minimized target acquisition time, rather than error. The verbal reports of subjects revealed no awareness of rapid amendments; control and computations were effected at subconscious level.

Figure 1 illustrates the significant finding that uncertainty of direction had a greater effect on the latency of correct responses, than doubt of extent. For example, four different extents could be demanded on a directionally unequivocal step, but only one extent was involved in a directionally improbable step. 'Correct' response latencies were 0·37 and 0·23 s respectively.

Psychological refractoriness

Data on the psychological refractory period are contained in the studies cited previously. In responses to two closely spaced, un-predicted stimuli, the latency of the second response is usually longer than that of the first. A decision to respond cannot be revoked immediately by a prompt indication of error. The amendment times of the present study were, in effect, the response latencies to the second of two closely spaced stimuli. In early practice, directional errors persisted for about 0·25 s and demonstrated the typical 'all-or-none' refractory effect, but the amendment time was reduced to 0·10 s in late practice.

By previous hypothesis, the reduction of delay is based on learned, serial probability relations which were not apparent initially. The subjects could learn the relations between step probability, response latency and errors; for example, that a latency of 0·28 s, on steps starting from positions 2 or 4, would produce an error percentage of 25 per cent. To this extent, errors became predictable. Once a response was initiated, the direction of any error was determined and time of detection would be set by a relatively small and uniform perceptual delay. There was no uncertainty of appropriate response when the error signal occurred; hence, visual attention and central decision were not involved in amendments.

The data show that one type of refractoriness can be reduced by practice. Learning permits prediction of the results of responses, and the delegation of monitoring from visual attention to proprioceptive mechanisms which function at subconscious level.

The alternative view

Whitteridge (1960) provides a concise, impartial account of the historic controversy between protagonists of the inflow and

185

outflow theories of movement control. In the former, precise, directed movements cannot be made without either exteroceptive or proprioceptive information (feedback), on the states of the controlled member. In the outflow view, proprioception has no important, central functions in control. Practice establishes learned patterns of motor impulses in the brain, and each is appropriate to nullify an error of specific extent. The incompatible relation could be learned, by the incremental, automatic reinforcement of 'correct' motor volleys, and the progressive inhibition of 'incorrect' patterns. At some stage of practice, conflicting volleys of motor impulses could be dispatched over the direct and the indirect motor pathways to muscle (Eldred, Granit and Merton, 1953). Known difference in condition time could produce rapid reversal of movements, and so account for the 0·1 s interval between successive movements, without invoking notions of feedback.

The proposed, differential reinforcement necessitates feedback, in order to discriminate between correct and incorrect responses, but the converse does not hold. The essence of inflow theory is that patterns of proprioceptive sensations, rather than motor impulses, form the content of learning. Notions of motor reinforcement are, at best, redundant, and have nothing to commend them except respectable antiquity. The hypothesis of automatic reinforcement implies a 'stamping in' process to ensure that the appearance of a familiar stimulus triggers its associated response. No provision is made for adaptive variability, demonstrated by subjects' compromise between the opposed needs to acquire the target quickly and to minimize error. In the outflow view, the appearance of either an improbable step from position 4 to 5, or an unequivocal step from 1 to 2 would trigger the same pattern of motor impulses. Hence, errors and response latency would be equal on steps of similar extent, in the same direction, irrespective of their probability. The data flatly contradict the predictions based on outflow theory. The subjects were undoubtedly learning the new directional relation between output and feedback, and the input–output serial probability relations that were present in the task.

References

ADAMS, J. A. (1961), 'Human tracking behavior', *Psychol. Bull.*, vol. 58, pp. 55–9.

ADAMS, J. A. (1962), 'Test of the hypothesis of psychological refractory period', *J. exp. Psychol.*, vol. 64, pp. 280–87.

CRAIK, K. J. W. (1948), 'Theory of the human operator in control systems. II. Man as an element in a control system', *Brit. J. Psychol.*, vol. 38, pp. 142–8.

DAVIS, R. (1956), 'The limits of the "psychological refractory period"', *Quart. J. exp, Psychol.*, vol. 8, pp. 24–38.

DAVIS, R. (1957), 'The human operator as a single channel information system', *Quart. J. exp. Psychol.*, vol. 9, pp. 119–29.

DAVIS, R. (1959), 'The role of "attention" in the psychological refractory period', *Quart. J. exp. Psychol.*, vol. 11, pp. 211–20.

DRESSLAR, F. B. (1892), 'Some influences which affect the rapidity of voluntary movements', *Amer. J. Psychol.*, vol. 4, pp. 514–27.

ELDRED, E., GRANIT, R., and MERTON, P. A. (1953), 'Supraspinal control of the muscle spindle and its significance', *J. Physiol.*, vol. 122, pp. 498–523.

GIBBS, C. B. (1954), 'The continuous regulation of skilled response by kinaesthetic feedback', *Brit. J. Psychol.*, vol. 45, pp. 24–39.

HELSON, H., and STEGER, J. A. (1962), 'On the inhibitory effects of a second stimulus following the primary stimulus to react', *J. exp. Psychol.*, vol. 64, pp. 201–5.

HICK, W. E. (1948), 'The discontinuous functioning of the human operator in pursuit tasks', *Quart. J. exp. Psychol.*, vol. 1, pp. 36–44.

HYMAN, R. (1953), 'Stimulus information as a determinant of reaction time', *J. exp. Psychol.*, vol. 45, pp. 188–96.

MATTHEWS, B. H. C. (1933), 'Nerve endings in mammalian muscle', *J. Physiol.*, vol. 78, pp. 1–53.

MOUNTCASTLE, V. B., POGGIO, G. F., and WERNER, G. (1963), 'The relation of thalamic cell response to peripheral stimuli varied over an intensive continuum', *J. Neurophysiol.*, vol. 26, pp. 807–34.

RUCH, T. C. (1951), 'Motor systems', in S. S. Stevens (ed.), *Handbook of Experimental Psychology*, Wiley.

VINCE, M. A. (1948), 'The intermittency of control movements and the psychological refractory period', *Brit. J. Pyschol.*, vol. 38, pp. 149–57.

WELFORD, A. T. (1952), 'The psychological refractory period, and the timing of high-speed performance: a review and a theory', *Brit. J. Psychol.*, vol. 43, pp. 2–19.

WELFORD, A. T. (1959), 'Evidence of a single channel decision mechanism limiting performance in a serial reaction task', *Quart. J. exp. Psychol.*, vol. 11, pp. 193–210.

WHITTERIDGE, D. (1960), 'Central control of eye-movements', in H. W. Magoun (ed.), *Handbook of Physiology, Vol. II: Neurophysiology*, American Physiological Society.

14 A. J. Dinnerstein, T. Frigyesi and M. Lowenthal

Delayed Feedback as a Possible Mechanism in Parkinsonism

Excerpt from A. J. Dinnerstein, T. Frigyesi and M. Lowenthal, 'Delayed feedback as a possible mechanism in Parkinsonism', *Perceptual and Motor Skills*, vol. 15, 1962, pp. 667–80.

Many aspects of human behavior may be viewed as the functioning of feedback control systems (Powers, Clark and McFarland, 1960). This paper is concerned with some temporal aspects of feedback factors, which might explain Parkinsonian disability.

Parkinsonism is a disorder involving a loss of normal synchrony between agonist and antagonist musculature and is characterized by motor signs such as muscle rigidity, tremor and slowness of movement. In advanced stages the patient can neither walk nor perform coordinated hand and arm movements for such activities as feeding or dressing himself. The disease is considered to be the result of malfunction of the extrapyramidal system but there is no complete neurophysiological explanation of the mechanism by which this malfunction produces the symptoms. It has been argued that the motor symptoms result from a loss of normal inhibition of antagonistic reflexive movement (Denny-Brown, 1950). The nature of the inhibition and disinhibition has not been elaborated, however. The present authors believe that the loss of at least some of the normal patterns of control might be explained by the hypothesis of a simple perceptual malfunction, an abnormal delay in proprioception. The theory which follows draws heavily on the analogies of experimentally induced disabilities and on evidence concerning normal perceptual delay. While possible neurophysiological mechanisms are described, the theory is justified on the grounds of parsimony and on successful experimental tests rather than on the grounds of excluding alternative hypotheses.

A. J. Dinnerstein, T. Frigyesi and M. Lowenthal

The Theory

Proprioceptive delay hypothesis

A common characteristic of the motor system, and of subunits of this system, is the normal balancing of tensions between antagonistic muscle activity. The balance of agonist–antagonist forces involves simple or complex coordinating centers which receive sensory information concerning the moment by moment state of the system. Blockage or other malfunction within the proprioceptive mechanism will almost inevitably produce some type of distortion of system function. Among the many possible sensory malfunctions, proprioceptive delay seems specifically plausible in Parkinsonism. The plausibility follows from analogous malfunctions produced experimentally and from the specific nature of Parkinsonian symptoms.

Analogies

Parkinsonian tremor has been compared with the oscillations found in electromechanical feedback systems (Wiener, 1950). More relevant to the present discussion have been experimental demonstrations that analogous behavioral disability can be induced by sensory delay.

The behavioral disabilities in Parkinsonism have analogies in the speech disabilities found in stuttering. The tremor in Parkinsonism is superficially similar to the syllable repetition of stuttering speech. Slowness and delay in movement in Parkinsonism is somewhat analogous to the slowness and tense pauses of speech in stuttering. While the normal mechanisms involved in stuttering are uncertain, stuttering can be induced experimentally by delayed auditory feedback. This is produced by having Ss speak or read aloud while listening to their own speech which has been recorded and played back via earphones after a delay of a fraction of a second. The speech disruption is dramatic, though Ss show some ability to learn to overcome the induced disability (Chase et al., 1959; Goldiamond, Atkinson and Bilger, 1962; Lee, 1950).

More directly related to the present concern is the fact that vacillation, repetitions, and pauses in writing and other visual–motor coordination tasks can be induced by experimentally

189

delayed visual feedback (Kalmus, Fry and Denes, 1960). The situations involved procedures similar to those employed in auditory delay. A visual display presented to *S* information concerning his movements, but the display lagged behind *S*'s movements. Again, the behavior disruption was dramatic.

The effect of auditory delay on a task normally utilizing auditory feedback, and the effect of visual delay on tasks normally employing visual feedback, suggest that a proprioceptive delay would produce analogous disruption of those motor tasks involving proprioceptive feedback. These analogies, in fact, were the starting point of the present theoretical activity.

Parkinsonian tremor

In addition to pointing to analogies between Parkinsonism and stuttering, one can argue that a proprioceptive delay, if it exists, should produce the *specific* outstanding Parkinsonian symptoms. The mechanism of Parkinsonian tremor might be as follows. A normal limb held unsupported in space has been reported to show tremor over a wide range of frequencies, most strongly in the 8 to 12 cycle range (Fossler, 1931; Travis and Hunter, 1931). These tremors serve to maintain muscle tone and to prime the limb for activity. Normally, these tremor movements are almost imperceptible because proprioceptive impulses, the afferent consequence of muscle contraction, arouse antagonistic muscles which oppose the tendency to movement or which return the limb to its original starting position. If the occurrence or transmission of the proprioceptive impulses were excessively delayed, the initial automatic movement would be larger because the antagonistic muscle contraction would be delayed. The movement to return the hand to the original starting position, once begun, would continue too long as the proprioceptive impulses indicating that the hand had reached the 'correct' position would be late in signaling the termination of contraction. The resulting sequence of new delayed proprioceptive impulses and the inevitably delayed and prolonged compensating muscle contractions would produce oscillating movement.

The frequency of normal, fine, limb tremor is apparently non-neurological in origin (Brumlik, 1962). It is possible that the amplitude of normal limb tremor reflects the inevitable degree of proprioceptive delay in any sensory system. Prolonged delays, if they occurred, would clearly produce large tremors such as are found in Parkinsonism.

Rigidity

A delay in the proprioceptive control of the normal muscle tone mechanism might produce muscle rigidity. This hypothesis involves no significant conflict with current notions of the mechanism involved in muscle tone.

The muscle is composed of two contractile systems, each with its own motor nerves and with the possibility of independent sensory feedback systems. The gamma motor neurons innervate the intrafusal muscle fibers of the muscle spindles and alpha neurons innervate the extrafusal muscle fibers. Two sensory systems exist within the muscle spindle to provide both spinal and supraspinal proprioceptive controls of motor outflow (Granit, 1955).

The functions and interrelation of the alpha and gamma motor systems are not fully understood. It is clear, however, that they have antagonistic effects on the tension of the intrafusal fibers. A current view stresses the likelihood of gamma-motor system control of muscle tone by means of evoked intrafusal fiber contraction which, in turn, results in reflexive extrafusal fiber contraction (Thomas, 1961). According to this view, muscle rigidity is the result of an excessive gamma activity, with the excessive activity being of unknown origin. If, however, the gamma system is subject to proprioceptive control, a possible source of excessive gamma activity could be a delay in transmission of the proprioceptive impulses which are utilized in this control. The delay would produce an oscillation in the tension of intrafusal fibers in much the same way in which limb tremor was hypothesized to follow from proprioceptive delay. Proprioceptive delay, if it exists, thus might produce hyperactivity in the gamma system with resulting muscle rigidity.

The notion that rigidity is due to a delay induced oscillation in the gamma system is attractive for another reason as well. While tremor may be due to a proprioceptive delay acting on the limb position control mechanism, as proposed earlier, it is also plausible that tremor is the result of the assumed oscillation in

191

the gamma system. Oscillations in the lengths of intrafusal fibers, if in phase with each other and of great enough amplitude to evoke a full stretch reflex, could drive the limb into gross oscillatory movement. Both tremor and rigidity may thus reflect the identical process, a delay in the proprioceptive control of the gamma system.

Hypokinesis

A slowing of behaviors is the most reliable outcome of experimentally induced delay of auditory or visual feedback. The mechanism is unclear but may indicate that, in behavior extending over time, the sensory feedback from one unit of the behavior contributes to the evocation of later behavior units. Delayed sensory feedback from early behavior units possibly causes those units which follow to wait for the 'normal' signal to appear.

Alternative hypothesis

Within the general view of motoric function as being a balancing of agonist–antagonist forces by a sensory feedback control system, the authors have argued that Parkinsonian symptoms appear to reflect excessive delay in the sensory systems. Such motoric functions, however, would show almost identical malfunction as a result of excessive speed in the efferent paths or of other events which reduce latency of muscle contractions.

While the proprioceptive delay hypothesis and the present alternatives are in one sense in opposition to each other, they share a fundamental similarity. Both hypotheses follow from the assumption that complex motor symptoms do not necessarily indicate a malfunction of specific motor-control center or disruption of pathways. The symptoms can result from such general factors as a change in speed of action of components of the sensorimotor system.

Present knowledge does not permit a true specification of the locus of the Parkinsonian malfunction. It may be perceptual, integrative or motoric. The present concern with proprioception follows from research and argument by others that the speed of motoric events in normals is set by the limits of afferent control (Bartlett and Bartlett, 1959). It also follows from observations that the slowing of performance in ageing is primarily due to perceptual rather than to efferent or muscular deterioration (Braun, 1959). As will be described below, moreover, there is ample evidence concerning the presence of both normal and pathological perceptual delays.

Perceptual Delays

Normal delays

While not often discussed in recent psychological literature, variable delays in the normal perceptual process are a common and well-established phenomenon (Boring, 1950). The existence of perceptual delays in normals was first noted in the early 1800s by astronomers. It appeared as disagreement between different observers in attempts to compare the time of the transit of a star across a point in the telescope field with the beat of a clock. Laboratory research directed to the problem, the complication experiment, soon showed that if, for example, an auditory and visual stimulus were presented at the same moment, either one or the other might be experienced as occurring first. The intermodal difference in perceptual speed varied among Os, and varied within a single O as a function of direction of attention. The modality to which one attends shows the shortened delay (Angell and Pierce, 1892; Stone, 1926).

Perceptual delays can also be produced by variations of stimulus intensity. One measure of such a delay appears in reaction time studies, in which decreases of stimulus intensity can drastically increase response latency (Cattell, 1885).

In summary, the study of perception in normals shows perceptual delay to be a common phenomenon. Delay varies as an inverse function of stimulus intensity within a modality. It varies between modalities as a function of direction of attention and of fairly stable aspects of individual difference.

Existence of pathological delay

The theory, that Parkinsonism involves proprioceptive delay, gains credibility from a report of a specific perceptual delay in another patient population (Sutton et al., 1961). Normal and schizophrenic Ss were presented with a series of stimuli at

193

intervals of a few seconds. Red and green lights and high and low tones were presented in an apparently random sequence, with instructions to release a single key no matter which one appeared. A given stimulus could be preceded by an identical one, by a different stimulus from the same modality or by a stimulus from another modality. In the shift from light stimuli to sound stimuli, the schizophrenics showed a disproportionately longer retardation than did normals.

The above research design controlled for the effects of general response speed, for level of attention and for the effects of motor set. By exclusion, therefore, the present writers infer that the prolonged response times were the result of a delay in perception. While this auditory delay appeared as a result of a specific stimulus sequence, the fact of a difference between schizophrenics and normals shows that perceptual delays can occur as aspects of a pathological condition.

Neurophysiology of Delay

Parkinsonism may be produced by anatomical lesions in the extrapyramidal system, by a variety of drugs or by metabolic disturbances (England and Schwab, 1961). Why should dissimilar events such as these all produce the same group of symptoms? The notion of a proprioceptive delay, as the source of the varied motor malfunctions, provides a possible unifying process. While the mechanism of the hypothesized delay is itself a problem requiring explanation, we now need explain only one event rather than many.

Obviously, a detailed mechanism of transmission delay can not be proposed at present. Knowledge concerning such a mechanism is lacking for the variable delays known to occur in normals, as well as for the hypothesized proprioceptive delay. In attempting to point the way to a neurophysiological explanation of delay, one can only describe a possibly relevant phenomenon, the observed functional inhibition and facilitation of neural conduction.

Reticular formation

The regulatory activity of the reticular formation on sensory conduction is itself dependent on ascending somesthetic input as well as on impulses from the sensory-motor cortex (England and Schwab, 1961). The brainstem reticular formation is a significant relay station of the extrapyramidal system. Unregulated motor activity can be produced by anatomical damage to the basal ganglia, by damage to certain parts of the reticular formation or by disruption of connecting pathways between basal ganglia and reticular formation (Himwich and Rinaldi, 1957). The reticular formation, therefore, provides pathways (and connexions between them) by means of which an imbalance might be produced between the ascending impulses and the descending extrapyramidal outflow.

Reticular activating system

The role of the reticular system in arousal is well established. Drugs and electrical stimulation that produce alerting may also produce tremor and rigidity. Conversely, those drugs that block arousal, and some lesions of the system, are often effective against extrapyramidal disorders. Moreover, extrapyramidal symptoms disappear in sleep and reappear on awakening. The function of the reticular system thus plays an important role in extrapyramidal disorders (Himwich and Rinaldi, 1957).

Biochemistry

Parkinsonism responds to, or is produced by, a number of compounds. The postulated central synaptic transmitter, acetylcholine, produces alerting and worsens Parkinsonism. Anticholinergics can prevent arousal and are used in the treatment of Parkinsonism (Himwich and Rinaldi, 1957). Two other compounds, serotonin and norepinephrine, have recently been implicated as also playing an active role in central synaptic transmission. Both of these compounds exert an influence on Parkinsonism and were found to be present in abnormal concentrations in Parkinsonian brain and urine (Barbeau, 1962). Reserpine and chloropromazine, used in the treatment of schizophrenia, were found to interfere with the utilization of serotonin and norepinephrine, respectively. Both drugs influence the reticular system and may worsen or even produce Parkinsonism. These latter observations suggest that an abnormal concentration or metabolism of serotonin and norepinephrine may be the biochemical requirements of the Parkinsonian state (Frigyesi, 1961). It is of interest that all of the biochemical mechanisms implicated in Parkinsonism are also implicated in synaptic transmission and in the functioning of the reticular activating system. They could thus act on these processes governing normal transmission delay.

It was mentioned earlier that schizophrenics reportedly showed a different pattern of perceptual delay than normals. This observation now gains in relevance in light of the fact that abnormal metabolism of serotonin and norepinephrine has been implicated in the etiology of schizophrenia (Wooley and Shaw, 1954).

In summary, present knowledge of the neurophysiology and biochemistry of Parkinsonism is incomplete. The existing data, while compatible with alternative theories as well, are clearly consonant with the notion of a changed speed of neural transmission. This mechanism could account for tremor and rigidity as due to anatomical damage or to chronic or drug-induced metabolic disturbances. Delay could, in principle, occur by a variety of neurophysiological processes and at various loci. The detailed mechanisms of delay, both normal and pathological, have yet to be discovered.

Symptom Variability and Delay Theory

The proprioceptive delay theory accounts for a number of generally puzzling aspects of Parkinsonian symptoms. Short-comings in the theory are also evident.

Behavioral paradoxes explained

Many patients who can no longer walk, can march or dance to music (Meyer-Koenigsberg, 1923). Patients examined in our laboratory, whose slowness and rigidity prevent them from feeding themselves, can often catch a ball. These apparent paradoxes in the behavior of patients with Parkinsonism become meaningful when viewed in relation to the present theory. In walking, the proprioceptive feedback from one step serves as a signal for the next step so that a proprioceptive delay would distort and abort the movement sequence, while in marching and dancing the beat of the rhythm signals each step. Ball catching, unlike feeding oneself, involves a brief movement in response to a visual signal. The oddly intact behaviors thus have a common characteristic. An external stimulus provided an alternative to proprioception.

Variability of tremor

Tremor is highly variable, tending to decrease during voluntary movements and to be subject to voluntary inhibition. In these situations the patient's attention is, in all likelihood, directed to proprioceptive stimuli. As indicated earlier, attending to a modality increased speed of perception in that modality, relative to the speed in other modalities. The reticular activating system is the likely neurophysiological mechanism. The decreased Parkinsonian tremor during volitional motor acts is thus in accord with the theory of proprioceptive delay.

Rigidity

Parkinsonian rigidity does not commonly decrease in response to the above events which reduce tremor. The theory of propriocep-tive delay, and of the effect of attention on delay, does not easily account for this aspect of rigidity. A similar difficulty appears in the effects of anti-Parkinsonism medications, where some drugs are more effective against tremor and others are more effective against rigidity (Frigyesi, 1961). The proprioceptive delay theory is thus, at best, incomplete. If proprioceptive delay is the com-mon mechanism in Parkinsonian symptoms, the theory must eventually be elaborated so as to explain how this delay varies independently within different functional units of the proprio-ceptive system.[1]

1. After this paper was completed, W. W. Hofman in two articles dis-cussed the role of the gamma system in the Parkinsonian state. These articles (*J. Neurol. Neurosurg. Psychiat.*, vol. 25, 1962, pp. 109–15, 203–7) describe electromyographic studies in man from which he concludes that an overdamping of the gamma system occurs in Parkinsonism.

The Role of Proprioception in Skill

References

ANGELL, J. R., and PIERCE, A. (1892), 'Experimental research upon the phenomena of attention', *Amer. J. Psychol.*, vol. 4, pp. 528–41.

BARBEAU, A. (1962), 'A new hypothesis concerning the pathomechanism of parkinsonism', *J. Canad. med. Assn*, vol. 87, pp. 802–7.

BARTLETT, N. R., and BARTLETT, S. (1959), 'Synchronizations of a motor response with an anticipated sensory event', *Psychol. Rev.*, vol. 66, pp. 203–18.

BORING, E. G. (1950), *A History of Experimental Psychology*, Appleton-Century.

BRAUN, H. T. (1959), 'Perceptual processes', in J. E. Birren (ed.), *Handbook of Aging and the Individual*, University of Chicago Press, pp. 543–61.

BRUMLIK, J. (1962), 'On the nature of normal tremor', *Neurol.*, vol. 12, pp. 159–79.

CATTELL, J. M. (1885), 'The influence of the intensity of the stimulus on the length of the reaction time', *Brain*, vol. 8, pp. 512–15.

CHASE, R. A., HARVEY, S., STANDFAST, S., RAPIN, I., and SUTTON, S. (1959), 'Comparison of effects of delayed auditory feedback on speech and key tapping', *Science*, vol. 129, pp. 903–4.

DENNY-BROWN, D. (1950), 'Disintegration of motor function resulting from cerebral lesions' (Hughlings Jackson Lecture), *J. nerv. ment. Dis.*, vol. 112, p. 1.

ENGLAND, A. C., and SCHWAB, R. S. (1961), 'Parkinson's syndrome', *New Eng. J. Med.*, vol. 265, pp. 785–92, 837–44.

FOSSLER, H. R. (1931), 'Range and distribution of tremor frequencies', *J. gen. Psychol.*, vol. 5, pp. 410–14.

FRIGYESI, T. (1961), 'Evaluation of UK-738 in the treatment of extrapyramidal disorders', *Neurol.*, vol. 11, pp. 1050–54.

GOLDIAMOND, I., ATKINSON, G. J., and BILGER, R. C. (1962), 'Stabilization of behavior and prolonged exposure to delayed auditory feedback', *Science*, vol. 135, pp. 437–8.

GRANIT, R. (1955), *Receptors and Sensory Perception*, Yale University Press.

HIMWICH, H. E., and RINALDI, F. (1957), 'The effect of drugs on the reticular system', in W. S. Fields (ed.), *Brain Mechanisms and Drug Action*, C. C. Thomas, pp. 15–43.

KALMUS, H., FRY, D. B., and DENES, P. (1960), 'Effects of delayed visual control on writing, drawing and tracing', *Lang. Speech*, vol. 3, pp. 96–108.

LEE, B. S. (1950), 'Effects of delayed speech feedback', *J. acoust. Soc. Amer.*, vol. 22, pp. 824–6.

MEYER-KOENIGSBERG, E. (1923), 'Die Beeinfluessung der Bewegungstoerungen bei der Encephalitis lethargica durch rhythmische Gefuehle', *Muench. Med. Wchschr.*, vol. 70, p. 459.

POWERS, W. T., CLARK, R. K., and MCFARLAND, R. (1960), 'A general feedback theory of human behavior', *Percept. mot. Skills*, vol. 11, pp. 71–88, 309–23.

STONE, S. A. (1926), 'Prior entry in the auditory-tactual complication', *Amer. J. Psychol.*, vol. 37, pp. 284–91.

SUTTON, S., HAKEREM, G., ZUBIN, J., and PORTNOY, M. (1961), 'The effect of shift of modality on serial reaction time: a comparison of schizophrenics and normals', *Amer. J. Psychol.*, vol. 74, pp. 224–32.

THOMAS, J. E. (1961), 'Muscle tone, spasticity and rigidity', *J. nerv. ment. Dis.*, vol. 132, pp. 505–14.

TRAVIS, L. E., and HUNTER, J. A. (1931), 'Tremor frequencies', *J. gen. Psychol.*, vol. 5, pp. 255–60.

WIENER, N. (1950), *Human Use of Human Beings*, Houghton Mifflin.

WOOLEY, D. W., and SHAW, E. (1954), 'A biochemical and pharmacological suggestion about certain mental disorders', *Science*, vol. 119, p. 586.

Part Five
The Mechanisms Underlying Skilled Performance

The basic ideas advanced by Craik (Reading 10) that man's behaviour in a control system could be modelled by an intermittent correction servo have been actively developed by many researchers. The three papers in this part represent three ways in which servo principles have been incorporated in theories of the mechanisms underlying perceptual–motor skill.

Paillard (Reading 15) shows the way in which various parts of the central nervous system are linked by tracts to make a series of closed loops – an essential condition for servo-control. The C.N.S. is organized hierarchically with an appropriate closed-loop system at each level. He shows how the teleological behaviour of organisms may be accounted for simply by the operation of a series of self-regulating mechanisms. The excerpt shows how engineering and physiology may combine to provide a basis for psychological explanation.

Gibbs (Reading 16), in a paper specially prepared for this book of readings and completed shortly before his untimely death, takes this idea further. He juxtaposes the expected performance of a control mechanism working according to the principles of servo-engineering with the ease with which subjects can transfer skills from one situation to another. He notes that the sophistication of the biological error-actuated control system is considerably greater than that of an engineering analogue, but that the essential features are the same.

Licklider (Reading 17) describes two servo-based systems as models of different kinds of tracking performance. Naturally the dominant concept is that of feedback but an attempt is made to describe a complete system involving both feedback loops and information transformation. The system is complex and described largely in engineering terms. One consequence of this analysis is to emphasize the critical differences between different forms of tracking behaviour.

15 J. Paillard

Mechanisms of Self-Adjustment

Excerpt from J. Paillard, 'The patterning of skilled movements', in J. Field (ed.), *Handbook of Physiology: Section I Neurophysiology*, vol. 3, American Physiological Society, 1960, pp. 1700–703.

For biologists, the most interesting control systems are those commonly called 'servo-mechanisms' or slave systems. Components and characteristics of servo-mechanisms are numerous and varied, but their common feature is that they possess some kind of controlling device able to appreciate continuously the discrepancy between the state of the machine realized at a given moment and the final aim assigned to it by its constructor. Through a 'feedback' circuit, the information collected from an error-detecting device is at every moment sent back to the servo motor controlling the output. By modifying the input command it permits the output to be corrected for the detected discrepancy. Thus the 'behavior' of a servo-mechanism is not governed by a blind obedience to the order of a predetermined program of action, but it presents a kind of self-adjustment by modifying the input command of the system as a function of its output.

Such 'telelogical' mechanisms (4) are designed to attain a given goal (such as attainment or maintenance of a given equilibrium or pursuit of a moving goal) by their operation despite unexpected changes occurring (within a certain range) in the field of external forces. They present a type of 'flexibility' of their performance.

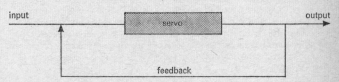

Figure 1 Schema showing the principle of organization of a servo-mechanism unit

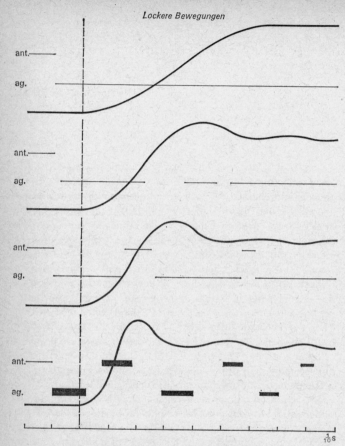

Lockere Bewegungen

ant.———
ag.

ant.———
ag.

ant.———
ag.

ant.———
ag.

$\frac{1}{10}$s

Figure 1 (cont.) Distribution of the muscular activity in two antagonizing groups of muscles, the agonists (ag.) and antagonists (ant.), at four stages of increasing speed of movement. The electromyographic activity of each group is schematized by a *line* the thickness of which varies with intensity. The *mechanographic record* shows the increasing tendency to oscillation when the speed of execution is increasing. The final position is achieved only by a transient oscillatory movement (from Wachholder, 10)

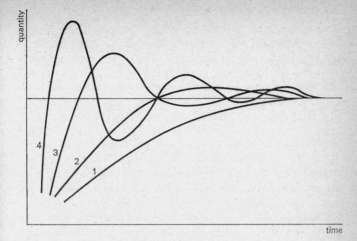

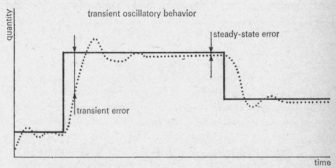

Top: Diagram showing transient stability of a physical system
with varying degrees of damping. Curves 2, 3 and 4 are progressively
underdamped and show increasing signs of oscillatory behavior. Curve
1 is overdamped and shows great stability at the expense of a long
response time. A servo-mechanism shows a similar mode of
functioning. Compare these curves with those recorded by
Wachholder (from Brown and Campbell, 1).
Bottom: Response of a human subject in a tracking experiment.
The diagram illustrates the several kinds of observed errors between the
response (dashed line) and the command (solid line) during a sudden
change in the latter. A steady state and transient errors, as well as
transient oscillatory behavior, are also characteristic of the
performance of a servo-mechanism (from Ruch, 9)

They give a clue to understanding how a simple physical system, the organization of which rests on unmodified rigidly connected working parts, can, thanks to the feedback action, present a certain range of freedom in the adjustment of its performance. Homeostatic processes and more general neural activities have been analysed in this way (6, 7).

Attempts also have been made to approach certain aspects of human sensorimotor behavior in the same way. Although too schematic and too simple to account for the complex total process involved in human behavior, the analogies with the physical systems just described provide a suggestive model for the dynamic aspects of human controller tasks (2, 3). Figure 1 shows some aspects of these analogies.

The analogies between the mechanisms of voluntary movements and those of servo-mechanism are also found to be close, although not complete (9). The stream of volitional impulses which initiates skilled movements may be seen as a programmed input which puts to work the cortical motor mechanisms considered as part of a complex servo-mechanism.

Several closed loops have been identified which modulate by feedback control the emission of corticofugal impulses. Some are long loops including either various proprioceptive or exteroceptive feedback circuits, more or less directly coupled with the organ of movement or with the outcomes of the action; they constitute, therefore, 'output-informed' feedback circuits. Others are shorter loops connecting the motor cortex to the cerebellum or to the other subcortical way stations. They do not include the peripheral output of the system, and hence constitute what Ruch calls 'input-informed' circuits (9). Organized close-loop controls have been found at all levels of the nervous system (see Figure 2).

The spinal machinery presents the closest comparison with the servo-mechanisms (8). Thanks to its many self-regulating circuits, it gives to its output, the contraction of muscle, smoothness and precision. Despite the classic view of reflexes as stereotyped reactions of a rigid prearranged apparatus, this reflex machinery taken as a functional whole appears as a self-adjusting mechanism of high flexibility. Such systems adapted to local regulations are included in larger functional units likewise organized as self-regulatory devices of a higher order of complexity. We know,

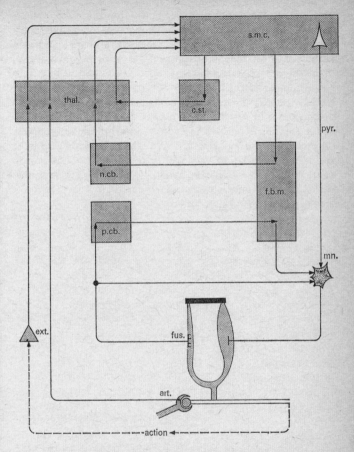

Figure 2 Simplified diagram showing some examples of output- and input-informed circuits playing part in the control of motor command. s.m.c., sensory–motor cortex; thal., thalamus; c.st., corpus striatum; pyr., pyramidal tract; n.cb., neocerebellum; p.cb., paleocerebellum; f.b.m., bulbomesencephalic formations; mn., motoneuron; fus., intrafusal receptors; art., articular receptors; ext., exteroreceptors

for instance, the astonishing flexibility of postural regulatory systems. Taken as a whole, such systems act like time-continuous error-detecting devices that position the body in space by varying the output of the muscle to counteract changes in gravitational force (9).

According to Ruch (9), the corticocerebellocortical circuit may also represent a part of a mechanism by which an instantaneous order of cortical origin may be 'amplified and extended forward in time'. It should be efficient in starting and in stopping a movement without jerkiness. This might be accomplished by a controlling feedback proportional to the velocity of the movement. In this view 'cerebellar tremor may be comparable to the oscillation of an undamped servo-mechanism in which the feedback is removed'.

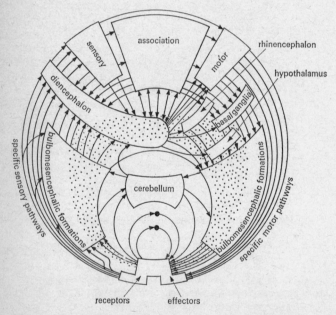

Figure 3 Highly simplified diagram of the chief sensory, associative and motor paths throughout the nervous system, which illustrates the circular organization of the sensorimotor relations at any levels. Only the 'output-informed' circuits are represented. Some direct sensory connexions to various higher structures have been intentionally omitted

Ruch likens the cerebellum to the 'comparator' of a servo-mechanism which receives from the cerebral cortex some representation of the command, and from the muscle and other exteroceptors representation of the resulting movement. These, compared, may result in a signal which when transmitted to the motor cortex alters its commands to the muscles so as to diminish the discrepancy.

The higher integrative levels themselves, which operate within a system of higher order, do not escape the same basic mode of organization. Thus, the whole nervous system will have to be viewed as a functional hierarchy of systems, each of which includes subsystems and so on, a view already stressed earlier by Weiss (11). At all levels of this hierarchy, we shall find the same common principle of organization of sensorimotor functional units.

A principle of circular regulation seems to govern the fundamental mode of relation which ties the efferent to the afferent portions of the nervous system either inside the body or through the external medium. Thanks to its self-regulating mechanism, each working unit of this system assumes, in a given range of flexibility, its own functional balance in accordance with the requirements of the general equilibrium which results in this internal unit contributing to the effectiveness of the organism as a whole.

We are then led to the older concept of 'senso-motility' of Exner, as well as to its more recent expressions (5), to conceive the dynamic patterning of nervous commands as a result of the continuous stream of nerve impulses which is carried along a variety of circular paths that form closed loops at various levels of an anatomically ordered structure and which flows continuously from sensory receptors to effector organs, as shown in Figure 3.

Space does not permit further discussion of the several functional implications and the necessary limitations of such a principle of organization in its theoretical as well as practical aspects. Although we may speculate concerning its broader significance for the analysis of living organisms as teleological systems of action (4), we will assert for our restricted field its undeniable explicatory power to account for the flexibility of motor performance which, in other respects, is dependent on a prearranged pattern of neuronal interconnexions.

References

1. G. S. Brown and D. S. Campbell, *Principles of Servo-mechanisms*, Wiley, 1948.
2. K. J. W. Craik, *Brit. J. Psychol.*, vol. 38 (1947), p. 56.
3. K. J. W. Craik, *Brit. J. Psychol.*, vol. 38 (1948), p. 142.
4. L. K. Frank, G. E. Hutchinson, W. K. Livingston, W. S. McCulloch and N. Wiener, *Ann. New York Acad. Sc.*, vol. 50 (1948), p. 187.
5. W. Gooddy, *Brain*, vol. 72 (1949), p. 312.
6. H. Hoagland, *Science*, vol. 109 (1949), p. 159.
7. W. S. McCulloch, *Elec. Eng.*, vol. 68 (1949), p. 492.
8. P. A. Merton, in J. A. Malcolm, J. A. B. Gray, G. E. W. Wolstenholme and J. S. Freeman (eds.), *The Spinal Cord* (Ciba Foundation Symposium), Churchill, 1953, p. 247.
9. T. C. Ruch, in S. S. Stevens (ed.), *Handbook of Experimental Psychology*, Wiley, 1951, p. 154.
10. K. Wachholder, *Willkürliche Haltung und Bewegung insbesondere im Lichte elektrophysiologischer Untersuchungen*, Bergmann, 1928.
11. P. Weiss, *Comp. Psychol. Monogr.*, vol. 17 (1941), no. 88.

16 C. B. Gibbs

Servo-Control Systems in Organisms and the Transfer of Skill

Original paper published here for the first time.

A large amount of biological data support the thesis that there are essential similarities between the methods used by organisms for controlling their movements and those developed, much more recently, by control engineers. Servo theory has important applications to the study of human behaviour. One major problem concerns the transfer of skill between two tasks; the initial learning of one task may help or hinder the subsequent learning of another to give respectively, positive or negative transfer of skill.

A hypothetical servo-model of tracking skill is developed below. It is shown that the self-adaptive characteristics of the servo-model correspond closely with variants of a tracking task among which a trained human operator shows high positive transfer of skill. Conversely, there is little or no positive transfer and indeed there may be negative transfer, between two tasks that differ in such fashion that a servo-mechanism designed to discharge the first task would need considerable modification to deal with the second.

From the theoretical viewpoint, there are many transfer effects (Burke and Gibbs, 1965; Gibbs, 1951, 1954), which appear as inevitable by-products of the control methods adopted by organisms in the course of evolution. Such effects may therefore provide valuable clues to the particular type of sensory organization that has been adopted by organisms for movement control, from the many that could be conceived.

The practical requirements for effective training devices and for machines that take full advantage of habitual skills can only be met by improving our present understanding of the mechanisms that underlie the transfer of skill.

In an attempt to achieve fuller understanding, biological data relating to movement control are presented and a relevant servo-model is later deduced. Similarities between the action of the model and transfer effects are then discussed.

The model is somewhat speculative, as is inevitable in the present state of knowledge. The present concepts justify discussion, however, in the absence of tenable alternative notions and the pressing need to develop a systematic, experimental approach to the problems of the transfer of skill.

The General Problem of Control

Common requirements for speed, precision and flexibility must be met by living organisms and by mechanical control devices that match or compensate for unpredictable changes in the environment.

In an open-chain system, an input signal effects direct control of the output or motor element. The method is effective in specific conditions, where the input control signal is faithfully reproduced in transmission by all elements in the chain but the requisite conditions do not exist in the human neuromuscular system. There are gross non-linearities of power amplification in the muscles and skeletal linkages. The input–output relation depends on the initial length and load on the muscle and also varies with fatigue. There is continuous variation in these influences. A given input signal cannot produce a consistent response and simple, open-chain control is thereby precluded. The alternative method of error-actuation must be used for effective control. The method is based upon an input signal which defines the required state of a system and a signal fed back from the controlled member, which relates to the actual, achieved state of the system. The two signals are compared in an error-sensing device and the difference or error is fed forward as a demand signal that determines the magnitude of the motor response. The difference between signals, rather than absolute values, determines the response of an error-actuated system, which therefore compensates to some degree for changes in signals and absolute states due to sensory adaptation and fatigue.

It is not possible to initiate a movement of definite extent without data on the initial state of the controlled member. In organisms, as in machines, positional data on initial states are needed for control.

There are appreciable delays in the transmission of neural impulses and in generating forces in muscles. Movements could not be halted at a required point on the basis of positional feedback data that a body member had reached that particular point. The above delays would cause large and consistent overshoot, if positional data were used exclusively in control. In such conditions, a simple but effective method of controlling the extent of movement is to move the controlled member at an average speed proportional to the intended extent and to maintain that speed for an approximately constant period of time. A direct analogy is to use the speedometer to maintain speeds of 60 and 30 m.p.h. in a car for one hour, to travel respective distances of 60 and 30 miles.

Control at Peripheral Level

The servo-control loop in muscle has been described by many writers, including Eldred, Granit and Merton (1953), Lissman (1950), B. H. C. Matthews (1933), P. B. C. Matthews (1964) and Merton (1953). The probable action of the loop is illustrated by Figure 1 which depicts a descending foot, rotated by the contraction of muscle A to meet the sloping ground. The structure marked 'spindle', lying in parallel with the main muscle, is a micro-muscle which receives gamma motor impulses from the brain. The spindle contracts and changes its shape from that shown in muscle B to that in A, i.e. the polar regions thicken and thus extend the equatorial region and an annulo-spiral, primary nerve ending carried upon it. Extension of the latter causes an increase in the neural discharge flowing around the spinal pathways from the micro-muscle to the alpha motor nerves, that act directly to produce contraction of the main muscle A. The resulting contraction of the main muscle shortens the micro-muscle and the primary nerve which lie in parallel. The discharge of the primary nerve ending is thereby reduced to its initial level, when the new length of muscle A matches the changed length of the micro-muscle that initiated the cyclic activity. Changes in the length of the micro-muscle are therefore faithfully reproduced at a far higher power level by means of an error-actuated system which responds to differences in the length of the main and the micro-muscle. Changes in load, mechanical advantage and power may momentarily slow the contraction of the main muscle relative to the contraction of micro-muscle but increased disparity automatically

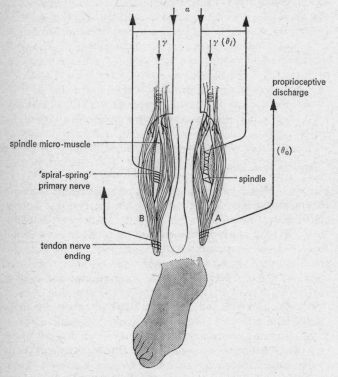

Figure 1 The servo-loop in muscles

increases the magnitude of the discharge that produces contraction of the main muscle. Similarly, when the foot meets the ground, the weight of the body will exert a levering action on the foot and apply a sharp stretch to muscle A and the primary nerve ending. The discharge to the main muscle is thereby greatly increased to produce massive contraction to support the weight of the descending body. The stretch reflex illustrates the important reversible property of error-actuated systems, i.e. proprioceptive feedback signals, like motor input signals, can produce contraction of muscles.

The muscles may be energized by the rapidly conducted alpha discharge through the direct routes shown in Figure 1 instead of by the slower gamma impulses which incur additional delays from transmission through the comparatively indirect pathways of the muscle loop. The cerebellum plays an important part in determining the relative use made of the rapid alpha discharge and the slower gamma impulses (Granit, Holmgren and Merton, 1955). The discharges may well be used in succession for the rapid primary movements and the slower secondary adjustments of discrete aiming movements that were distinguished by Woodworth (1899).

The delays in the muscle servo must be compensated for in walking, so that adequate force is available to support the body when the foot touches the ground. The discharges from proprioceptors in muscles and tendons, shown in Figure 1, are related to the rate of change of muscle length and tension respectively and these derivative data are used in the repetitive activity of walking, for predicting needs for future output of force. Appropriate demands are despatched from the cerebellum to muscle in time to compensate for neuromuscular delays (Higgins and Glaser, 1964), i.e. extrapolation from past motion compensates for system delays.

The contraction of the agonist muscle A stretches the antagonistic muscle B and its primary nerve. The increased discharge of the latter will produce some co-contraction of muscle B by the action described previously. The total discharge depends partly on the extension of the primary nerve that is related to the absolute length of the main muscle B. This component of the total discharge is related to the position (λ) of the limb. The primary ending is connected to the main muscle by visco-elastic attachments however, and there is much greater extension of the primary ending during rapid stretch than slow extension. This effect contributes a rate of stretch component (μ) to the total discharge. The total discharge is therefore related to the states that are controlled by a position plus rate servo, sometimes named a rate-aided or a quickened system. At slow rates of stretch, the discharge is correlated mainly with the length of muscle but the rate component (μ) increases with increased rate of stretch and becomes dominant in rapid movements. In organisms, the ratio of λ to μ is variable whereas it is constant in the mechanical rate-aided systems designed by control engineers.

The muscle loop deals automatically with the rapid fluctuations in external conditions that arise in walking over uneven ground and the servo eliminates the need for visual attention to detailed control. In organisms, such servo mechanisms are important because they are self-adaptive in operating conditions that are new in experience, i.e. they provide positive transfer between different operating conditions.

There are receptors in joints that can continuously indicate initial position, rates of angular movement and also signal, at least intermittently, the angular positions of moving limbs (Boyd and Roberts, 1953).

Data from primary nerves and tendon organs are transmitted in rapidly conducting fibres to the cerebellum but not, it appears, to the cerebral cortex. Data from joint receptors are conducted relatively slowly to the thalamus and the cortex (Mountcastle and Rose, 1959), thus supporting the view of Goldscheider (1889) that joint receptors are mainly responsible for conscious sensations of position and movement.

Control at Corticocerebellar Level

Figure 2 is a highly simplified diagram of some neural arrangements that are used in the control of movement. Visual input data go to zone 1, representing the thalamus, that also receives proprioceptive feedback signals via the spino-thalamic tracts. It is hypothesized that this zone produces an error signal, based upon the required and actual positions of the body member and that this signal is transmitted onward to zone 2 which represents the cortex. The cortical demand signal to muscles may be transmitted via the pyramidal pathways that are used in effecting fine, positional adjustments. This pathway excites but does not inhibit muscular activity. A representation of the cortical order goes to the cerebellum (zone 3) and the extrapyramidal motor pathways

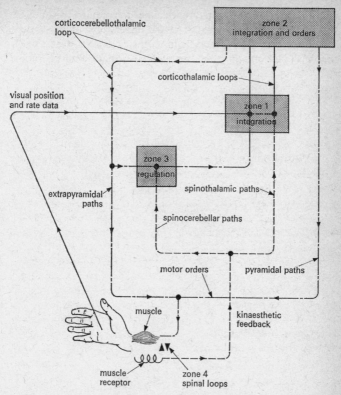

Figure 2 Diagram of the central nervous system relating to movement control

continue down to subserve reflex activity and long-sustained, relatively gross movements. These pathways may either excite or inhibit muscular activity and they may well be part of a system that generates and regulates a required rate of movement.

Model of Movement Control

Figure 3 shows a model of neural arrangements and functions that are depicted in Figure 2.

The pick-up element (left) detects the position (λ) and speed

(μ) of a target. The λ-signal that defines the required position is transmitted to the differential at the upper right of the figure, that also receives feedback defining the actual position of the motor. A rack and pinion moves a sliding contact along potentio-

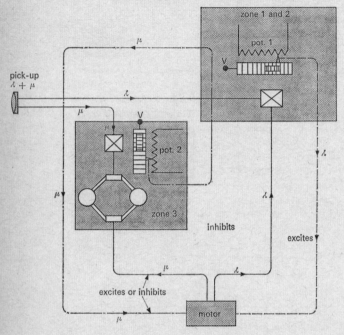

Figure 3 Servo-model of placing reaction and tracking responses

meter 1 by an amount proportional to the difference between the required and actual positions of the motor. The motor runs until this difference is eliminated by movements of the λ feedback shaft which return the slider on potentiometer 1 to its zero or null position.

The required speed (μ) of the system is also detected and transmitted from the pick-up element to move a sliding contact along potentiometer 2. The position of the slider is also affected by a feedback signal defining the actual speed of the motor, that is transmitted via a conventional speed governor. The latter maintains the required motor speed.

Essential features of the model are a λ-pathway that transmits an input discharge which is always excitory and a corresponding feedback path which always inhibits and halts movements. The feedforward and feedback pathways that define required and achieved speed respectively, are used to generate and monitor speed. They can either accelerate (excite) or decelerate (inhibit) the speed of the motor.

Despite its simplicity, the model is compatible with many data. The speed regulator of the model corresponds to the cerebellum and here, injury or ablation produce deficiencies in movement that would also occur after damage to the regulator of the model. The fact that monkeys rush headlong into clearly visible objects may be due to movements that are weak and slow or not restrained by the right amount at the right time.

The positional differential of the model represents the thalamus, a centre of known importance in controlling the position of body members. The model shown in Figure 3 has a connexion to convey data on the 'present position' of the controlled member to the differential that represents the thalamus. This pathway provides negative feedback that always inhibits movement. The model is therefore consistent with findings that stimulation of the thalamus can halt an animal's movements in a frozen posture.

Advantages of Rate-Aided Control

Figure 4 illustrates the advantages of a rate-aid system, which provides simultaneous corrections to errors of both position and speed, over systems which control only position or else speed alone. The figure illustrates the problems involved in tracking an accelerating target where a constant speed of following may be adequate for brief periods but soon becomes stale and leads to a positional error. The positional error may be corrected, as shown in Figure 4, without necessarily correcting the basic error in speed. In such a case, further positional errors rapidly develop. Similarly, a correction of the speed error alone will not correct positional error. Figure 4 also shows simultaneous correction of

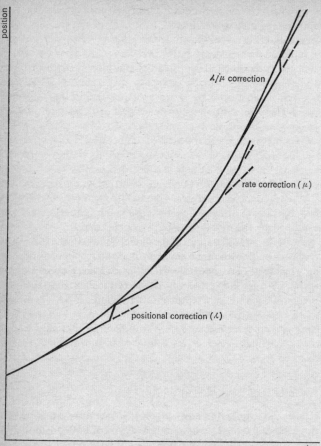

Figure 4 Corrections in tracking an accelerating target

a positional error (λ) and the rate error (μ) that caused it and so illustrates the typical correction of a rate-aid system.

In mechanical rate-aid systems there is a fixed ratio between the magnitude of a positional adjustment and the resulting change in system speed. Usually, a target is acquired by means of a large positional adjustment that may in turn generate unduly high system speed in a specific direction. On acquisition, the speed of the tracking system rarely matches that of the target. A number of successive corrections are then needed to nullify the error in initial speed. In contrast, a position plus rate correction can be made with considerable speed and accuracy by a finger when first pointed at a moving target, irrespective of the relative values of the two components. On acquisition, the finger settles almost immediately to the correct tracking rate. The control methods adopted by organisms over some hundred million years still have considerable advantages over those developed by modern control engineers.

Some Characteristics of Servo-Control

In an open-chain system, a specific input signal produces a stereo-typed, highly invariant output. The system cannot provide the adaptability needed in a highly variable environment. Stimulus–response theorists tend to assume that a main function of learning is to provide open-chain control; such theories are entirely inappropriate in the context of perceptual–motor skills that demonstrate marked variability and adaptability in dealing with changes in the environment.

From the servo viewpoint, skill is based largely on learned relations between the output of body members and propriocep-tive feedback that defines their position, force output, direction and rate of movement (Boyd and Roberts, 1953; B. H. C. Matthews, 1933; Mountcastle, Poggio and Werner, 1963). The extent of movement is probably determined by monitoring a required rate of movement, as defined by proprioception, for a definite time. Learning would be minimized by maintaining all movements for a relatively constant period and making move-ment speed proportional to the extent of movement required, rather than using several combinations of different times and speeds for each required extent. There is in fact, relative time con-stancy in primary, aiming movements of different extent when the same proportional accuracy is required in all movements (Fitts, 1954) and this characteristic would be provided by the servo-model shown in Figure 3.

The muscle servo shown in Figure 1 provides automatic

compensation for different terrains or loads. Such adaptability, or positive transfer, is a major characteristic of control by error actuation.

The Hierarchy of Control Systems

There is a hierarchy of control loops in the central nervous system. The loops are far more numerous and complex than those shown in Figure 2. Transfer of skill effects vary with the control loop in use. The inadequacy of current theories of the transfer of skill stems largely from the failure to make this distinction.

It is hypothesized that exteroceptive feedback is dominant in the early learning of all tasks and skills. A main function of learning is to permit the use of lower loops in the hierarchy by delegating detailed duties of monitoring from exteroceptors to proprioceptors. A major function of such delegation is to reduce demands on visual attention. The relations between the output and proprioceptive feedback must be learned to permit delegation of monitoring. The duration of delegation depends on the predictability of the effects of a given activity upon the environment.

In the tasks of continuous tracking or tracing, close visual attention is needed and monitoring can only be delegated to proprioceptors for very brief periods. The environmental effects of such activity cannot be reliably predicted long in advance of its execution. There is considerable positive transfer between many variants of tasks that are monitored in the main by exteroceptive feedback. The skill of tracing transfers highly among different templates, scale of movements, limb segments and limbs. Similarly, in continuous tracking, skill transfers highly between task variants that differ in respect to target motion, control gain, control lever, limb segment and limb. In one study (Gibbs, 1954) there was about 90 per cent of positive transfer in both directions between a conventional free-moving control lever and a pressure-operated lever, although the effects of a given deflection of the two levers differed in the ratio of 40 to 1. The explanation is that in continuous tracking the operator deflects the control lever by whatever amount is needed to nullify the visually perceived error. The procedure is identical, irrespective of the size of the error or the corrective adjustment that is made, so that automatic compensation is provided for changes of gain.

Controller motion is paced by the target in continuous tracking and it is often slow enough to be monitored closely by vision, but in step-input tracking a common criterion of performance is the time taken to acquire a target with a specified degree of precision. Rapid movements are needed but cannot be visually monitored, so that monitoring must be delegated to proprioceptors. The hypothetical basis for control is that a particular rate of contraction is maintained for a definite time. The free-moving and the pressure-control levers were deflected, respectively, by the isotonic and isometric contraction of muscle. The discharges and their feedback were completely different and they provided no basis for positive transfer between two levers in a task that by hypothesis, was monitored by proprioceptive feedback. In this case, the relevant prediction was that there would be no positive transfer between the levers. This prediction was confirmed in a study of step tracking with a positional control system with no lag, using eight adult subjects (Gibbs, 1965). One group of four subjects had 5 days of practice on the moving control and then transferred to the pressure control for a further 5 days. This group showed about 40 per cent of negative transfer on exchanging controls. The other four subjects learned and transferred between the controls in the opposite order. There was no positive transfer from the pressure-operated joystick to the moving control lever.

The skill of writing is a development of copying and tracing and it can be delegated and monitored by proprioception because of the highly predictable effects of this bodily activity. Programmes of movement, based on highly invariant relations between output and proprioceptive feedback can therefore be established. Occasional visual checks are needed on size, slope and margin but fairly extensive passages can be written with the eyes closed. The skill is usually learned by practising with the fingers and wrist but there is high positive transfer to some limb segments that are not usually practised directly. Arm movements are used for writing on a blackboard and it is possible to write with a pencil held between the toes. There is little positive transfer of writing skill however, from the preferred to the non-preferred hand. This phenomenon is compatible with the hypothesis of proprioceptive monitoring. Groups of proprioceptors in specific muscles and joints that signal a right to left movement of one arm are activated by the opposite direction of movement of the other arm. Two directionally opposed codes for programmed movement appear to co-exist in the brains of ambidextrous subjects but it may be reasonably assumed that the adoption of a single code would reduce interference and increase the number and speed of the programmes that could be established. The assumption finds some support in the fact that most people develop a dominant hand.

Habitual Output–Feedback Relations

The everyday activities of pointing and placing objects establish consistent relations between the movements and feedback data from exteroceptors and proprioceptors. The 'expected' relations that develop provide support for the theory that organisms make extensive use of servo methods of control. Habitual relations have great practical importance also, because it is difficult to learn to control a machine with relations that are incompatible with those that obtain in everyday skills.

The habitual directional relation between control and display movements is developed because in pointing and placing, the proprioceptive and visual data are compatible in signalling the same direction of movement. Some machines have an incompatible relation however, where the controlling limb and the display index move in opposite directions and there is a conflict between the directional data fed back from proprioceptors and exteroceptors. The same situation arises in mirror tracing. There are well-known difficulties in learning incompatible directional relations, because there is no positive transfer, indeed there may well be negative transfer, from habitual skills.

In habitual skills, there are similar, concomitant changes in the discharge from exteroceptors and proprioceptors that both define limb motion and the beginning and cessation of movement. These relations are retained in a positional servo-system but not in control systems of higher order. For example, when the foot on an accelerator pedal ceases to move, the car may still be in motion with the changes registered by exteroceptors. Again, there is little or no positive transfer from habitual skills to high-order control systems which are much more difficult to learn than positional systems.

Finally, there are transmission delays in the central nervous system but these are relatively uniform. They are learned and compensation is provided for in the exercise of everyday skills. However, the time delays in many machines impose additional delays between proprioceptive and exteroceptive feedback, that produce well-known difficulties in learning.

Incompatible relations provide a valuable tool in research because they force a return to the tactics and the exteroceptive control loop that were used in the initial learning of everyday skills. It then becomes possible to observe the delegation of monitoring to proprioceptors as the incompatible relation is learned (Gibbs, 1965).

Conclusions

The model and the various hypotheses presented here provide bases for functional and mechanistic explanations of phenomena of the transfer of skill. It is clearly important to classify skills and task variants that produce different transfer effects despite considerable similarity, as in the remarkable example of pressure-operated and free-moving controls.

At the present time, even the descriptive distinctions made between different types of activity, e.g. 'voluntary' and 'involuntary' movements are woefully inadequate. The use of these terms connotes control by the will and begs all possible questions of control. Activities that are monitored mainly by vision demand close attention, whereas proprioceptive monitoring occurs mainly in the cerebellum that is not a centre of consciousness. The terms 'attentive' and 'programmed' activities are suggested to provide a verbal distinction that is useful in practice, although theoretical views on the nature of movement control will probably differ for a considerable time.

References

BOYD, E. A., and ROBERTS, T. D. M. (1953), 'Proprioceptive discharge endings in the knee joint of the cat', *J. Physiol.*, vol. 122, pp. 38–59.

BURKE, D., and GIBBS, C. B. (1965), 'A comparison of free-moving and pressure levers in a positional control system', *Ergonomics*, vol. 8, pp. 23–9.

ELDRED, E., GRANIT, R., and MERTON, P. A. (1953), 'Supraspinal control of the muscle spindle and its significance', *J. Physiol.*, vol. 122, pp. 498–523.

FITTS, P. M. (1954), 'The information capacity of the human motor system in controlling the amplitude of movement', *J. exp. Psychol.*, vol. 47, pp. 381–91.

GIBBS, C. B. (1951), 'Transfer of training and skill assumptions in tracking', *Quart. J. exp. Psychol.*, vol, 3. pp. 99–110.

GIBBS, C. B. (1954), 'The continuous regulation of skilled response by kinaesthetic feedback', *Brit. J. Psychol.*, vol. 45, pp. 24–39.

GIBBS, C. B. (1965), 'Probability learning in step-input tracking', *Brit. J. Psychol.*, vol. 56, pp. 233–42.

GIBBS, C. B. (1965), Proprioceptive functions in control and learning, *Unpublished Ph.D. thesis, University of London*.

GOLDSCHEIDER, A. (1889), 'Untersuchungen über den Muskelsinn', *Arch. Ant. Psychol.*, pp. 369–502.

GRANIT, R., HOLMGREN, B., and MERTON, P. A. (1955), 'The two routes for excitation of muscle and their subservience to the cerebellum', *J. Physiol.*, vol. 130, pp. 213–24.

HIGGINS, D. C., and GLASER, G. H. (1964), 'Stretch reflexes during chronic cerebellar ablation. A study of reflex instability', *J. Neurophysiol.*, vol. 27, pp. 49–62.

LISSMAN, H. W. (1950), 'Proprioceptors', in *Physiological Mechanisms of Animal Behaviour* (*Soc. exp. Biol. Symp.*, no. 4), Cambridge University Press, pp. 34–59.

MATTHEWS, B. H. C. (1933), 'Nerve endings in mammalian muscle', *J. Physiol.*, vol. 77, pp. 1–53.

MATTHEWS, P. B. C. (1964), 'Muscle spindles and their control', *Physiol. Rev.*, vol. 64, pp. 219–88.

MERTON, P. A. (1953), 'Speculations on the servo-control of movement', in *The Spinal Cord*, Ciba Foundation Symposium, Churchill.

MOUNTCASTLE, V. B., POGGIO, G. F., and WERNER, O. (1963), 'The relation of the thalamic cell response to peripheral stimuli varied over an intensive continuum', *J. Neurophysiol.*, vol. 26, pp. 807–34.

MOUNTCASTLE, V. B., and ROSE, J. E. (1959), 'Touch and kinaesthesis', in J. Field (ed.), *Handbook of Physiology*, vol. 1, pp. 387–428, American Physiological Society.

WOODWORTH, R. S. (1899), 'The accuracy of voluntary movement', *Psychol. Monogr.*, vol. 3, no. 2.

17 J. C. R. Licklider

Conditional Servo-Models

Excerpt from J. C. R. Licklider, 'Quasi-linear operator models in the study of manual tracking', in R. D. Luce (ed.), *Developments in Mathematical Psychology*, Free Press, 1960, pp. 266–72.

In the foregoing sections, we have suppressed two considerations that we must now bring into the discussion. The first is the dual input to the operator in pursuit tracking. The second is the larger role of proprioceptive feedback – feedback not confined to the motor centers but extending to the perceptual centers as well. These are closely related, because the proprioceptive feedback gives the compensatory tracker to some extent the same information that the pursuit tracker derives from his display.

A concept useful in thinking about these problems is the 'conditional servo'. It is a feedback arrangement discussed by Ham and Lang (1955) and suggested as a model for tracking by Elkind (1955). It has the feature of functioning as an open-loop system as long as the output agrees with an 'intention', but of subjecting any discrepancy between output and intention to negative feedback.

A simple conditional servo is represented schematically in Figure 1. G is a network to be stabilized. P is its inverse: $PG = 1$. For the sake of simplicity, we assume that P is correctly designed and stable. If G is correctly designed and stable, also, and if $N = 0$, then $Y = X$, and there is no error E and therefore no feedback. However, if the parameters of G change, or if there is a disturbance N at the output, the deviation of Y from X is subjected to negative feedback through the amplifier k, and the discrepancy is reduced to the fraction $1/(1 \pm kG)$ of the value it would otherwise have had.

This concept is useful for us because in some (particularly pursuit) situations the human operator tends to run freely in more or less open-loop fashion as long as all is going well, but to operate as a servo-mechanism when his responses cease to be

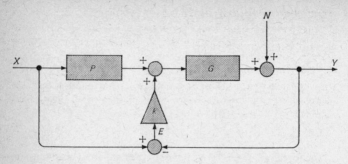

Figure 1 Schema of a conditional servo. If P is the inverse of G (i.e. if $PG = 1$), and if $N = 0$, $Y = X$ and there is no feedback. If G becomes different from P, or if there is a disturbance, $N \neq 0$ at the output, $X - Y = E$, and E is fed back with gain k. Since the feedback is negative, it stabilizes the output against variations in G and against disturbance N, without affecting the desired response

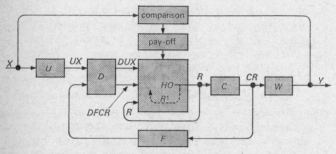

Figure 2 Schematic diagram showing various feedbacks that operate in a pursuit tracking situation. The output of the control is fed back through F and displayed to the operator as $DFCR$. The operator sees his hand move the control. This gives him R and therefore a chance to learn something about DFC. Internally, he has proprioceptive feedback from the movement. Putting this together with the visual information about R, he can in principle discover the input impedance of C. In simple cases, that may determine also the transfer function of C. The feedback path for 'knowledge of results' involves comparing Y with X and selecting pay-off or reinforcing stimuli on the basis of the comparison. The shaping of the human operator is governed by the pay-off and by information, derived from the other feedbacks, about the external situation. There is usually an 'instruction' channel into the operator

appropriate. The simple schema has to be adapted, of course, but it makes a useful component for models of the human operator.

A second useful concept might be called feedback control of parameters. It appears that the adjustments of the parameters of the human operator are made in part on a trial-and-error basis, and that the optimization and stabilization of behavior depend largely upon the preserving or discarding of trial adjustments under the influence of feedback. Ashby (1952) has developed this idea in detail.

Conditional Model for Pursuit Tracking

With the aid of those concepts, we may consider building a fairly literal model of the human operator in a visual–manual pursuit tracking situation.

First, we should distinguish among the several feedbacks represented in Figure 2. (a) A feedback signal $DFCR$ is presented to the operator via the display. (b) The manual response R usually is seen directly by the operator. (c) There is kinesthetic and somesthetic return R' from various parts of the hand, arm and body. There often is, or often should be, feedback concerning the effectiveness of the performance of the over-all system or the section of it within which the operator is working.

Next, referring to Figure 3[1] we should note that the target signal UX, the system feedback signal FCR, and the incidental visual signal R from arm, hand, etc., are delivered in parallel to the multichannel visual system. They are kept separate and at the same time interrelated in the process of visual perception.

For convenience, we may divide the over-all processing into (perhaps largely arbitrary) stages. First, we have the visual sensory process (*Vis*) culminating in a display of data to the perceptual mechanism. The perceptual mechanism predicts, from the display data, where the target is going. (It probably also predicts where the follower and the hand are going, but the schema will be complex enough without that.) In a separate operation, the perceptual mechanism measures the difference

1. To simplify the discussion, we shall assume that the display D may be represented by unity.

between the displayed target and displayed error. This difference is filtered and used as a conditional feedback and also as a 'knowledge-of-results' signal K to supplement the reinforcement P provided by the pay-off system.

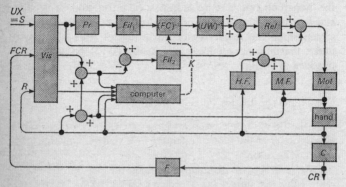

Figure 3 Semi-detailed schema showing some of the signal paths in pursuit tracking. The target signal UX and the two feedback signals are delivered to the visual system. The perceptual system operates in part on the target system signal and in part on its relation to the fed-back signals, trying to predict (Pr) ahead enough to neutralize the processing time delay. $(FC)^{-1}$ and $(UW)^{-1}$ are envisaged as networks developed in so far as possible to be inverse to FC and UW. The 'computer' shares in guiding the development of $(FC)^{-1}$, since there is some basis in the feedback channels for discovering the nature of the control-feedback dynamics. $(UW)^{-1}$ can be developed, however, only on the basis of pay-off (see Figure 2). The relay Rel passes the perceptual output on to the motor system, which is envisaged as a servo-loop, with feedback $M.F.$ from the contractions of the muscles and $H.F.$ from the resulting displacements of the hand. The two filters (Fil_1 and Fil_2) are developed in part to represent inversely the dynamics of the motor system and in part to suppress tendencies to oscillation that may result from the predictor's failure to neutralize the time delay. Fil_2 has high gain at low frequencies and acts as a conditional feedback path

Following the predictor is a cascade of filters. The first filter, Fil_1, adjusts itself to be the inverse of the relay and motor dynamics of the operator. Presumably he comes to the task with this network partly formed, since it is the component that translates the sensory signal into motor terms. The adjustment is refined by K and P. The second filter, $(FC)^{-1}$, adjusts itself in so far as possible to be the inverse of the cascaded control C and feedback network F. The required dyamics are computed from FCR and R, and the adjustment is refined by K and P. The third filter, $(UW)^{-1}$ adjusts itself in so far as possible to be the inverse of U and W, which are external to the loop. The only aid to that adjustment is P, and there appears to be little hope of accomplishment unless U and W are simple. However, if the system were set up with $U = 1$ and $W = -1$, for example, the operator should in due course learn to reverse his reaction.

The order of Fil_1, $(FC)^{-1}$ and $(UW)^{-1}$ as linear operators is of course immaterial. In the human operator, there doubtless is either a preferred sequence or a combining into one network.

In so far as the networks we have discussed are perfectly adjusted, there is no need for feedback and, since the feedback is conditional, there is none. The adjustments will not be perfect, however. For one thing, there is no perfect, physically realizable inverse to a time delay. The error signal K is therefore continually in action, feeding back into Rel, the relay to the motor system, in such a way as to bring the response into line with the target.

The motor system is represented in Figure 3 as a follow-up system, paced by control signals from the relay. The two feedback paths represent the relatively unimportant distinction between the kinesthetic and other purely internal receptors, on the one hand, and tactile receptors, etc., that gain information from the surface of the control, on the other.

The complexity of the arrangement just described almost precludes experimental analysis. In principle, however, analysis is possible, and work in the general area continues at such a pace that it may eventually be made for a few tracking situations. The basic problem, stated in terms of quasilinear models, is to find transfer functions for $(Pr)(Fil_1)(FC)^{-1}(UW)^{-1}$ and for Fil_2 that, taken together with high-frequency factors appropriate for Vis, Rel and the motor feedback loop, will check with experimental results. There is of course no need to analyse the cascades into separate blocks. It would be of considerable theoretical interest to trace the adjustment of parameters during learning. Tracking appears to offer an excellent setting for such study.

Conditional Model for Compensatory Tracking

A variation of the model just described lets us bring compensatory tracking into the same general paradigm. In compensatory tracking, only the error is displayed to the operator, but he has his hand on the control and therefore has direct visual and/or proprioceptive access to R. In Figure 4, the feedback signals from

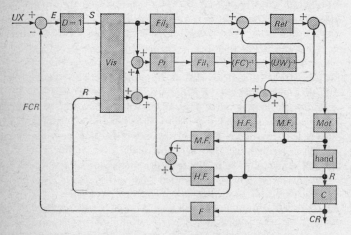

Figure 4 Semi-detailed schema for the compensatory tracking, corresponding to Figure 3 for pursuit tracking. Here the visual system does not see the target motion UX. The predictor and the several 'inverse' networks can function effectively, therefore, only to the extent that UK can be recaptured through joint analysis of R and S. If $D = 1$, $S = E$ and $UX = E + CR$. The main hope is for the 'computer' (not shown here in the interest of relative simplicity; see Figure 3) to solve the dynamics of C and to form CR from R. Then the chain Pr, Fil_1, ..., can operate on $UX = E + CR$ and the system can function, as in Figure 3, as a conditional servo. In practice, of course, the human operator does the necessary computing and circuit arranging imperfectly. Evidently the task of reconstructing UX from E and R is particularly difficult for him

R, and from within the motor system, are added to the sensed error signal, with the aim of re-creating X, the target motion. If the control, feedback and other external dynamics are unity, this is operationally a very simple matter. And experience in compensatory tracking suggests that one can and does to some extent figure out what the target is doing in more or less the way suggested. With that information, the operator can in principle proceed just as he does in pursuit tracking.

It is clear, however, that even the simple task of adding the error and feedback signals together is in practice very difficult, particularly if the feedback is mainly proprioceptive and the error visual. Even when the operator sees his response directly, he does not make very effective use of the possibility that lies open to him. The conditional servo is therefore usually in operation as a feedback system.

In most practical tracking situations, the control and other elements in the external dynamics involve integrations. This further complicates the problem by requiring the operator to match the integrations by adjusting his own feedback paths. This requires very much time and practice. Probably the development of the appropriate networks accounts for a large part of the experienced operator's skill.

There is one idealized situation, however, in which the operator might rather easily take full advantage of the possibility of reconstructing the target motion. Let all the external dynamics be unity, and let the control be located directly on the display. Then, if the control is truly compensatory – if an error to the right is corrected by a control motion to the left, and vice versa – the target position is given directly by the geometry. All the operator has to do is to examine as a function of time the distance between his control and the error dot. That is the target signal.

Even if the control is not immediately adjacent to the display, the operator may be able to use this geometrical aid to some extent. The thought suggests itself, therefore, that this notion may have a bearing on the question of display–control compatibility (e.g. Clutton-Baker, 1951; Grether, 1947; Mitchell and Vince, 1951). It is very much easier for an operator to learn to operate a compensatory control that has to be moved away from the error dot than one that has to follow the dot. The widely accepted theory that explains this sometimes quite dramatic difference is sometimes called the 'principle of the moving part'. As applied to simple situations with only one moving element, the principle states that the element in the display that moves with respect to the display's coordinate system should correspond to, and move in the same direction as, the element in the real situation that moves with respect to the earth's coordinate system. The principle leads, however, to a paradox: according to the theory, a pilot's view through his windscreen is a poor display, for, relative to the frame of the windscreen, the earth moves and the aircraft stands still. It seems possible that the distinction between pursuit and compensatory control may be basic to the whole problem, and that display–control compatibility in the case of compensatory control may be in large part a matter of approaching pursuit control as closely as possible.

References

ASHBY, W. R. (1952), *Design for a Brain*, Wiley.

CLUTTON-BAKER, J. (1951), *Some Alternative Control Lever Arrangements in a Compensatory Tracking Task*, Report RNP 51/655, Royal Naval Personnel Research Committee.

ELKIND, J. I. (1955), Personal communication.

GRETHER, W. F. (1947), *Direction of Control in Relation to Indicator Movement in One-directional Tracking*, Memo, Report no. TSEAA-694-4G. Engineering Division, Air Material Command. Wright Field, Dayton, Ohio.

HAM, J. F., and LANG, G. (1955), 'Conditional feedback systems: a new approach to feedback control', *Trans. Amer. Instit. elec. Engrs.*, vol. 74, part 2, pp. 152–61.

MITCHELL, M. J. H., and VINCE, M. A. (1951), 'The direction of movement of machine controls', *Quart. J. exp. Psychol.*, vol. 3, pp. 24–35.

Part Six The Acquisition of Skill

Two main problems are posed by the acquisition of a new skill. What are the conditions which promote acquisition and what changes take place in the underlying mechanisms when skill is acquired? The Hullian S–R approach to learning a skill emphasizes the association of responses to stimuli, some of which could be proprioceptive. Though not a necessary consequence of this view, many researchers have considered that such a theory would predict the development of relatively stereotyped chains of responses instead of the flexible, pragmatic behaviour which characterizes skilled performance (see Reading 16).

Miller, Galanter and Pribram (Reading 18) advance the theory that organisms more often learn guiding principles, programmes or Plans rather than specific responses. They draw heavily on the analogy of a computer programme which guides in a flexible manner. It may be that the chain of stimulus–response associations provides the best description of learning in simpler organisms but in man an emphasis on planning and strategy would appear more appropriate.

Learning a new skill depends upon feedback or knowledge of results which tell the learner how successful he is. Holding (Reading 19) presents a classification of different forms of knowledge of results. Experimental evidence is presented to show how manipulating feedback affects skill learning and performance. It is unusual for a new skill to be approached without some kind of initial guidance which usually constrains the ways in which the learner approaches his task. Guidance may range from a few verbal hints to exact physical guidance which ensures that the controls are never incorrectly manipulated. Holding (Reading 20) describes a number of different kinds of guidance and the relative efficiency of introducing them into a course of training.

Crossman (Reading 21) presents a mathematically expressed model of the selective development of skilled behaviour in which it is assumed that less successful approaches to the task are progressively eliminated. The model predicts that skill will continue to develop though improvements will become progressively less marked as the period of practice increases. This prediction is verified for a number of tasks including cigar-making performance over a period of seven years.

18 G. A. Miller, E. Galanter and K. H. Pribram

Motor Skills and Habits

Excerpts from chapter 6 of G. A. Miller, E. Galanter and K. H. Pribram, *Plans and the Structure of Behavior*, Holt, 1960, pp. 81–92.

Consider for a moment the family record player. It is a machine with a routine, or program, that it follows whenever it is properly triggered. The machine has a routine for changing records. Whenever the appropriate stimulus conditions are present – for example, when the arm is near enough to the spindle or when a particular button is pushed – the routine for changing the record is executed. There is even a 'sense organ' that discriminates between 10-in and 12-in records and there are effectors that push the next record into place and lower the tone arm gently into the groove of the record. The entire performance is obviously voluntary, for no matter how we curse the machine for failing to play the record we want, we will not alter its sequence of operations. The routine for changing records is built into the machine, locked in, and it never guides the actions of any other machine.

However, the record that is played by the machine is also a program. It is a program that controls the small movements of the stylus and, simultaneously, the larger and audible movements of the diaphragm of the loudspeaker. But the record is a *communicable* program. It can be played on any one of a large class of different machines. Machines that can use communicable programs, that can share them with other similar machines, are obviously more flexible than those that cannot. The fixed cycle of the record changer makes it far less flexible than the phonograph stylus, which can follow an indefinite number of different patterns of movement. Communicability is an extremely important property that a program – or a Plan – can have. Communicable programs are not limited to the mechanical world; the chromosome is an example of a communicable program in

237

biological form. At the behavioral level, of course, communicable Plans play the central role in our educational processes.

Habits and skills are Plans that were originally voluntary but that have become relatively inflexible, involuntary, automatic. Once the Plan that controls a sequence of skilled actions becomes fixed through overlearning, it will function in much the same way as an innate Plan in instinctive behavior. The description of the conditions under which various skilled components will be triggered, or released, is much the same in both cases. The new problem that we must consider when we move from instincts to habits and skills concerns how learned Plans become automatized.

When an adult human being sets out to acquire some new skill, he usually begins with a communicable program of instructions. Another person, either verbally or by exemplification, communicates more or less schematically what he is supposed to do. But just having the basic strategy in verbal form does not mean that the learner can correctly develop and elaborate the tactics on the first try to execute the Plan. For example, when a man learns to fly an airplane he begins by getting a communicable Plan from his instructor. The Plan – or a rough, symbolic outline of its strategy – is communicated through some such message as this:

To land this plane you must level off at an altitude of about ten feet. Then, after you have descended to about two feet, pull back on the elevators and touch down as you approach stalling speed. You must remember that at touch-down the control surfaces are less sensitive, and any gust may increase your airspeed. That may start the plane flying again, so be prepared to take corrective measures with the throttle and elevators. And if there is a cross-wind, lower the wing on the windward side, holding the plane parallel to the runway with the opposite rudder.

That is the strategy for landing airplanes. When skilfully elaborated and executed it will serve to get pilot and craft safely back to earth. It is a short paragraph and could be memorized in a few minutes, but it is doubtful whether the person who memorized it could land a plane, even under ideal weather conditions. In fact, it seems likely that someone could learn all the individual acts that are required in order to execute the Plan and still be unable to land successfully. The separate motions, the separate parts of the Plan, must be fused together to form a skilled performance. Given the description of what he is supposed to do, the student still faces the major task of learning how to do it.

There is a kind of complementarity between the teacher and the student. It is easy for the teacher to describe the general strategy, but difficult for him to communicate the detailed tactics that should be used. For the student, on the other hand, each of the muscular movements involved can be made in isolation, but it is difficult for him to combine those tactical details into a larger motor unit, into a feedback mechanism that will effortlessly guide his movements to reduce the differences between his intended and his actual performance. In order to be able to execute the Plan by a smooth, controlled motor unit, the aspiring aviator must find many small, intercalated acts not specified in the instructor's original description of the Plan. The general strategy provided by the teacher says nothing about the activities of individual muscle groups – the instructor 'knows' these intercalated acts because he knows how to fly, but they are locked in, implicit, tacit, rather than explicit and communicable. Thus, we get a picture of the instructor working from the strategic toward the tactical in his efforts to communicate the Plan, while the student is working from the tactical toward the strategic in his efforts to carry it out.

Even when an instructor does recognize a possible intercalated act, it may actually be better pedagogy to let the student invent his own idiosyncratic tactics for carrying the Plan into his muscles.

On take-off the throttle should be opened slowly so that rudder-control can be introduced smoothly to overcome the tendency of the plane to turn as a result of increased torque. Open the throttle continuously so that it is completed by the time you count to five; when you reach three start to apply some right rudder.

The instruction to count is an attempt to provide a more detailed integration of the successive parts of the Plan and it is bad teaching. The student is, or feels, terribly tense and terribly busy. Telling him to count to five is almost certain to interfere with his performance of other parts of the Plan. Counting might work for some people, but for the entire sample that we studied it was a dismal failure – he found a trick of his own that he liked far better. As he pushed the throttle forward to the panel he kept one finger of the hand on the throttle extended, and when the extended finger hit the panel he began to apply the right rudder. This simple device provided the feedback that enabled him to convert a sequence of discrete acts into a coordinated unit of behavior.

Since a learner must discover these little tricks that can connect the successive parts into a smoothly running skill, it might appear that he is merely *chaining* one activity to the next, not building a hierarchical Plan. But if the skill is simply a chain of reflexes, each one hooked to the next, then it is difficult to understand why, in the preceding example, the instructor's method of chaining was not satisfactory. Unless there is some over-all pattern to the skill, a pattern that the instructor sees one way and the student sees differently, why would one intercalation, *ceteris paribus*, be better or worse than another?

What would happen if all the details of a sequence were worked out by the coach and imposed with rigid insistence on the learner? If skills were nothing but chains of reflexes, a detailed account of the correct sequence should be an efficient way to teach them. Probably the most intensive effort to specify exactly what a person must do with each movement is the work of 'motion-study' experts. On an assembly line in a factory there may be a task that consists of, let us say, assembling three washers on a bolt. The analysis of this task into 'micromotions' will specify the exact time at which each hand should move and the operation it should perform. For the left hand, the instructions may read 'Carry assembly to bin', 'Release assembly', 'Reach for bolt', etc., while at the same time the right hand is instructed to 'Reach for lock washer'. 'Select and grasp washer', 'Carry washer to bolt', etc. For each of these motions a fixed duration is specified. This is about as near as anyone can come to writing programs for people that are as detailed as the programs we write for computing machines.

The description of the task can be transformed in various ways in an attempt to find a sequence of motions that achieves the result most efficiently, with fewest movements and in least time. The men who make this kind of analysis have developed certain general rules about how sequences of action can be formed to run off smoothly and rapidly. For example, the two hands should begin and complete their movements at exactly the same time. Motions of the arms should be opposite and symmetrical. There must be a fixed position for all tools and materials. And on and on. Following these rules, motion-study engineers are able to develop chains of responses that can be executed with nearly maximal efficiency. But, unfortunately, workers may not acquire the strategies possessed by the engineers – they frequently object to being so tightly regimented and seem to feel that the boss is trying to exploit them unfairly.

When people have time to develop the skill themselves, that is to say, when they form a Plan to guide the gross actions – even an inefficient Plan – they find for themselves the interposed elements that produce the skill. Finding these elements is essentially a test of the adequacy of the strategy. Once a strategy has been developed, alternative modes of action become possible, and we say that the person 'understands' the job that he is to do.

In most natural situations, the development of skills involves the construction of a hierarchy of behavioral units, each unit guided by its own Plan. This fact is seldom recognized in the motion-study analysis, which is rather puzzling because the hierarchical character of skills was pointed out explicitly by Bryan and Harter at least as early as 1897, when they demonstrated the successive levels of skill involved in telegraphy.[1] In 1908 Book wired a typewriter to record the time of occurrence of successive key-strokes and then collected data while people learned the 'touch method' of typing. People first memorized the positions of the different letters on the keyboard. Then they would go through several discrete steps: look at the next letter in the material that was to be copied, locate this letter in their image of the keyboard, feel around on the actual keyboard for the key corresponding to the remembered position, strike the key and look to see if it was correct. After a few hours of practice these components of the Plan began to fit together into skilled movements, and the learner had acquired dependable 'letter habits'. Further speed resulted when they began to anticipate the next letter and build up small subroutines to deal with familiar sequences like -*ing* and *the*. By then dependable 'word habits'

1. For a short but representative summary, see Woodworth and Schlosberg (1954), pp. 809–13.

were developing. Finally, the experienced typist read the text several words ahead of the letters he was typing at the moment, so that one could say he had developed 'phrase habits'. He learns, one might say, to put feedback loops around larger and larger segments of his behavior. This sequence of stages in the acquisition of typing skill is familiar to anyone who has gone through it, who has watched the units at one level of skill come smoothly together to form units at a higher level, until eventually a skilled typist can concentrate on the message and let the muscles take care of the execution of details.

Typewriting, however, is a rather special case. The final components, the key movements, are very discrete and atomic. Probably most of the skills we have to acquire are much more fluid in their execution, but these are correspondingly more difficult for a psychologist to collect data on.

We have assumed that the human being who is acquiring a new skill is aware of the strategy that he is attempting to follow. At least, he is aware of it in the sense that he can talk about it or point to examples of it. It is quite possible, of course, to build up skills without verbalizing the strategy, the way a baby learns.

Almost no one – including physicists, engineers, bicycle manufacturers – can communicate the strategy whereby a cyclist keeps his balance. The underlying principle would not really be much help even if they did know how to express it: 'Adjust the curvature of your bicycle's path in proportion to the ratio of your unbalance over the square of your speed.' It is almost impossible to understand, much less to do. 'Turn your handle bars in the direction you are falling,' we tell the beginner, and he accepts it blindly, not understanding then or later why it works. Many teachers impart no rule at all, but perform their service by running alongside the bicycle, holding it up until the beginner 'gets the idea'.[2] It is not necessary, fortunately, to know explicitly the rules that must be observed by a skilful performer – if it were, few of us would ever be able to sit up in our cradles. Sometimes we can help a learner do the right thing for the wrong reason,

2. The bicycle is borrowed from Polanyi (1958). Chapter 4 in that remarkable book emphasizes the importance of our inarticulate skills for all branches of knowledge and the extent to which we blindly accept a frame of reference that we cannot justify when we acquire a skill.

as when we tell a skier to make a left turn by imagining that he is putting his right hand in his left pocket or when we tell a golfer to keep his eye on the ball. But for the most part we must rely upon inarticulate guiding and demonstrating until the pupil 'catches on' or 'gets a feel for it'.

Animals acquire skills, of course, without memorizing verbal descriptions of what they are supposed to do. When we train an animal to execute a series of responses in order to attain a valued outcome, the strategy is not carried in the animal's memory. Only the experimenter needs to know the total Plan. The animal is required merely to build up the smooth transitions that chain one action to the next. That was probably the goal of the motion-study experts.

For example, if we wish to train an animal to press a lever in order to get a ball, then to push the ball into a funnel, and after that to return to the food magazine to be fed, we could build up the chain in many different ways. Any of the components could be taught at any time. Then when they are put together the consequences of one action become the occasion for the next action, and each new segment is released as it becomes appropriate. Probably we would choose to build up the chain of responses backwards, starting first with the approach to the food tray, then with the ball down the funnel, etc. Many psychologists are quite skilful at training animals to perform such long and elaborate stunts. But we would argue that the animals seldom acquire the total Plan; the strategy is in the trainer, or in his mechanical substitute, the experimental equipment. The animal has learned a number of different components that enable it to perform as though it had a larger Plan. The critical test occurs when some particular outcome in the long chain fails to occur on schedule. The animal will not continue with the next step. Tolman and his students have argued that rats are capable of mastering a total Plan as well as its component parts, but a rat's skills in this direction are difficult to demonstrate in a laboratory situation.[3] In any

3. The evidence indicates that rats, and probably most other inarticulate creatures, are much more proficient in mastering Plans when the Images that support them can be spatially organized. The well-known observation by Lashley (1929) that rats that had learned a maze could still negotiate it even though Lashley had, by surgical operations, made it impossible for them to

case, rats are so vastly inferior to human beings in their ability to remember elaborate Plans that it is difficult to see why psychologists have felt that valid generalizations about cognitive structure could be extended from rats to men. A central feature of the difference, of course, is that men have language to communicate their Plans from expert to novice and from one generation to the next.

The verbal Plans with which a beginner tackles a new job – the look-remember-hunt-hit-check Plan for typing, or the move-right-rudder-when-extended-finger-touches-panel Plan for taking off – get turned over to the muscles that carry them out when the skill is acquired.[4] The verbal form of the Plan is a learner's crutch which is later discarded when he learns to walk alone. The entire pattern of movements, guided continually by perceptual feedback, can then be represented in other Plans as if it were a unitary, independent act. The same procedure of welding these new units together to form still larger skilled units may repeat at the higher level, until eventually the typist is planning whole paragraphs or the aviator is planning whole trips, secure that when the time comes to execute the Plan the subdivisions will be prepared to carry out orders in a rapid, efficient manner.

The verbalized strategies of a beginner may achieve the same result as the involuntary, habitual strategies of an expert, so there is a sense in which we recognize that they are the 'same' Plan. But the beginner's plan is carried out in a way that is voluntary, flexible and communicable, whereas the expert's version of the Plan is involuntary, inflexible and, usually, locked in. One can say that the development of skill frees the verbal planner to work with larger units of the Plan.

The implication of this attitude toward skills and habits is that man is assumed to be capable of building up his own 'instincts'. Lower animals come with strategies wired in; man wires them in

---

use the customary sequence of movements, must mean that new motor tactics could be substituted into the same general strategy; certainly the maze skill was not a learned chain of movements. When the organization cannot be represented spatially, however, as in Hunter's (1920) temporal maze, the rat has great difficulty. Cf. Campbell (1954).

4. For a discussion of the integration and symbolization of overlearned responses, see Mandler (1954).

deliberately to serve his own purposes. And when the Plan is highly overlearned, it becomes almost as involuntary, as resistant to change depending upon its outcome, as if it were innate. Take a skilled typist, who for years has triggered off a muscular pattern for striking t, then h, and finally e whenever he wants to write 'the'. Offer him money to type a page with the word 'the' always transcribed as 'hte', then watch him work. Probably he will not be able to do it. If he does, he will do it by slowing down, by trying to reinstate letter habits instead of word and phrase habits, thus abandoning his usual Plan for typing. If you put pressure on him to work fast in order to earn the money, he will certainly not be able to inhibit his usual Plan of action. Your money is quite safe. But one word of caution: do not let the offer stand too long, for habits are not completely resistant to change. If you take the time, you can replace them with new habits. Let him practice enough and he will build up the action unit needed to win your money.

A good typist has constructed a set of inflexible strategies with most of the properties of instincts, a fact that non-psychologists often recognize when they speak of habitual actions as 'instinctive'. The human being is frequently the victim of releasers for his skilled acts, just as the lower animal is for his instinctive acts. A trained athlete, for example, waits for the starting gun before he begins to execute his Plan for running the race. But he does not have his starting completely under volitional control, for otherwise he would never make a false start or 'jump the gun'. The human being's advantage lies in the fact that his releasers are more complicated and that, moreover, he can usually determine the conditions under which a releasing stimulus will be presented, whereas in the case of the animal's instinctive act the trigger is usually simple and is provided by an environment that is not under the animal's control.

The construction of integrated strategies for skilled acts through long practice and repetition has a further consequence for the kind of planning that the adult human can do. The construction of these subplans enables a person to deal 'digitally' with an 'analogue' process.[5] The input to an aviator, for ex-

5. In the language of computing machines, an analogue device is one in which the magnitudes involved in the computations are represented by

ample, is usually of a continuously varying sort, and the response he is supposed to make is often proportional to the magnitude of the input. It would seem that the good flier must function as an analogue device, a servo-mechanism. The beginner cannot do so, of course, because his Plans are formulated verbally, symbolically, digitally and he has not yet learned how to translate these into the continuous, proportionate movements he is required to make. Once the subplan is mastered and turned over to his muscles, however, it can operate as if it were a subprogram in an analogue computer. But note that this program, which looks so continuous and appropriately analogue at the lower levels in the hierarchy, is itself a relatively stable unit that can be represented by a single symbol at the higher levels in the hierarchy. That is to say, planning at the higher levels looks like the sort of information processing we see in digital computers, whereas the execution of the Plan at the lowest levels looks like the sort of process we see in analogue computers. The development of a skill has an effect similar to providing a digital-to-analogue converter on the output of a digital computing machine. (It may also be true that the perceptual mechanism provides an analogue-to-digital input for the higher mental processes, but we shall not explore that possibility here.) When an action unit has become highly skilled it can be executed directly without being first expressed in a digital, or verbal, form, and even without focal awareness.[6]

---

physical quantities proportional to those magnitudes, e.g. by a voltage, a duration, an angle of rotation, etc. Thus, continuous variation in the input to the machine will result in a correspondingly continuous variation in the magnitude of the processes that represent it inside the machine and in the output of the machine. A digital computer, on the other hand, represents the magnitudes with which it works by symbols corresponding to discretely different states of the machine, e.g. by a relay that is closed or open, or a dial that can assume any one of ten positions, etc. Thus there is no simple resemblance between the input to a digital computer and the processes that represent that input inside the machine. If you multiply by writing the numbers on paper, you are using a digital procedure. If you multiply by using a slide rule, you are using an analogue procedure. See Neumann (1958).

6. Pavlov's well-known distinction between a first signal system, concerned with directly perceived stimuli, and a second signal system, devoted to verbal elaborations, seems, in so far as we understand it, to parallel the present distinction between analogue and digital systems. See Simon (1957).

A reader who resents such crudely mechanistic analogies and hypotheses has the authors' sympathy, but it is difficult to know how to express more accurately the difference between the strategic and tactical levels of skilled and habitual Plans. The argument could, of course, be phrased in neurological terms that might sound a bit less offensive. The cerebellum, for example, which has been considered the regulator and integrator of voluntary movements, may play the role of the digital-to-analogue converter. In a discussion of the cerebellum as a feed-back mechanism, T. C. Ruch (1951, p. 204) commented that 'slowness of voluntary movement is characteristic of cerebellar patients and of normal individuals executing unpracticed movements'. The problem for most theories of the neural basis of skilled movements is that the skilled movements run off so very rapidly that there is little time for proprioceptive feedback from one movement before another must occur. Any simple conception in terms of feedback, or error-correcting, circuits must cope with the relatively slow transmission rates that are possible over neural paths. Ruch suggests that 'a time-tension pattern of muscle contraction' is instituted, projecting into the future, and then he notes that for such 'planning movements' the nervous system would have to have some way, presently unknown, of storing impulses for fixed delays.

The cerebral–cerebellar circuit may represent not so much an error-correcting device as a part of a mechanism by which an instantaneous order can be extended forward in time. Such a circuit, though uniformed as to the consequences, could, so to speak, 'rough-in' a movement and thus reduce the troublesome transients involved in the correction of movement by output-informed feedbacks (Ruch, 1951, p. 205).

These suggestions correspond remarkably well to the kind of hierarchical Plans we have been considering here, particularly if we can consider Ruch's 'instantaneous order' as an instruction generated by a digital device and issued to an analogue device for the execution of planned movements. A Plan, either stored in or transferred to the cerebellum, would provide the roughed-in movement in advance of its actual execution.

With proper scientific caution, Ruch comments that such

analogies between neural systems and servo-systems are 'essentially allegorical'. Yet it is difficult to see how we can get along without them. The first thing we must know about any machine we might want to study is that it really *is* a machine, and the second is a shrewd guess as to what it is supposed to do. Given that much guidance, it is then possible to analyse in proper scientific spirit how the parts work to accomplish their purpose. But without a guess to guide him, the scientist may waste his beautifully precise descriptions on irrelevant aspects of the problem. It is in that spirit that one ventures a guess that the cerebellum is a machine to provide analogue Plans for regulating and integrating muscular coordinations, that is to say, that the cerebellum is a critical component in a digital-to-analogue converter on the output of the neural system for processing information.

References

CAMPBELL, D. T. (1954), 'Operational delineation of "what is learned" via the transposition experiment', *Psychol. Rev.*, vol. 61, pp. 167–74.

HUNTER, W. S. (1920), 'The temporal maze and kinaesthetic sensory processes in the white rat', *Psychobiol.*, vol. 2, pp. 1–17.

LASHLEY, K. (1929), *Brain Mechanisms and Intelligence*, University of Chicago Press.

MANDLER, G. (1954), 'Response factors in human learning', *Psychol. Rev.*, vol. 61, pp. 235–44.

NEUMANN, J. VON (1958), *The Computer and the Brain*, Yale University Press.

POLANYI, M. (1958), *Personal Knowledge*, University of Chicago Press.

RUCH, T. C. (1951), 'Motor systems', in S. S. Stevens (ed.), *Handbook of Experimental Psychology*, Wiley, ch. 5.

SIMON, B. (ed.) (1957), *Psychology in the Soviet Union*, Stanford University Press.

WOODWORTH, R. S., and SCHLOSBERG, H. (1954), *Experimental Psychology*, rev. edn, Holt.

19 D. H. Holding

Knowledge of Results

Excerpt from chapter 2 of D. H. Holding, *Principles of Training*, Pergamon, 1965, pp. 21–35.

A Classification

We must next inquire what kinds of knowledge of results there are and how well they serve the purposes of incentive or information, and of action or learning feedback. There are a number of distinctions to be made. To make it easier to appreciate the classification which is proposed these distinctions have been set out in the form of a 'family tree' in Figure 1.

Knowledge of results may be *intrinsic* or *artificial*. In other words it may be present in the usual form of the task or else it may take the form of extra information added in for training purposes, like a buzzer which sounds all the time a rifle is on target. This second kind is often called 'augmented' knowledge of results.

Artificial knowledge of results may be *concurrent* or *terminal*. This rather ugly piece of jargon is intended to convey the distinction between information which is present all the time a person is responding, as in watching a pointer while adjusting a control knob, and information which arises as a result of a completed response like the score of a dart throw. It will have occurred to many readers that intrinsic knowledge of results may also be concurrent or terminal. This is true. Similarly, most other distinctions shown in Figure 1 may also be subdivided. The diagram only shows one set of branches for the sake of clarity.

Terminal, and concurrent, knowledge of results may be either *immediate* or *delayed*. These types in their turn may be *verbal* or *non-verbal*; that is to say they may take the form of words or scores, or else appear as physical indications like pointers or buzzers. Knowledge of results in a verbal form may be called knowledge of score. This or its physical counterpart may be given after each response as *separate* knowledge or else *accumulated* over several attempts and presented at the end of the series.

This classification is merely a convenience. Nevertheless, most practical examples can be adequately described in terms of these distinctions and, somewhat surprisingly, examples can be found to fit into most of the 'spaces' it provides. For instance, accumulated, verbal, immediate, concurrent, artificial knowledge of

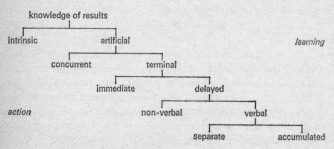

Figure 1 Different kinds of knowledge of results

results is given by a trainer shouting integrated error scores to a person trying to follow a moving target, although we shall avoid these concatenations of adjectives wherever possible. More importantly, it makes possible some generalizations concerning the functions of different kinds of knowledge of results. As shown in the diagram, the nearer an artificial item is to the left-hand side of the tree the more likely it is to function as action feedback; and of course the nearer it is to the right the more likely it is to be learning feedback. Furthermore there is probably a tendency for greater incentive value to follow the lines of learning feedback, although this is less clear.

Intrinsic or Artificial

The difficulty about putting in artificial knowledge of results is that its effects may not last after its removal. Eventually the learner must come to rely upon the intrinsic cues. There is no point in learning to rely upon information which will not be there when training is finished. The success of techniques of augmenting feedback will depend upon whether they call attention to the intrinsic cues or make possible control of the relevant responses in a way which can later be taken over by the intrinsic cues. Of course intrinsic cues may contribute to the original learning, but by definition the trainer has no control over them. It is important here that he draws attention to them in various ways.

One problem which arises is that tasks exist in which the intrinsic feedback does not relate directly to the object of the activity. It may be clear *whether* we have achieved what we intended to do, but not whether *what* we intended to do was correct. If we are asked to give the Dutch equivalent for 'stork', intrinsic auditory feedback will help us to approximate to the sound 'ooievaar', but will not indicate whether we have used the right word. In such cases learning will not take place without knowledge of results, which must be injected artificially. More exactly, what the trainer must do is to provide *standards* against which we can assess our performance. It has already been pointed out that the learner must know what he is to do. Where this information is not available, it is essential to provide it. In this kind of situation the trainer is, in a sense, giving artificial knowledge of results indirectly by providing the standards which transform feedback into real knowledge of results.

Artificial feedback might be useful in training operators to appreciate cues of which they are not usually aware, as in the case of kinaesthetic sensitivity. Seymour (1954) discusses the handling of electrical pottery. Before firing, porcelain insulators must be held firmly as they are moved but not so firmly as to crush them. Seymour describes the use of dummy insulators with spring-loaded sides bearing on micro-switches; the right amount of finger pressure flashes on a white light, while pressing too hard switches on a red light. Operators then build up familiarity with the necessary pressures by transferring the dummy insulators rapidly from tray to tray, all the time attempting to keep the white light in view and to avoid even momentary flashes of the red light.

However, withdrawing artificial feedback may give disappointing results. Goldstein and Rittenhouse (1954) provide an example in training for air-to-air gunnery. Practice was carried out on a simulator, target aircraft being projected on to a curved screen in front of the gunsight assembly. With the 'pedestal' sight which they used, pointing the gun in the right direction for azimuth and elevation presents less difficulty to trainees than the problem of ranging. Setting to the correct range, by the method of 'framing', consists of squeezing a spring mechanism until a circle of dots just encloses the wing tips of the target aeroplane. The artificial feedback was a buzzer which sounded whenever the gun was on target. In similar work a filter which reddens the appearance of the aircraft has also been used for this purpose.

As Figure 2 shows, the control group who worked without the buzzer made no real improvement after the first seven trials. A

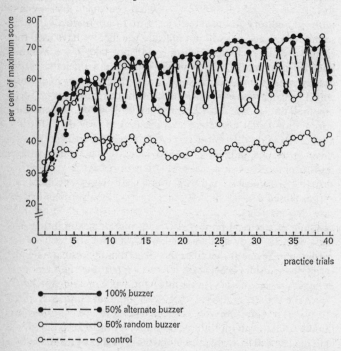

Figure 2 Artificial knowledge of results. Performance in the two middle curves fluctuates as the buzzer is used or withheld. From Goldstein and Rittenhouse (1954)

group getting buzzer information on 100 per cent of the trials appeared to improve, but showed a drop on the fortieth trial when the buzzer was withheld. In a later experiment this drop continued until the sixtieth trial, at which stage no significant difference remained. In yet another experiment, when the trainees were transferred to a different kind of gunnery apparatus the buzzer group tended actually to perform worse than the control group.

The results of two other groups are also shown in Figure 2. Both of these received buzzer information on 50 per cent of the trials, randomly chosen in one case and on alternate trials in the other. In each case the scores moved up and down depending upon whether or not the buzzer was used – this is what gives the 'zigzag' appearance to the middle scores. The experimenters conclude that the effects of adding the buzzer were not permanent and they do not recommend the use of this kind of artificial feedback. It is worth noting that the buzzer feedback is essentially of the concurrent type and will tend to behave as action feedback; the trainees tend to use it continuously to guide their responses rather than to evaluate their results.

Concurrent or Terminal

At first sight the distinction between concurrent and terminal feedback may appear completely to determine whether action or learning is helped by a particular kind of information. The example of the kitchen scales which was used to illustrate the difference between the two functions contrasted the *concurrent* technique of watching the pointer moving with the *terminal* technique of making a reading when the push is complete.

However, there are many ways in which the operator can make later use of information which he gains during action feedback, so that it is unlikely that his performance will not improve at all. Also, the use he can make of terminal cues may be limited since, as we have seen, a number of psychological stages intervene between one response and the next. The mere presence of terminal knowledge of results will not by itself guarantee a fast rate of learning. It remains true on the whole that, where the task is relatively simple, we may expect the results of terminal feedback to be the more permanent.

The comparison is clearly made in an experiment by Annett (1959). His subjects practised pressing the handle of a plunger, receiving artificial knowledge of results for the first thirty attempts. The plunger was wired up to an oscilloscope so that concurrent visual feedback, in the form of a moving light, resulted from pressing the plunger. Roughly the same effect could also be produced by a neon light which came on as the subject attained the target pressure. Alternatively the experimenter could make the knowledge of results take a terminal form by covering the oscilloscope face until the subject had attempted to get the right amount of pressure. The experimenter could then expose the oscilloscope, upon which there was a printed scale, or else announce the error verbally.

What happened was that the subjects with concurrent feedback were able to reproduce the correct pressure with each response, while the terminal procedure gave fairly large errors at the outset which gradually reduced towards the end of the learning period. Next, the subjects were tested with no feedback. The subjects with terminal feedback did get worse, but only gradually. On the other hand, removing the concurrent feedback led to immediate and drastic loss of accuracy. After twenty 'blind' trials responses became so wild that the apparatus was damaged several times. The average error scores for the first twenty test trials are represented in Figure 3, which shows that the best condition of all was the verbal form of feedback.

One might imagine that giving concurrent feedback only intermittently would help to maintain performance. For instance, if a subject is given knowledge of results every other trial he can use the feedback during any trial as a kind of terminal knowledge of results at one remove from the previous 'blind' trial. In another pressure-learning test Annett did compare intermittent with continuous knowledge of results. Despite the fact that knowledge of results on alternate trials only gives half the informed practice that continuous feedback offers, it did appear that there was an advantage in the intermittent procedure. However, the difference was not large and other studies of the same problem like the gunnery work of Goldstein and Rittenhouse (1954) have given negative results.

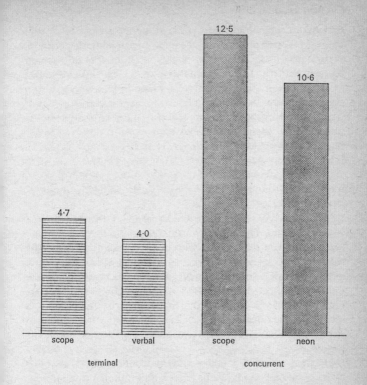

Figure 3 Errors after learning with terminal or concurrent knowledge of results. The effects of terminal knowledge of results are more permanent, giving smaller errors on the 'blind' trials. After Annett (1959)

Immediate or Delayed

The effects of delay differ markedly between concurrent and terminal feedback. When the feedback is concurrent any delay or lag makes performance more difficult. With terminal knowledge of results the evidence suggests that mere delay is ineffective, or even conducive to learning, although it is true that the delay may offer an opportunity for interference from other sources.

Lag in concurrent feedback from continuous motor skills disrupts performance (Conklin, 1957). The longer a delay between moving a control and the corresponding movement of an indicator the worse performance becomes. In fact some deterioration occurs even if the delay is so slight that operators do not consciously notice it. The effects of this kind of lag are most dramatic in delayed feedback of speech (Lee, 1950). In these experiments a person speaks into the microphone of a tape recorder assembly, which stores his speech and replays it into his earphones about a quarter of a second later. The sound of his ordinary speech is masked off by the earphones and his effective feedback is the much louder delayed speech. In these circumstances the average person stutters, slurs his words or omits whole syllables, as if in a state of intoxication. Similar effects occur with delayed handwriting (van Bergeijk and David, 1959).

When the knowledge of results is terminal a rather different situation arises. The subject has merely to complete a response and attend to the relevant feedback in due course. It was originally thought that delay of knowledge of results was similar in its effects to the delay of reward with animal subjects, whose learning is adversely affected. An experiment by Greenspoon and Foreman (1957) did appear to show that increasing the delay up to 30 seconds caused decreasing learning, but many other studies of delayed terminal feedback have given negative or conflicting results.

One reason for the confusion is that several quite different time intervals are involved. We have seen that although the information arises as a result of a previous response it supplies learning feedback for the *next* response. It seems likely therefore that the delay before the next response will be at least as important as the delay before knowledge of results is given. The position is shown in Figure 4. If the response (R1) which produces the knowledge of results (KR) is followed by the next response (R2) at a constant time interval, both kinds of delay are affected by a shift in the timing of knowledge of results. Changing from case (a), with short delay of KR to the longer delay in case (b) has had the effect of reducing the delay before the second response, so that what is lost on the swings is gained on the roundabouts.

When we consider case (c), where the interval between responses is longer, the implications are different. Both delays are long and we may expect some decrement in learning. Bilodeau and Bilodeau

(1958) have shown that this is true, and it is also true that, if anything, the delay *after* knowledge of results is more important than the delay beforehand. In order to find any substantial effects of delay they were led to investigate delays of as long as 24 hours or 1 week. Clearly, if the subject can make a response on one day and receive knowledge of the results of that response the following week, we may conclude that the mere passage of time is of little importance. Presumably what matters is whether or not the knowledge of results is unambiguously seen to belong to the appropriate response. In some cases we may even expect delay to be beneficial, forcing the learner to attend to the intrinsic cues.

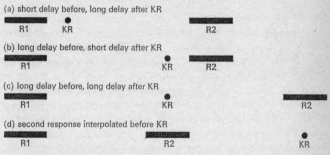

Figure 4 The timing of knowledge of results. R1 is a first response; K R is the knowledge of results resulting from R1; R2 is a second response

On the other hand, if the feedback from the first response is withheld until *after the next response* as in case (d) of Figure 4, the interpolated response may interfere so that learning will suffer. Lorge and Thorndike (1935) first showed this effect, using subjects whose task was to throw balls over one shoulder at a target. In a simple lever-pressing task Bilodeau (1956) showed that the amount of learning depended upon the number of intervening responses – the more intervention, the less appeared to be learned.

Even so, we must be cautious in drawing conclusions. Again and again in considering the effects of knowledge of results it is easy to observe the effects on immediate performance or apparent learning, while forgetting that retaining the skill will depend upon the intrinsic cues when extra feedback is removed. Lavery and Suddon (1962) have recently shown the importance of tests of retention with reference to our present problems, the effects of delay with interpolated responses. Comparing delays of nought and five responses, they showed that thirty training trials seemed to produce slower learning in the delayed group. However, after ninety trials the performance level was the same for both of the groups. What is more, removing knowledge of results left the delayed group *more skilled* than those trained with no delay. It may often be worth sacrificing speed of learning to ensure permanence.

Verbal or Non-verbal

Verbal knowledge of results tends to have lasting effects. However, it is difficult to find comparisons of verbal and non-verbal forms of information in which the other conditions have been equivalent, and it is possible that its advantages appear because it is usually terminal and often delayed.

For example, Karlin and Mortimer (1963) fed three kinds of artificial knowledge of results back to subjects carrying out a kind of tracking. In this task a target blip on an oscilloscope face moved backwards and forwards unless the operator corrected its position by turning a control knob, his aim being to keep the target stationary on an illuminated centre line. Verbal cues, or scores, were more effective both in training and on a subsequent test than were visual or auditory cues. A control group which received no supplementary cues performed worst.

Unfortunately, the verbal feedback consisted of time-on-target scores given after every trial and was thus terminal, while the auditory cue was the now familiar buzzer which sounded whenever the subject was approximately on target and was thus effectively concurrent. The visual cue was not feedback at all, but consisted of two extra lines delineating the target area which were presented the whole time. We can therefore draw no firm conclusions from this experiment on the effects of verbal treatment. Annett's (1959) study discussed earlier shows a much clearer difference between terminal verbal and non-verbal knowledge of results, but the effect is rather small. It might be suspected in this case that the information presented on the oscilloscope was somewhat less easy to assimilate.

Some of the work by Goldstein and Rittenhouse (1954) in the experiments on gunnery training discussed earlier introduces yet another factor. The verbal knowledge of the results which they compared with the buzzer treatment gave far more stable results. During training the level of scores for the groups with verbal feedback were lower, but did not fluctuate in the same way as those of the buzzer groups. After training, when all artificial feedback was removed the scores of the verbal group remained almost constant. However, it is important to notice that the verbal feedback, in addition to being terminal, carried far more information than did the buzzer. After each trial subjects were told what proportion of time they had remained on target, performance at different parts of each aircraft attack were compared and the current score was compared with the previous record. This is widely different from the buzzer treatment, and far more elaborate.

Clearly one of the advantages of the verbal method is the fact that it provides a convenient and flexible means for the trainer to convey a wide range of information to the subject. After any trial he may communicate a detailed analysis of responses and their effects, hints on form and stance, on what to look for in the task stimuli and information about standards of performance. In fact he may give a variety of types of information which shade into and out of knowledge of results. Also, basically factual feedback may be phrased in normative or emotive terms – 'you're slipping; why not wait for the signal or have you got a train to catch?' – with resulting effects on motivation.

Of course, non-verbal methods may also be far more elaborate than appears in the buzzer example. Often the trainer will need detailed records of performance, which may be made available to the learner. Graphical methods for instance are often more efficient than verbal coaching when tricky movement sequences are to be taught. English (1942) showed that recruits may be taught to squeeze the trigger of a rifle by comparing recordings of each squeeze with those made by an expert. Quite clear and explicit verbal instructions were far less effective. Howell (1956) found similar results, using the force–time graphs of a runner's front foot movement to teach efficient sprint starts. It is obvious then that the kind of knowledge of performance which is given must

259

depend upon analysis of the skill concerned, with insight into its points of difficulty.

The information given, whether verbal or non-verbal, may take many forms. The error or mismatch between the result of an action and its target may be transformed in many ways. It may be magnified or distorted, or a constant may be added (Bilodeau and Bilodeau, 1961) and behaviour will usually be regulated accordingly, although the effects may be transient. Denny and others (1960) successfully used a verbal scale consisting of imaginary units called 'glubs'; such a scale has an internal consistency which averts the disruptive consequences of the nonsense syllables mentioned earlier. The fact that such information may be imprecise seems not to matter greatly.

Precision, like delay, is a factor which experiments show to be less important than one might expect. For example, varying the size of the target seen by the subject while scoring him to closer limits makes very little difference (Green, 1955). What matters most is the relation between the precision of any artificial feedback and the intrinsic or internal feedback. Over-precise artificial feedback may act as a 'crutch' during training, again with the danger that performance sags after its withdrawal, as in an experiment on the accuracy of line-drawing by Holding and Macrae (1964).

Of course, there are cases in which the basic task contains very few or not any intrinsic cues. Trying to make judgements of the amount of time which has passed is an example (Waters, 1933). In this kind of work, where the subject has little else to go on, the efficiency of learning seems to vary directly with the accuracy of the knowledge of results.

Separate or Accumulated

On the evidence so far available it is not easy to decide what is the best length of performance upon which to report, but several kinds of information may all be available. The accumulation factor may vary from piecemeal movement-by-movement correction to the vastly condensed knowledge of results afforded by a degree examination after several years of study.

The effects of more accumulated knowledge of results may be lasting and appear to have incentive value, but if accumulated over too long a period the effect on performance is so slight that its permanence has no attraction. A tracking study by Smode (1958) suggests that training with separated feedback is superior to accumulated verbal feedback, but the separated form contains both visual and auditory elements so the conclusion is not clear cut. Separate or item-by-item correction is very effective in teaching machines [see ch. 8 of *Plans and the Structure of Behavior*] or in the learning of Morse code (Keller, 1943).

There is no doubt too that accumulated knowledge of results can be extremely valuable. An elaborate experiment on accumulated verbal feedback was carried out by Alexander, Kepner and Tregoe (1962). This study attempted to modify the learning of groups rather than individuals, by giving information to air defence radar crews at 'debriefing' exercises held after training exercises. The job of each crew of thirteen men was to detect and follow the movement of any aircraft in their operational area, to report hostile aircraft to adjacent radar sites and to control tactical action by interceptor pilots where necessary.

During training a number of exercises were held, providing data on the efficiency with which each crew detected and kept contact with the aircraft they were to track. This information was discussed at extensive debriefing meetings with some of the crews at the end of each exercise, the crews being encouraged to identify problems arising in the exercise and to work out revisions of their operational methods. After training, crews were tested on a 'unique problem' offering relatively stressful situations which had not previously been encountered. The proportion of aircraft tracks during certain critical flights which were established and maintained by the crews who had debriefing throughout training are compared in Figure 5 with the performance of two uniformed control crews. Debriefing gave results twice as good as the control figures.

Fortunately there is usually no reason why separate and accumulated results should not both be given. The combination of separate, response-by-response information with periodic progress reports or knowledge of score is unexceptionable. Knowledge of progress is usually a kind of 'second-order' knowledge of results. That is to say it consists of relating the accumulated knowledge of results of many individual actions to some kind of composite goal and is thus knowledge of results, of results. Care is needed in setting up the goals against which progress is matched since these will determine the success or failure experienced by the learner.

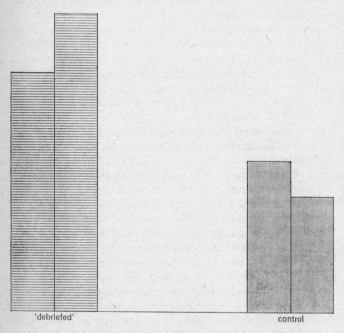

Figure 5 Accumulated verbal knowledge of results. The percentages of 'tracks' established and maintained by radar crews with and without 'debriefing'. After Alexander, Kepner and Tregoe (1962)

Failure affects a measure called the 'level of aspiration', which has little to do with aspirations but indicates how well the learner thinks he will do on his next attempt. At present, studies of this kind of estimate seem to provide little of interest with reference to permanent learning, although it is easy to show disturbances of performance as a result of failure. An example is provided by Willingham (1958), who examined the records of 2500 flying trainees. After failures on a check flight, these students, particularly the better ones, obtained lower training marks for 1 or 2 days. However, little effect remained only 4 days later.

The effects of failure are complex, and the relation of failure to learning is indirect. Nevertheless it does seem desirable on commonsense grounds to make knowledge of progress as favourable as possible, an effect which can be arranged by manipulating the target set for the learner. One way of keeping failure to the minimum is to set him to better his own previous performance, rather than to reach an arbitrary standard. Like other training procedures, such techniques should be evaluated in actual practice.

Summary

We have seen that active behaviour is constantly regulated by the feedback of information conveying knowledge of the results of his actions to the learner. Some kinds of feedback are *intrinsic* to the task to be performed, while the task may also be augmented by *artificial* feedback. Sometimes the task itself is artificial, in which case no progress will be made unless the trainer provides *standards* against which performance may be seen to be right or wrong. It will always pay the trainer to draw attention to the intrinsic cues and to the use which can be made of them, but the value of artificial kinds of knowledge of results needs more examination.

Terminal. It is important to distinguish between changes in immediate *action* and performance and changes which give rise to more permanent *learning*, since quite dramatic manipulations of action feedback may have only temporary effects. The terminal knowledge of results coming after an action is more likely to assist in learning than is concurrent feedback, whose function is rather to regulate the actions during which it occurs. Giving concurrent feedback only intermittently is of possible assistance.

Delayed. Lags in action feedback are disruptive, but learning is relatively unaffected by the delay of terminal knowledge of results. The time interval between feedback information and the next response is of some importance, but the major factor is the total interval between responses. Interpolating other responses between knowledge of results and the action from which it stemmed seems inadvisable, although at least in simple tasks the effects may again be temporary.

Verbal. Knowledge of *score* is likely to help the learner, although the design of experiments using verbal feedback has often been unsuited to direct comparisons with non-verbal equivalents. Verbal knowledge of results can convey a variety of types of information and persuasion. Points of technique which are obscure to the learner may be made clear by non-verbal methods.

Accumulated. Separate knowledge of results gives the learner the information he needs for step-by-step correction of his actions. Knowledge of *progress* is gained by relating accumulated knowledge of results to long-term goals. Particularly when linked to analysis and discussion, accumulated knowledge of results is likely to improve training. Changing the long-term goals of the learner will affect his experience of success and failure.

References

ALEXANDER, L. T., KEPNER, C. H., and TREGOE, B. B. (1962), 'The effectiveness of knowledge of results in a military system-training program', *J. appl. Psychol.*, vol. 46, pp. 202–11.

ANNETT, J. (1959), 'Learning a pressure under conditions of immediate and delayed knowledge of results', *Quart. J. exp. Psychol.*, vol. 11, pp. 3–15.

BILODEAU, E. A., and BILODEAU, I. McD. (1958), 'Variation of temporal intervals among critical events in five studies of knowledge of results', *J. exp. Psychol.*, vol. 55, pp. 603–12.

BILODEAU, E. A., and BILODEAU, I. McD. (1961), 'Motor-skills learning', *Ann. Rev. Psychol.*, vol. 12, pp. 243–80.

BILODEAU, I. McD. (1956), 'Accuracy of a simple positioning response with variation in the number of trails by which knowledge of results is delayed', *Amer. J. Psychol.*, vol. 69, pp. 434–7.

CONKLIN, J. E. (1957), 'Effect of control lags on performance in a tracking task' *J. exp. Psychol.*, vol. 53, pp. 261–8.

DENNY, M. R., ALLARD, M., HALL, E., and ROKEACH, M. (1960), 'Delay of knowledge of results, knowledge of task, and the intertrial interval', *J. exp. Psychol.*, vol. 60, p. 327.

ENGLISH, H. B. (1942), 'How psychology can facilitate military training – a concrete example', *J. appl. Psychol.*, vol. 26, pp. 3–7.

GOLDSTEIN, M., and RITTENHOUSE, C. H. (1954), 'Knowledge of results in the acquisition and transfer of a gunnery skill', *J. exp. Psychol.*, vol. 48, pp. 187–96.

GREEN, R. F. (1955), 'Transfer of skill on a following tracking task as a function of task difficulty (target size)', *J. Psychol.*, vol. 39, pp. 355–70.

GREENSPOON, J., and FOREMAN, S. (1957), 'Effect of delay of knowledge of results on learning a motor task', *J. exp. Psychol.*, vol. 51, pp. 226–8.

HOLDING, D. H., and MACRAE, A. W. (1964), 'Guidance, restriction and knowledge of results', *Ergonomics*, vol. 7, pp. 289–95.

HOWELL, M. L. (1956), 'Use of force–time graphs for performance analysis in facilitating motor learning', *Res. Quart.*, vol. 27, pp. 12–22.

KARLIN, L., and MORTIMER, R. G. (1963), 'Effect of verbal, visual and auditory augmenting cues on learning a complex motor task', *J. exp. Psychol.*, vol. 65, pp. 75–9.

KELLER, F. S. (1943), 'Studies in international Morse code. I. A new method of teaching code reception', *J. appl. Psychol.*, vol. 27, pp. 407–15.

LAVERY, J. J., and SUDDON, F. H. (1962), 'Retention of simple motor skills as a function of the number of trials by which knowledge of results is delayed', *Percept. mot. Skills*, vol. 15, pp. 231–7.

LEE, B. S. (1950), 'Effects of delayed speech feedback', *J. acoust. Soc. Amer.*, vol. 22, pp. 824–6.

LORGE, I., and THORNDIKE, E. L. (1935), 'The influence of a delay in the after-effect of a connection', *J. exp. Psychol.*, vol. 18, pp. 186–94.

SEYMOUR, W. D. (1954), *Industrial Training for Manual Operations*, Pitman.

SMODE, A. F. (1958), 'Learning and performance in a tracking task under two levels of achievement information feedback', *J. exp. Psychol.*, vol. 56, pp. 297–304.

VAN BERGEIJK, W. A., and DAVID, E. E. (1959), 'Delayed handwriting', *Percept. mot. Skills*, vol. 9, pp. 347–57.

WATERS, R. H. (1933), 'The specificity of knowledge of results and improvement', *Psychol. Bull.*, vol. 30, p. 673 (Abstr.).

WILLINGHAM, W. W. (1958), 'Performance decrement following failure', *Percept. mot. Skills*, vol. 8, pp. 199–202.

20 D. H. Holding

Guidance

Excerpts from chapter 3 of D. H. Holding, *Principles of Training*, Pergamon, 1965, pp. 38–53.

Types of Guidance

There are many methods for minimizing errors in early learning and experiments have been carried out in an attempt to see how effective these techniques are. 'Guidance' is the description traditionally assigned to these methods. The term is not particularly explicit, and we must make some further distinctions before surveying the results.

Physical restriction. To prevent overt errors from appearing, we can often 'block off' incorrect movements, by making them physically impossible. A harness for controlling a golfer's swing makes use of this principle for instance. In this kind of guidance, the learner provides the power, while the direction or extent of the movement is externally controlled. Sometimes, physical restriction may take the form of providing support for part of an activity, so that the remainder may be practised freely. The use of floats and belts in swimming practice is an example of this partial guidance.

Forced response. Another method, the most direct, is to control a pattern of movement by actively transporting the limb or the whole body of the subject; it appears, for instance, that the Balinese use this method in passing on the movements of their dance gestures and other ritual activities (Bateson and Mead, 1942). Dual control devices may take this form, although these are usually employed more for reasons of safety than of training. The forced-response learner does not actively initiate his responses but remains overtly passive. In the early experimental work, the guidance was usually given by hand, although nowadays a number of mechanical methods have been developed.

Visual guidance. As we have seen, most skills are controlled in the early stages by external cues, predominantly visual cues. Often, visual materials may be laid out in such a way as to show the learner what to do at each point. The plan view of a maze, which is eventually to be traced blindfold, may be laid out before the learner to give him preliminary visual guidance; he may either trace through using the plan or store the visual information for later use, taking no immediate action.

Verbal guidance. The giving of verbal instructions is another way of making sure that the learner does not have to use trial-and-error methods. As Annett (1959) has pointed out, we may often regard guidance techniques as giving 'knowledge before' a response, rather than 'knowledge after' in the form of feedback. Not all verbal methods can be considered guidance techniques, of course, and the use of words in training raises a number of other issues which are best dealt with in a later chapter. [. . .]

Adjustive Skills

The kind of operation which calls for continuous, adjustive movements is typified by the 'tracking task'. Driving a car, turning a cube on the lathe or catching a ball, all require some kind of moment-to-moment adjustment of responses to a target. If the target is stationary and the operator's responses are directed towards correcting deviations from the target, the task is *compensatory*. If the target is changing and the operator is required to locate and keep pace with the target, his task is one of *pursuit tracking*. Steering a car on a steady course down a straight road requires compensatory tracking; steering it round a bend involves pursuit tracking. Other things being equal, pursuit tracking tends to be the easier (Poulton, 1952). No data are available on guidance in compensatory tracking. Such guidance would consist only of control movements, giving only kinaesthetic information. This occurs because the indicators in a self-tracked compensatory task would remain stationary, so that no visual cues would be available.

An evaluation of forced-response guidance in pursuit tracking was attempted by Holding (1959). Two different target courses were used, generated by a cam which moved the pointer up and down a vertical scale. Under normal conditions the subject used a large control knob to follow the target movement with a second pointer. For guidance runs, the motion of the target course cam was geared directly to the control knob and the two pointers, so that subjects merely gripped the knob lightly while the apparatus tracked itself. Only short amounts of guidance were given, as the learning curve flattened out very quickly and it would have been difficult to evaluate large amounts. The effect of 2 min guided tracking was to reduce the error scores to the same level as normal practice produced in the same time. This learning was not specific to the target course for which guidance was given, because transferring guided and unguided subjects to the other course resulted in equivalent amounts of saving.

The next step was to split the guidance into separate components. Full guidance, of the kind described above, was compared with visual guidance and kinaesthetic guidance. The kinaesthetic training group were blindfolded while feeling the rotation of the control knob, and the visual group folded their arms while watching the pointers tracking in unison. The contribution to learning due to visual guidance was about 60 per cent of the error saved by full guidance, while kinaesthetic guidance seemed to account for only 20 per cent. Melcher's (1934) results on children's maze learning, while incomplete, seem to parallel these findings. Possibly these proportions would have differed, had guidance been given after some preliminary practice. Kinaesthetic maze guidance appeared better after some exposure to the task, in the experiment by Ludgate (1924); and in the tracking case it may give information before the subject is ready to make use of it, while visual guidance permits the learner to see at the outset what is required.

Guidance in turning a handwheel at a constant rate was compared with knowledge of results by Lincoln (1956). During learning, three methods were used. The handwheel might be turned by a motor at the standard speed of 100 r.p.m.; it might be turned at a rate corresponding to the error on the subject's previous trial and the subject told whether this represented a negative or a positive error; finally, the previous error might be given verbally. Although the verbal method appeared slightly better during training, when performance was measured later without any supplementary cues, the accuracy of the three groups was about the same.

The other form of guidance – the restriction method – was tried out in two-handed tracking of a clover leaf pattern (Bilodeau and Bilodeau, 1958). Subjects could either track along a flush surface or along a recessed path which restricted their movements. Transferring from restrictive guidance to free tracking saved about one day's practice, as did transferring from free movement to the guided version of the task. Clearly, restriction training has some value in continuous adjustive skills, although no direct comparison with forced-response methods is available.

Graded Movements

Further evidence on the results of physical manipulation of human responses comes from work on single adjustive movements. Holding and Macrae (1964) adapted the line-drawing experiment to permit the comparison of forced-response and physical restriction with two kinds of knowledge of results. Six groups of subjects were blindfolded and instructed to move a knob along a rod for a distance of exactly 4 in. After a set of twenty attempts, nine sets of training trials were given by different methods, followed by a test set of a further twenty trials. Learning was measured in terms of the difference in error score between the first and final test sets.

A control group received no guidance or feedback throughout the experiment. Another group received guidance in all the training trials, from a modified door-spring which towed the hand along, decelerating to a stop at 4 in in a manner resembling an ordinary human movement. The problem of accurate simulation in guided movements is probably important but has hardly received experimental attention. A third group received 'distributed guidance'; that is to say, guidance was alternated with normal practice for successive sets of training trials. For the fourth group, restrictive guidance was provided by a stop screwed into the rod at the 4-in mark. The training method for a further group was 'right–wrong' knowledge of results, the last group receiving detailed knowledge of results in terms of the amount and direction of error.

Figure 1 shows the results obtained. The two kinds of forced-response training had some effect, but restriction gave a greater gain, and was quite as effective as knowledge of results. The superiority of restriction was unexpected, although the activity

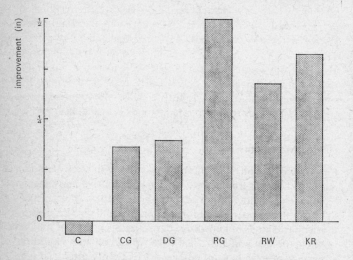

Figure 1 Comparing knowledge of results with different kinds of guidance. Each bar shows the amount learned during training. 'C' was a control group; CG learners had forced response guidance throughout; DG was forced response on alternate trials; RG was guidance by restriction; RW was right–wrong information. KR was full knowledge of results. After Holding and Macrae (1964)

it allows to the subject may be beneficial, and hitting the stop may have some emphasis value which the forced deceleration lacked. Again, just as restrictive guidance materially altered the maze-learning task for the subject, so forced-response guidance alters the character of discrete movements. If anything, the learner is pulling against the door-spring, a movement opposed to the push required in the test trial. Thus, while the movements required in training and testing are identical for restriction, they are antagonistic in the forced-response case. Of course, this is only true when the task is to push; in a pulling, or releasing, task we might expect the advantage to be reversed.

This last prediction has been tested with a further modification of the previous apparatus (Macrae and Holding, 1965). Figure 2 shows the results of two groups repeating the restriction and guidance conditions of the first experiment, compared with the

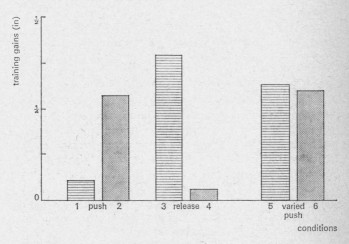

Figure 2 Restriction, forced-response and knowledge of alternatives. 1 Forced response (push task). 2 Restriction (push task). 3 Forced response (release task). 4 Restriction (release task). 5 Varied forced response (push task). 6 Varied restriction (push task). Plain bars are forced response; hatched bars represent restriction

results of these training methods on a releasing task. The new test conditions resembled the 'deadman's hand' mechanism of the tube train; the control knob was pulled along at a constant speed when gripped by the subject, and stopped when he released it at his estimate of 4 in. For this new task, forced-response training appeared to be superior to restriction, as predicted.

At the same time, a further idea was tested. Guided subjects, while prevented from learning errors, are usually deprived of the chance to build up a range of experience by making a wide selection of responses. However, guidance is a flexible technique and it is equally possible to give guided experience of a range of responses. Two further groups were therefore given guidance and restriction at 2, 3, 4, 5 and 6 in, before testing on the 4-in pushing task; these results also appear in Figure 2. Forced response appears to be improved, although the restriction group does not. It seems likely that this multiple restriction technique, together with simple restriction and knowledge of results in the previous experiment, have encountered a limit on learning. It is difficult to better the final error scores, and wider differences between experimental conditions might only appear with fewer training trials.

Knowledge of Alternatives

These multiple guidance techniques give the learner what might be called *knowledge of alternatives*, with the important proviso that the subject knows in advance which is the correct alternative. In two earlier experiments (Carr, 1921; von Wright, 1957) on visual guidance, described more fully in the next chapter [not included here], it emerged that showing the learner the full range of possibilities gave better results than merely showing him the correct path. These findings give us a clue towards assembling a great deal of what has gone before.

We began by considering how far reducing errors might contribute to learning. However, if this is done in such a way as to reduce the information available to the learner the learning will suffer. Knowledge of the correct response is incomplete if there is no opportunity to define it against the alternatives, just as we cannot be said to understand 'red' if we have never identified other colours. On the other hand, Kaess and Zeaman's (1960) experiment suggests that it is inefficient to present the learner with a number of possibilities without indicating which of them is correct. Giving both correct and incorrect alternatives while ensuring correct responses seems to be the best solution.

In the two visual studies (Carr, 1921; von Wright, 1957), giving information about incorrect alternatives was an improvement. Similarly, Koch's animals learned well, having a view of the incorrect alley through a glass partition; her discrepant results with humans have already been considered. Naturally, knowledge of alternatives may be acquired before guidance is given, with some benefit. For this reason, Ludgate's (1924) results were better after some unguided trials had provided contrast. Again, purely kinaesthetic guidance (Holding, 1959; Melcher, 1934) was relatively poor if given at the outset, but not when interspersed with free activity (Lincoln, 1956).

Of course, mere knowledge of the alternatives to the correct response need not encourage errors, as might appear at first sight. Kaess and Zeaman (1960), for instance, whose work on punchboard learning has been described, showed that merely reading wrong answers did not fixate them as errors. On the other hand, if the wrong answers were actually punched then later unlearning was needed. It is easy to see, therefore, that the methods of visual guidance lend themselves readily to the presentation of incorrect alternatives; but we might imagine that the danger of error learning prohibits the giving of extra information by the physical methods of guidance. Forcing a subject to commit an 'error' might be undesirable. However, a subject guided into an alternative response pattern has not made a mistake – he has merely practised a response slightly different from the one finally required. Thus, the apparent success of guiding a range of movements, including both correct and 'incorrect' items (Macrae and Holding, 1965; Waters, 1931), also falls into place.

It is clear, too, why training by knowledge of results is often preferred. At the expense of some errors, knowledge of alternatives is acquired automatically, becoming more precise as the correct response is neared, by successive discrimination. However, it is possible to build knowledge of alternatives into guidance procedures and, as we have seen, these techniques may often considerably shorten the course of learning.

Summary

The fact that efficient performance depends upon knowledge of results does not imply that all learning must take place by trial-and-error. The methods of physical, visual and verbal guidance are all directed towards limiting the learning of errors which must later be eradicated. The present chapter reviews the evidence on the physical methods of restriction and forced response.

Forced response. In these methods the trainer takes complete charge of the response. Thus the exact form of the guided response is probably critical, although this has not received attention. In humans there is substantial learning of mazes and some benefit to discrete and continuous adjustive tasks. When the forced response is finally acquired, the restriction technique is more effective.

Restriction. Here the learner initiates and controls the speed and force of the response under spatial guidance. Restriction is effective in maze learning and in adjustive tasks. No direct comparisons with forced response are available except in discrete adjustive skills, where restriction compares favourably with knowledge of results. Reversing the required movement favours forced response.

Amount and position. Early conclusions recommending small amounts of guidance in the first stages of learning are not really borne out by the data, which show the issue to be rather complex. There is no doubt that for practical purposes guidance will often be used to teach the basic requirements, leaving final learning to the action of knowledge of results if only because the necessary refinements to guidance methods would be uneconomic. Some preliminary experience of unguided trials seems desirable.

Alternatives. Training by guidance methods may restrict the information offered to the learner by withholding knowledge of alternatives. When this difficulty is not overcome by preliminary experience or the design of the task explicit practice with alternatives may be given. A learner practising alternatives is not learning errors if he knows which is the correct response.

References
ANNETT, J. (1959), 'Learning a pressure under conditions of immediate and delayed knowledge of results', *Quart. J. exp. Psychol.*, vol. 11, pp. 3–15.
BATESON, G., and MEAD, M. (1942), *Balinese Culture: A Photographic Analysis*, New York Academy of Science.
BILODEAU, I. McD., and BILODEAU, E. A. (1958), 'Transfer of training and physical restriction of responses', *Percept. mot. Skills*, vol. 8, pp. 71–8.

CARR, H. A. (1921), 'The influence of visual guidance in maze learning', *J. exp. Psychol.*, vol. 4, pp. 399–417.

HOLDING, D. H. (1959), 'Guidance in pursuit tracking', *J. exp. Psychol.*, vol. 47, pp. 362–6.

HOLDING, D. H., and MACRAE, A. W. (1964), 'Guidance, restriction and knowledge of results', *Ergonomics*, vol. 7, pp. 289–95.

KAESS, W., and ZEAMAN, D. (1960), 'Positive and negative knowledge of results on a Pressey-type punchboard', *J. exp. Psychol.*, vol. 60, pp. 12–17.

LINCOLN, R. S. (1956), 'Learning and retaining a rate of movement with the aid of kinaesthetic and verbal cues', *J. exp. Psychol.*, vol. 51, pp. 199–204.

LUDGATE, K. E. (1924), 'The effect of manual guidance upon maze learning', *Psychol. Monogr.*, vol. 33, no. 148.

MACRAE, A. W., and HOLDING, D. H. (1965), 'Method and task in motor guidance', *Ergonomics*, vol. 8, ppl 315–20.

MELCHER, R. T. (1934), 'Children's motor learning with and without vision', *Child Develpm.*, vol. 6, pp. 315–50.

POULTON, E. C. (1952), 'Perceptual anticipation in tracking with two-pointer and one-pointer displays', *Brit. J. Psychol.*, vol. 43, pp. 222–9.

VON WRIGHT, J. M. (1957), 'A note on the role of guidance in learning', *Brit. J. Psychol.*, vol. 48, pp 133–7.

WATERS, R. H. (1931), 'The effect of incorrect guidance upon human maze learning', *J. comp. Psychol.*, vol. 12, pp. 293–301.

21 E. R. F. W. Crossman

A Theory of the Acquisition of Speed-Skill

E. R. F. W. Crossman, 'A theory of the acquisition of speed-skill', *Ergonomics*, vol. 2, 1959, pp. 153–66.

1. Introduction

Training is an art which can be successfully practised with little or no scientific backing, but as in other fields, really reliable and reproducible results flow only from a sound basic theory. Since training serves to facilitate the natural process of acquiring skill by practice, the most important theoretical question is: how and why does a learner acquire skill in ordinary practice?

This paper is concerned with manual speed-skills and dexterities, a class of skills which is both common and important in industry today. Its aim is to put forward a theory of their acquisition suggested to the writer by the results of some recent experimental work carried out by Seymour at Birmingham University and by de Jong at the Berenschot Bureau, Amsterdam. The theory stems essentially from the trial-and-error view of learning put forward by Thorndike more than 50 years ago (see Hilgard, 1948, p. 409). Though this view has since been elaborated by many students of animal learning, and concepts of drive, reward, habit strength, etc., introduced, no serious attempt seems to have been made to build up a quantitative account of the acquisition of skill from it. The writer has taken up its basic premise that a learner faced by a new task tries out various methods, retains the more successful ones and rejects the less successful ones, and has constructed from it a formal theoretical model to explain the experimental findings. While the model is presented here in a skeleton form, it agrees quite satisfactorily with experiment, and interesting new questions are raised.

2. Skill and Learning

Recent researches on manual skill have been largely concerned with the *general* features of skilled performance; the importance of perceptual and central organizing activities, the temporal interlacing of receptor and effector actions and the role of feedback or knowledge-of-results have all been stressed. But when studying industrial operations the writer has been struck by the highly *specific* nature of most skills. The expert's ability seems to lie rather in knowing exactly the right method to use in each

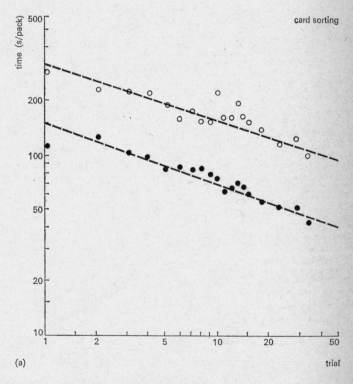

(a)

Figure 1 Learning curves on log–log scales for two subjects each on five tasks (data of Blackburn, 1936)

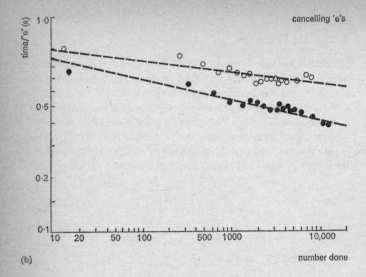

(b)

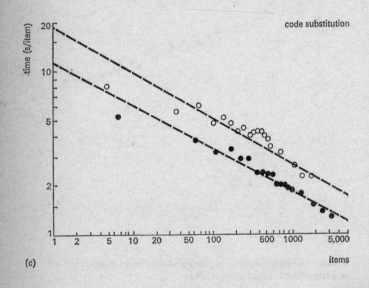

(c)

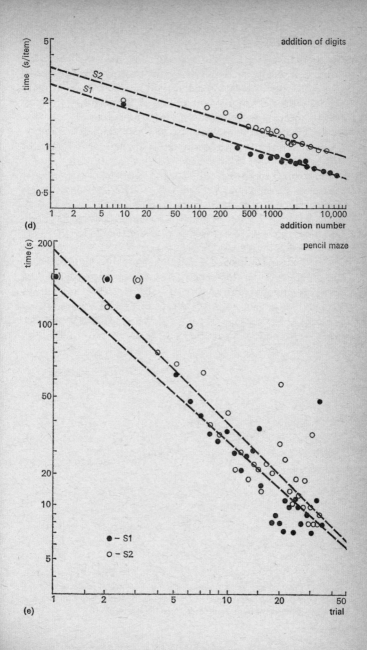

addition of digits

time (s/item)

(d)   addition number

pencil maze

time (s)

● – S1
○ – S2

(e)   trial

situation that arises in the task, than in having superior co-ordination, acuity or timing. He can select the right source of signals to attend to, choose the right course of action, make precisely the right movements and check the results by the most reliable means. In other words, his behaviour is closely 'adapted' to the situation in the same sense in which animals are said to become adapted to their environment by natural selection; he possesses only 'fit' behaviour patterns.

For manual speed-skills, the operator's degree of adaptation is measured principally by his speed of performance, once success can be taken for granted. It increases gradually and continuously over long periods of practice, as many experimental learning curves have shown (Blackburn, 1936). De Jong (1957) has recently put forward a rational equation which fits the results of several industrial studies. He finds that cycle time plotted against cycle number on log–log paper shows a linear decrease followed by an asymptotic approach to an 'incompressible' cycle time; the relationship may be called' de Jong's Law'. De Jong has not provided statistical support for his argument, and some data are given here both to remedy the omission and by way of example.

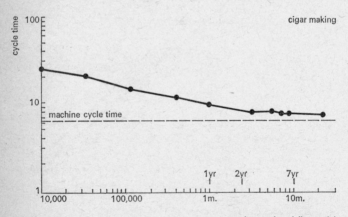

number produced (log scale)

Figure 2 Practice and speed in cigar making. Each point is the average cycle time over one week's production for one operator. The ordinate is the total production by the operator since beginning work

Practice and speed in five simple tasks

Results given by Blackburn (1936) on card-sorting, cancelling 'e's in nonsense French, adding digits, code substitution and maze learning have been re-analysed. Figure 1 (a to e) shows the learning curves and Table 1 a statistical test of de Jong's Law. The law clearly describes the data for the first four tasks well, but the fifth is doubtful.

Table 1

A Statistical Test of de Jong's Law on Data given by Blackburn (1936) for Subjects Learning Five Simple Repetitive Tasks

Task	Subject	Regression coefficient b	Correlation coefficient r	Variance ratio F	Time for First trial predicted (s)	Time for First trial actual (s)
Sorting forty-two cards into individual compartments	1	—0·326	—0·95	1·40	149	111
	2	—0·300	—0·91	1·35	322	279
Cancelling 'e's in nonsense French	1	—0·137	—0·94	4·67†	14·1	2 (est.)
	2	—0·064	—0·76	2·68*	11·5	,,
Substituting code symbols for letters	1	—0·261	—0·99	2·12	11·4	10 (est.)
	2	—0·250	—0·95	2·65*	16·1	,,
Adding pairs of digits	1	—0·147	—0·97	0·56	2·47	3 (est.)
	2	—0·144	—0·94	2·52*	3·34	,,
Tracing a pencil-maze blindfold	1	—0·949	—0·84	1·79	222	>180
	2	—0·959	—0·88	1·05	266	>180

* Significant at 5 per cent level.   † Significant at 0·1 per cent level.

Notes: (1) Each subject performed thirty-five periods of about 180 s each, on successive days.

(2) The logarithms (to base 10) of cycle-time have been correlated with the mean logarithm of the number of cycles performed up to and during each trial

(3) The significance of the departure from linearity has been tested by Analysis of Variance, grouping the last five blocks of five readings together in order to estimate error. In each case the variance ratio F is based on 13 and 20 df.

(4) The times for the first trial are only known in two cases; in the others an estimate has been made.

Long-period improvement in cigar making

A study was made of the speeds of production of several girls in the same shop, operating special-purpose, cigar-making machines (Crossman, 1956, ch. 10). The job had a very short cycle, but considerable variation was experienced in the raw materials, and there was high 'perceptual load'. Figure 2 shows the weekly average cycle time for operators of various lengths of service. Only after two years and about three million cycles does the curve depart appreciably from a straight line.

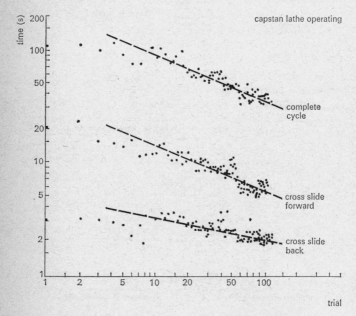

Figure 3 The effect of practice on element and cycle times for the simulated capstan lathe operation (data of Seymour, 1954). The results of one subject are shown and each point represents one cycle of practice

Improvement of the elements within a motion cycle

Data provided by Seymour (1954) on learners operating a capstan lathe have been re-plotted and are shown in Figure 3. It is clear that the two elements obey de Jong's Law as does the complete cycle.

The steady decrease in cycle time shown by de Jong's Law is accompanied by considerable variation from cycle to cycle.

Studies of cycles and element times have shown quite clearly that the average does not decrease by a proportionate change in all times but by a change in frequency distribution. Early in practice this is symmetrical; it becomes more and more skewed with practice, and finally J-shaped. Different elements show

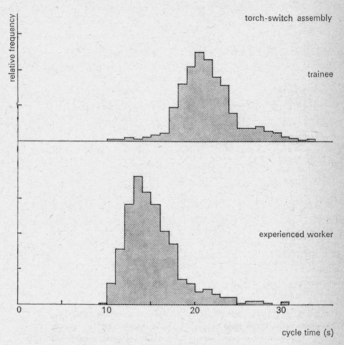

Figure 4 The distribution of cycle times for a learner and an experienced worker at torch-switch assembling (data of Dudley, 1955)

different initial distributions; very short ones (1 to 2 s) tend to the rectangular or J-shaped, longer ones tend more and more to the Gaussian form. Figures 4 and 5 show typical results from an industrial assembly operation (15- to 20-s cycle) and a laboratory assembly task (2-s cycle). The scatter of element times does not appear to be due to varying levels of effort, and must presumably be attributed to variations of method. Unfortunately we have little direct evidence on the distribution of motion patterns (but see de Montpellier, 1935, p. 251) and still less about that of perceptual activities. Lewis (1954) has, however, shown in car driving that more skilled performers behave more consistently from occasion to occasion.

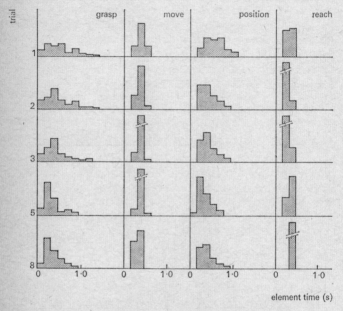

element time (s)

Figure 5 The distribution of element times for a simple assembly operation (the three-hole connector). The four elements – reach, grasp, move and position – are shown. Each histogram represents 100 cycles for one subject and there was no interpolated practice (data of Seymour, 1954)

3. A Theory of the Selective Process

These findings strongly suggest that practice exerts a selective effect on the operator's behaviour, favouring those patterns of action which are quickest at the expense of the others. In order to examine how this might work, a mathematical model of the selection process has been constructed, and will now be formally stated and discussed.

Let us consider an operator learning a repetitive task. For each trial or 'cycle' he will adopt some particular combination of sensory, perceptual and motor activities, partly from deliberate choice, partly from habit and partly by chance; these activities could, in principle at least, be completely described by an observer. In successive cycles he will use either the same or more or less different combinations. Let us call each such distinguishable action pattern a 'method' (M) and identify each by a subscript (e.g. M_1). The operator can be imagined to possess a repertoire or stock of r different methods, from which he picks one by chance for each cycle. The methods will each have a different 'habit strength', availability or probability of use; let M_i occur with probability p_i where $\sum_{i=1}^{r} p_i = 1$. At the outset of practice the repertoire will normally include some wholly unsuccessful methods, but let us imagine that these have been eliminated, and that the repertoire includes only successful ones. From this point on, practice produces a steady decrease in the average cycle time. At any one cycle, say the nth, the average cycle time $T(n)$ is the time for all the methods, M_i, weighted according to their probabilities p_i of occurring, i.e.

$$T(n) = \sum_{i=1}^{r} t_i \times p_i(n) \qquad 1$$

where $t_i =$ time taken by Method M_i.

We assume that a selective effect takes place, increasing the availability of 'fit', i.e. quick methods, and reducing it for 'unfit', i.e. slow ones. To be precise, the speed of any method which happens to be used is measured in relation to the current average, and its probability of occurrence then changes in proportion to the result. Algebraically, let method M_i whenever it occurs have its future probability of being chosen increased by δp_i where

$$\delta p_i = -k\{t_i - T(n)\} \qquad 2$$

(where k is a small positive constant). Since M_i occurs on the average $p_i(n)$ times per cycle, the average chance in its probability on one cycle is

$$p_i(n) \times \delta p_i = -k p_i(n) \times \{t_i - T(n)\} \qquad 3$$

and its probability for the next $(n + 1)$th cycle is,

$$p_i(n+1) = p_i(n) + \delta p_i = p_i(n)[1 - k\{t_i - T(n)\}]. \qquad 4$$

The average cycle-time for the next or $(n + 1)$th cycle can now be calculated

$$T(n+1) = \sum_{i=1}^{r} p_i(n+1) \times t_i = T(n) - k(\text{variance of the } t_i). \quad 5$$

(It is a convenient property of expression 4 that the sum of the $p_i(n+1)$ remains unity, hence no 'normalizing factor' is needed.)

Ideally the next step would be to express $T(n)$ as an explicit function of n, and plot the resulting learning curve; this can be done but the expression is complicated and involves high order moments of the initial distribution of the t_i. Instead, a learning curve has been computed numerically for an imaginary task where the learner starts with ten equiprobable methods, whose times are the integers 1 to 10, and practises with a selective constant $k = 0.1$. The distributions for the first twenty cycles are given in Table 2 and plotted in Figures 6, 7 and 8.

Table 2

The Learning Performance of the Theoretical System

Time taken by method (units)	Probability of method Cycle							
	1	2	3	5	8	11	15	20
1	0.1	0.145	0.198	0.315	0.476	0.607	0.733	0.839
2	,,	0.135	0.171	0.230	0.264	0.253	0.205	0.140
3	,,	0.125	0.146	0.164	0.140	0.097	0.050	0.020
4	,,	0.115	0.123	0.114	0.069	0.030	0.101	0.002
5	,,	0.105	0.102	0.075	0.031	0.010	0.002	—
6	,,	0.095	0.082	0.047	0.013	0.003	—	—
7	,,	0.085	0.065	0.028	0.005	—	—	—
8	,,	0.075	0.050	0.016	0.002	—	—	—
9	,,	0.065	0.037	0.008	—	—	—	—
10	0.1	0.055	0.026	0.003	—	—	—	—
average time	5.5	4.68	3.92	2.80	1.98	1.59	1.39	1.19

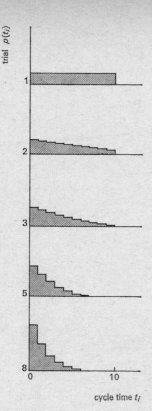
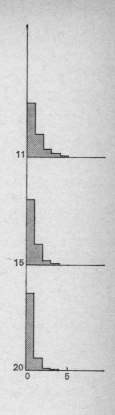

cycle time t_i

distributions derived from equation **5** with

$$\begin{cases} i = t_i = 1 \text{ to } 10 \text{ units} \\ k = 0{\cdot}1 \end{cases}$$

Figure 6 The distributions of cycle times at successive cycles as predicted by the theoretical model (equation **5**) for an imaginary task with ten methods in the operators' repertoire

By comparing Figure 1 with 7, and 5 with 6, the reader will see that the model does fit the experimental findings. There is only one clear discrepancy: the first few cycles of practice should be faster than de Jong's law suggests, and on this point there are

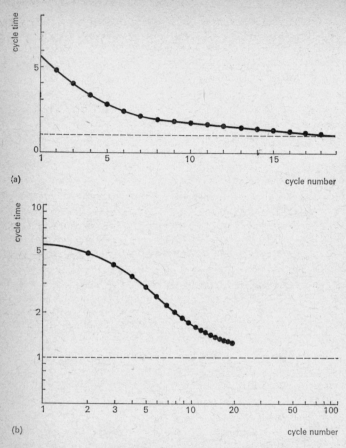

Figure 7 The learning curve given by the theoretical model, plotted (a) on linear and (b) on double logarithmic coordinates

indications (see e.g. Figure 1) that the model gives a rather better fit to the experimental data than de Jong's formula. The theory could be tested more rigorously by applying it to the actual starting distribution for an element or cycle and testing the agreement between the predicted and actual learning curves.

The curve of Figure 8 shows that some individual methods may increase in strength at first, and only later decline towards zero; this recalls what does not seem to have been shown experimentally but can easily be seen in industrial practice, that certain methods may be learned at first, only to be discarded again as the average speed increases.

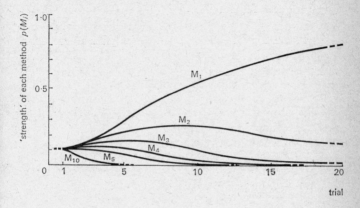

Figure 8 The change of availability of methods as practice proceeds according to the theoretical model equation **5**

Several complications which arise in the real situation have been ignored, and a few of them will be briefly indicated:

1. It has been assumed that only one repertoire is being subjected to selection. In a real task there will be one for each different work situation or subtask that arises. Thus in reality several largely independent selection processes must be going on at once.

2. Selection may act on elements rather than on the complete cycle. In order to find the distribution of cycle times, one must then combine those of the element times by *convolution*. The combined distribution may be quite unlike the separate ones (Figure 9), and tends to be more and more Gaussian as the

289

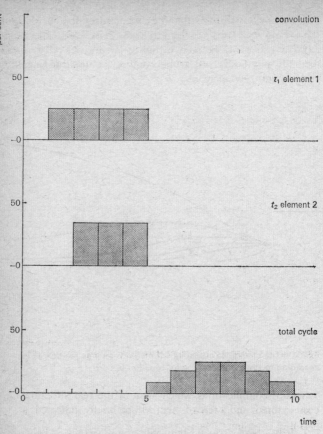

Figure 9 The frequency distributions of times for the two elements combined by convolution to give the distribution of cycle times

number combined increases (by the central limit theorem). The element times for a long cycle must be highly skewed before the cycle time is appreciably so.

3. The time for any one method may not be constant, but affected by chance variations in the work. This complicates but does not essentially change the picture.

4. The operator's repertoire may gain or lose methods during practice, by deliberate or chance invention, by instruction, or by forgetting. The rate of learning is then affected in proportion as the variance of method times is changed (equation 5), sometimes abruptly so.

5. The availability of methods may change for reasons other than selection. For instance, fatigue may be expected to reduce availability for any method which is used. The selection process would then be progressively distorted as any one practice period proceeds.

Despite the complications, certain conclusions follow from the theory. First, the rate of learning for a subtask will depend on the size of the learner's repertoire for it; on the variance within it, which in turn depends on the amount of previous selection; and on the selection pressure. Secondly, the over-all learning period will increase steeply with the number of subtasks to be learned and with the initial variance of the repertoire for each; tasks whose subtasks are independent of each other will be more rapidly learned than those in which they interact. Third, transfer of skill from one task to another will take place where methods appropriate to one are almost appropriate to the other, but the amount of transfer will depend on the *selectivity* that has been established rather than on the mere coincidence of methods.

The particular model given is only one out of a class of such models. The principle of selective processes in general can perhaps best be set out in a diagram (Figure 10). The learner possesses a 'pool of methods', each with a certain strength, but no means of choosing particular ones; they differ in various respects, producing a variance in any given characteristic. The pool may have its variance increased or diminished as practice proceeds. The most important cause of reduction is selection in favour of methods more closely adapted to the work-situation. A parallel to this process is to be found in the genetical theory of natural selection (Fisher, 1930); here the genetic variance of a population is increased by mutation and reduced by natural selection. Unfortunately Fisher's mathematical treatment deals with two-factor (Mendelian) inheritance, and cannot be applied directly to this multifactor problem.

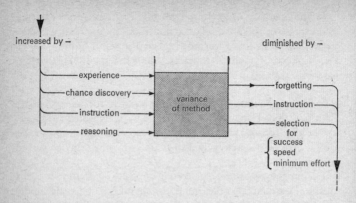

increased by →   diminished by →

experience →
chance discovery →   variance   → forgetting
instruction →   of method   → instruction
reasoning →   → selection
                                                for
                                                { success
                                                  speed
                                                  minimum effort

Figure 10 A diagrammatic representation of the selective processes in the acquisition of skill

4. The Selective Mechanism

Although selection of methods for their relative speed has been postulated to account for the acquisition of speed-skill, it is not at all easy to see how the psychological and neural mechanisms could produce this result. At each trial the operator would have in some way to retain data about what method had been used, measure the time it took and then alter its 'strength' in proportion. But judgement of short time intervals is very inaccurate and externally given knowledge-of-results, such as the time taken for so many pieces, is not detailed enough to be effective. Instead of *time* the selective variable might well be *work* for if the operator exerts a constant level of effort, the work done to complete a cycle by any particular method would be proportional to its duration. If this were so, one would regard the gradual speed-up with practice as being secondary to the operator's pursuit of the minimum (physiological) 'cost' to himself, and the acquisition of speed-skill could be seen as an instance of the more general biological principle of 'least effort' (see Zipf, 1949). Unfortunately there is even less indication that a mechanism exists for measuring physiological cost than one for measuring time.

A plausible case might be made for a mechanism based on the time-course of the decay of short-term memory. The method used for any given trial must necessarily be remembered to some extent, if any selective reinforcement is to take place at all, and it is obviously not permanently and perfectly remembered. If, as other experiments suggest, the memory of what has been done decays in a regular way with time, this might provide the necessary time scale for the selective process. If the memory could be in some way 'fixed' by the successful completion of the element or cycle, then the sooner this happened, the more memory would remain to be fixed and the more chance there would be that the precise method would be recalled and repeated. Since most motion elements seem to require a perceptual completion signal of some kind, its arrival could cause the memory to be fixed.

5. Implications for Training

If the acquisition of speed-skill depends primarily on a selective process, it follows that training should aim at deliberately strengthening the selection pressure, while taking steps to ensure that the best 'methods' are in the learner's repertoire to be selected. The trainer must first know what is to be selected, i.e. what methods (both perceptual and motor) give fast performance; secondly, he must ensure that the learner can do them; and thirdly he must set up conditions in which they are consistently more successful than all others.

Verbal or visual instruction and demonstration are of use for putting the best methods into the repertoire, but for selection systematic practice under pressure for speed is probably the only effective way. Breaking down the task into elements increases selective efficiency, but the trainer must ensure that by so doing he does not find wrong methods being selected, that is ones that are optimum in the isolated element but not in the complete task. These elements which have most variation of method need most selection and should be isolated; they are usually the ones which are highly specific to the particular job and so have not been selected by previous practice. Training for transfer, except where there are many identical elements, should presumably be aimed at giving the learner a good power of selection.

6. Further Research

Studies of the distribution of methods rather than of times should show more clearly what is happening, and just how certain methods are selected; and tasks might be set up in which different sorts of selective pressure could be applied. Further mathematical analysis is also needed to make possible a proper comparison between theory and experiment.

References

BLACKBURN, J. M. (1936), 'Acquisition of skill: an analysis of learning curves', *I.H.R.B. Report*, no. 73.

CROSSMAN, E. R. F. W. (1956), The measurement of perceptual load in manual operations, *Unpublished Ph.D. Thesis, Birmingham University*.

DUDLEY, N. A. (1955), Output patterns in repetitive tasks, *Unpublished Ph.D. Thesis, Birmingham University*.

FISHER, R. A. (1930), *The Genetical Theory of Natural Selection*, Oxford University Press.

HILGARD, E. R. (1948), *Theories of Learning*, Appleton-Century.

DE JONG, J. R. (1957), 'The effects of increasing skill on cycle-time and its consequences for time-standards', *Ergonomics*, vol. 1, pp. 51–60.

LEWIS, R. E. F. (1954), 'Consistency and car-driving skill', *Brit. J. industr. Med.*, vol. 13, pp. 131–41.

DE MONTPELLIER, G., (1935), *Les Altérations Morphologiques des Mouvements Rapides*, Eds. Inst. Sup. Philos., Louvain.

SEYMOUR, W. D. (1954), 'Experiments on the acquisition of industrial skills', *Occup. Psychol.*, part I, vol. 28, pp. 77–89; part II, vol. 29, pp. 82–96; part III, vol. 30, pp. 94–104. (Also personal communication, 1956.)

ZIPF, G. K. (1949), *Human Behaviour and the Principle of Least Effort*, Addison-Wesley.

Part Seven **The Breakdown of Skill**

Once thoroughly learned, skills are very resistant to disuse, though there is some deterioration after a long period without practice. The conditions which do cause the performance of a skill to deteriorate are studied to discover the range of conditions under which the skill can be performed, the way in which breakdown occurs and to examine the nature of the mechanisms underlying the skill which may be revealed in its impairment.

In his Ferrier Lecture in 1943, Bartlett (Reading 22) describes some of the main findings from the Cambridge cockpit experiments which were conducted to examine the consequences of prolonged performance of a complex skill – controlling a flight simulator. This research not only showed the ways in which performance changes with fatigue but it also pointed to the fundamental nature of skill and provided a basis for the ideas advanced by Craik (Reading 10) and Poulton (Reading 7). Bartlett stresses the very marked change in the temporal co-ordination of responses. He reports a splintering of stimulus and response patterns combined with increased tolerance of errors.

Broadbent (Reading 23) reviews a number of experiments conducted on the effects of heat, noise and lack of sleep. All these variables impair skill but by examining more than one variable at a time it has proved possible to show that they act in different ways. Both too high and too low a level of arousal impairs skill. Loss of sleep appears to result in too low a level of arousal while noise produces too high a level. Environmental temperature appears to act in a different way since its effects do not interact with the other forms of environmental stress.

Drugs may also cause performance to deteriorate. This is particularly true of drugs which depress central nervous system activity. Drew, Colquhoun and Long (Reading 24) studied the effects of small doses of alcohol on a skill resembling driving. Impairment was found to follow absorption of alcohol into the blood stream such that the larger the blood–alcohol level, the larger the effect. There was no sign of a threshold level which had to be exceeded before impairment was manifested.

Skilled performance also declines with advancing age. Welford (Reading 25) reviews some of the experimental results showing how older subjects tend to be slower in making decisions and to take longer to interpret visually presented information. The older subject has less spare capacity to deal with new problems and his deteriorating short-term memory may also limit his performance. Welford indicates some of the industrial significance of these changes with age.

22 F. C. Bartlett

Fatigue Following Highly Skilled Work

Excerpt from F. C. Bartlett, 'Fatigue following highly skilled work', *Proceedings of the Royal Society*, B, vol. 131, 1943, pp. 248–57. (Ferrier Lecture.)

When people began to try to apply experiment to the study of tiredness produced by the exercise of skill, they seem to have lost forthwith all their capacity for realistic imagination. They thought, and have continued to think, almost solely in terms of exactly repeated activity. Thus Kraepelin – who did far more harm than good, I think, in this field – introduced his method of the reckoning test: a person must add, or subtract, or multiply, or divide simple digits for hours on end. Others have embroidered on the same theme. They have exposed colours, or words, or easy drawings in long series, asking all the time for recognition, or naming, or both. They have required letters, or letter combinations, words or word combinations, to be written, or perhaps to be cancelled, over and over again. They have set their victims to copy line diagrams, or designs, so often that one would think that all but the most faithful must have been reduced to profanity or to tears, at least through boredom if not through fatigue. Through it all runs one great, unverified guess: fatigue must consist of diminished efficiency of specific performance due to the repetition of that performance.

Suppose, instead of rather blindly taking over methods which were just and correct when applied to the case of simple muscular fatigue, that people had honestly asked themselves what looks to be the character of the skills involved when we say we get tired in the pursuit of complex activities in daily life, in industry, or in the practice of specialized skill in the fighting services. They would have got a picture wholly different from that of repeated movements set up in response to recurrent and unvarying stimuli. They would have found co-ordinated actions the constituents of which can, and frequently do, change places. They would have found a type of behaviour in which it has become of enormous importance to *time* the constituents correctly, so that each can flow readily into its neighbour. They would have found interruptions and rests no more uniform than actions. They would have seen stimuli to such co-ordinated action which are not a repetitive succession but a field, a pattern, an organized group of signals capable of changing their internal arrangement without loss of their identity as an organized group.

This is the situation which must be brought within full experimental control if the tiredness, or fatigue, or strain following highly skilled work is to be understood.

It has proved possible to do this, but for various reasons I cannot now so describe the setting designed to investigate these fatigue effects that it may be exactly identified, for it had a very strong and realistic interest, bearing on current affairs.

The subjects of the experiment sat comfortably, surrounded by instrumental controls and faced by a panel containing all the main signals for action. These signals were in three chief groups: in the middle a group important throughout the whole period of the test; to one side a group important only at certain stages, especially at the beginning and the end; to the other side a group intermittently important indicating occurrences calling for prompt, but only occasional, action. Above and below were stimuli which could be brought in at the experimenter's will, each calling for a specific response, but still less closely bound up with the central task.

To all of these signals the operator must respond by co-ordinated movements of hands, feet, eyes and understanding. Moreover, with the exception of the very occasional stimuli, the significance of no signal was detached or isolated from that of any other. All the main stimuli were of the common form, for instrumental maintenance or control, of pointers moving across dial faces at different speeds and in different directions. Some of the subordinate stimuli were lights of varied colour. Each stimulus had a determinate relation to every other, so that both how and when any happened were by no means matters of chance. Also the response required itself helped to determine the next following pattern of stimuli, just as it usually does in real life. Consequently the skilled operator did not need to examine the signals one by one, in a regular order, but could take his cues from the whole pattern, with certain constituents always playing the dominant parts, again as happens in the skill of daily life. Since all stimuli and all reactions were moving in determinate relationships, the whole instrument was after the style of a rather complex calculating machine, and it became possible to record accurately the amount, direction and, most important of all – as it turned out – the timing of the essential elements in the operator's skill.

There is one thing more. At the beginning of the experiment this was what Ferrier would certainly, and correctly, have called an unverified guess. If one looks fairly at the tiredness which follows skill it is hard to resist the view that abstentions are as important as performances. When work begins, and the central nervous system is alert, keen and high in vigilance, its inhibitory activities are in perfect trim. Additional, irrelevant, unwanted and distracting stimuli are not within the effective field at all. But as work continues and fatigue grows, the inhibitions perhaps relax, until the skill-tired man is doing, not less work, but more, much more.

The instrumental setting was so designed that when the operator used his hands and feet to manipulate levers and switches, his eyes to follow moving pointers and flashing lights, he could – and in fact he did – interpret the result, not in terms of revolving wheels, engaging cogs, shifting currents, vibrating rods and pistons, but, just as any man does when he drives a motor car, in terms of the whole machine. The machine, though in fact stationary all the time, seemed as if it could move, change direction, vibrate, and no single skilled operator of the men who have attempted the task has failed to experience the effect of his skill as a total, combined performance of the machine.

When a man moves with a machine there are inevitably set up a mass of proprioceptive impulses coming from changes of stress and tension at various points of the body surface, from underlying tissues and from other bodily sources. These are not original conditions of the acquisition of the skill concerned, but they are inevitable additional stimuli occurring while the skill is being acquired and when it has been mastered. Sometimes they have the character of distractions, and it may be that the fresh and the tired nervous system react differently towards them. They conform to the principle which ought to be observed in all experimental study of additional or distracting stimuli: they are an integral part of the situation itself, and not merely disconnected signals put in at the whim of an experimenter. The neglect of this principle has led to much unfortunate misunderstanding about the functions and manner of operation of distractions. In the experiment as designed it was not difficult to introduce the required proprioceptive impulses at the appropriate points. The guess was that they might act differently as strain, or fatigue, increased.

Such was the experimental setting. There was little or nothing sheerly repetitive in the stimuli or the behaviour, and nothing at all demanding strong physical effort. The task was one requiring skill and, as it proved, of absorbing interest. That the experiment was possible at all was due mainly to the brilliant mechanical inventiveness of Dr K. J. W. Craik, and that noteworthy results were achieved was due to the patience and high experimental competence of Mr G. C. Drew, both of these being members of the Psychological Department of the University of Cambridge.

I turn now to a description of the main results. The picture which emerges may, I think, fairly be said to be the first reasonably complete representation that has been drawn of the fatigue following highly skilled work. All the phenomena to be described were obtained from a large group of operators. They are statistically reliable to a high degree. There is less than one chance in a hundred that they represent mere accidental occurrences.

We may, perhaps, see the beginning of skill when nervous mechanisms acquire the character of 'graded' response, adjusting the amount of their action to the variable intensity of the stimulus. As skill develops into concerted action, where all subordinate constituents are organized around a few outstanding ones, a new kind of 'grading' appears. Effective stimuli now acquire an 'indifference range' within which stimulus changes, though they may be appreciated, do not call for compensating activity. Variations outside that range at once set central control awake and compensating reactions appear. In the experimental setting two of the instruments were generally central, or dominant. One recorded the extent of deviation of the machine from any given course and the other the speed of movement in any direction. At the beginning the operator, watching the pointer which showed extent of deviation, allowed it to move two or three degrees on either side of the vertical and then began at once to make the necessary control reactions. A little later he was letting it move five degrees in either way, then ten degrees and finally it could swing from side to side over a wide range before anything was done. Exactly the same happened in the case of the speed indicator, and in fact with every other important recording device in the total group of stimuli, I think that everybody who drives a motor car will be able to observe just this same type of widening indifference range of stimuli as he becomes more and more tired.

One way of putting this is to say that skill fatigue is marked by a progressive lowering of standards of performance. But if this is so the standard is certainly not normally formulated, not one of which the operator need be aware. It is a truly physiological function of the central nervous system. It means that at any moment in the continuous exercise of skill every leading stimulus has a range of variation within which the central nervous system exercises no direct and overt control over the local responding mechanisms, and that this range has no fixed limits, but increases progressively as work continues. A large majority of the experimental operators finished their task satisfied that they had improved steadily all the time, though in fact the increase in large errors over small ones, in the case of deviation from a wanted course was 400 per cent as between the first and last periods of a two-hour experimental run, and 92 per cent in the case of speed control. Actually, in relation to their unformulated standards, they *were* doing as well at the end of their task as at the beginning, and perhaps even better.

Now suppose that one element of the response, the simple control, for example, of direction or speed, were taken out of its skill setting and required merely as an element at any stage of the experiment from beginning to end. It showed no deterioration. The absolute efficiency for the element remained unaffected. It is therefore no wonder that an experimental method which has taken elements out of skill has produced results which are strikingly at variance with everyday observation. It is not the local response that has lost its accuracy or its power. It is the central control which has functionally, but without knowledge, expanded the limits of its indifference range.

We can go farther than this with our analysis of the large errors which bunch up as fatigue increases. It will be recalled that the operator was faced with a group of changing signals from which he must select the most significant ones and time his response to these correctly. An instrument may, for example, record an unwanted change of direction. Then the operator may use a control which accelerates that very change, and if he does he has performed the wrong action at the right time. Or he may make delayed use of a control which neutralizes this unwanted change. Or yet again he may manipulate a control which itself produces a consequential change of direction, and then bring in the counteracting control too soon. That is, he can do the right actions at the wrong time, either too late or too soon.

The over-all results of the experiment showed a non-significant increase in wrong actions done at the right time, but a highly significant increase in right actions done at the wrong time. And this same type of deterioration was shown in another way as well. The whole task has to be performed to a time schedule and to help the operator to keep to this he had a clock in his instrument panel and a stop-watch at his side. As the task proceeded the clock and the watch faded out and might almost as well not have been there at all. Of the result the operators were, apparently, faintly aware, for most of them said that their timing might have become a little erratic at the end. In fact the time estimates made by them could be as much as 200 per cent wrong.

So much for some of the facts concerning the deterioration of the skill response. Now let us see what happened as regards the organization of the group of stimuli. It has already been said that all the instruments on the panel were related in a determinate manner. When an operator was fresh a glance at the dominant signals meant an interpretation of the whole panel, and a movement of a controlling lever meant something that the machine was doing, or would very soon begin to do. As the task continued the panel split up, so that it became twenty or so separate recording instruments. And the controlling movements split up also, so that when any one was made it was not pictured in a pattern of machine control, but only as the correction of a particular instrument reading.

When this stage was reached it appeared as if central nervous control tended to slacken either momentarily or finally. The operator's temperament surged up and took charge of his behaviour. For the reaction to one instrument only, when reaction to many was called for, generally set a lot of the others beyond their limits of indifference range. Either there was a moment of flurry and then central control reasserted itself, or there was panic and the operator, dashing from one control to another, pulled his machine to disaster.

The splitting of the stimulus field and the corresponding progressive dissociation of actions did not occur in a haphazard manner. The field contained a central sector important all the time, side sectors important at specific intervals and other signals calling for action at irregular and occasional moments. With some individual differences of detail, the splitting up proceeded regularly from margin to centre. The merely occasional stimuli were the first to break away from the rest. There was a phase during which they were met by delayed, and often hurried, response. At length they were very frequently indeed ignored, to use psychological language they were 'forgotten', and there was a definite and, as it might be called, 'stupid' lapse of action. The machine control was, for example, constructed as if it were maintained by an internal combustion engine. A device indicated the amount of petrol available at any time during a trial and replenishment was required irregularly. At first the petrol gauge was never neglected. As time went on it became common for the operator to put off replenishment and eventually to snatch hurriedly at the control lever. With increasing fatigue, over and over again, the petrol signal was ignored until the machine stopped and the experiment reached a temporary inglorious end.

I must make a brief comment on the initial guess about additional, or distracting cues. When the proprioceptive impulses which would normally be set up by movement of the machine were given to the alert operator, in by far the greater number of cases (75 per cent) they were at once interpreted in terms of the machine. There was first a deterioration in most aspects of the performance: but this was temporary only. Before long the impulses fell into place as additional and helpful stimuli, and the performance improved significantly. If, however, they were given to the tired operator, most of these (70 per cent) treated them as unwanted and disagreeable stimuli of bodily origin. There was now a temporary improvement, followed, more quickly as the operator was more tired, by marked deterioration. They were, in fact, not now additional cues for action, but merely signs of growing weariness. Their first effect was to rouse the operator to greater effort, but this could not be maintained, and then they became only an obsessive awareness of bodily discomfort, and impeded the performance.

It has been shown that the normal course of the experiment demonstrated a regular and progressive tendency on the part of the subject to lower his standard. This could be checked at any stage by introducing new instructions of a difficult type, the result of which was that while the operator was in fact doing just the same as before, it appeared to him that the whole task was made harder. When the alert subject had these instructions, he quickly improved and the improvement was maintained for a long time. If the tired operator were set the apparently more difficult task, he too improved, but only temporarily. Soon he slipped back to a lower level than before. In other words he could, within the limits of fatigue set by the experiment, still carry out the local actions of control as well as or better than ever; but he could not maintain the organized, co-ordinated and timed responses for more than a short period.

Side by side with all these changes, recorded quantitatively and objectively, went some striking subjective phenomena. Three of these are of primary importance.

First the operator's reports of what actually happened during the experiment became less and less reliable as his fatigue increased. His falsifications were of all kinds. Events which actually happened failed to be observed. Changes that never happened at all – loud noises, uncontrollable variations of the instruments – were reported. Levers and switches were said to have become 'sticky', or 'heavy', or 'sloppy', or 'ineffective', though there was no change from beginning to end of the experiment. When the operator realized that he was making mistakes, he regularly maintained his belief that he himself was doing just as well as ever by blaming the experimenter or the machine.

Secondly, as already indicated, awareness of physical discomfort increased enormously. Appliances worn by the operator were charged with being very heavy, or uncomfortably tight. The temperature was said to be too hot or too cold. Postural discomfort came into the front of the picture, and again and again bodily cramp was reported. All the proprioceptive signs became more pressing and at the same time their interpretation became less accurate.

Thirdly, this experiment demonstrated conclusively that the everyday observation which associates growing irritability with increasing fatigue of the central nervous system is correct, and that all those masses of experiments which, concentrating upon some simple, repeated mental task, have failed to reveal this are wrong. When the operator began, absorbed in his task, he was usually silent. As he went on, sighs and shufflings emerged from the machine. Then mild expletives took the place of sighs. By the end of the experiment, which lasted for two hours or more, most operators kept up a flow of the most violent language they knew. And all the time their handling of the controls became more and more rough, so that they were doing more work, and not less, as the task went on. It was at this stage that the tendency to project all errors on to the experimenter or the machine reached its height.

Here, then, in broad outline, is the picture of fatigue following highly skilled work. It was necessary to draw this picture before anything certain or convincing can be said about the fatigue specific to prolonged exposure to loud noise or to vibration, to extremes of temperature, to lack of oxygen, to drugs or to the many other special circumstances which are reasonably suspected to make the skilled man tired.

I must now try to bring together all these points and see what they tell us about how the central nervous system reacts to a complex environment when a man is growing weary. Central nervous fatigue cannot be evaluated in terms of a lessening of total effort, or, except in extreme stages perhaps, by any determination of the efficiency of the local reaction mechanisms. Its signs are indirect ones and are concerned with how the task is done, not with how much of it is done. As everybody knows, it is possible to take any mode of sensorial reaction – visual, auditory, tactual, thermal, proprioceptive – and find out the minimal value of effective stimulus necessary to evoke it and its changes. These are the sensory thresholds. As the senses and their modes of operation combine, under the guidance of central control, a new threshold emerges, a threshold of range or of limits, depending not upon the sensitivity of the special organs, but upon the place of the response in the task which is the combined expression of them all. This threshold of range appears as a standard, developed by the brain and used by it at every moment of every skilled performance. Yet it need not be formulated and the operator may remain as unaware of it as are the eye or the ear of their thresholds. When the operator tires, his standard drops, or, in other words, the threshold of effective range widens and becomes, in fact, the best of all single measures of his fatigue.

We can, perhaps, now begin to see how it is that timing is of tremendous importance as a sign of fatigue of this type. Time is not of great significance in relation to the single reaction. It is true that this has its history; it begins, rises to its maximum and fades away. But time does not matter much unless the single reaction must be followed by another and the two together have to achieve a practical fit. As tasks become more important than single actions, and central control dominates local performance, the temporal relations of activities acquire a practical importance equal to that of the facility of the constituent responses themselves. Time is a discovery, running side by side with that of the co-ordination of actions and achieved by the same central control. If the threshold of effective range for any leading constituent of skill is raised, other constituents will be pushed further off from it in the order of successive performance and then these other constituents will perhaps be hurried or forgotten or the whole performance will take longer. So it is the timing that goes wrong more easily than the efficiency of the local reactions. The rhythm of sequence of the activity is lost or broken, and performance becomes irregular, a story of spurts and delays.

All skill exhibits a number of constituent reactions which fit together. Some skills, when they are unrolled, are normally regarded as complete in themselves, forming, so to speak, a single unit of performance. Others involve critical points that are something like changes of direction in a journey and then the changes that occur in the skill at these critical points come to be treated as the finish of one unit in the complete accomplishment or the beginning of another. Now the standard, involving the threshold of range, operates in every unit of skill; but the combination of several units into a total accomplishment represents a still more advanced achievement.

When, many years ago, Hughlings Jackson introduced the notion of 'levels' of function of the central nervous system, he pointed out that certain very high levels seemed to require a process which he called 'formulation'. It appears to be fair to hold that the successful maintenance of a fluent spacing of units of skill in a complex accomplishment is at this high level, so that what is an unwitting tribute to time in the unit becomes a conscious and controlling schedule of time in the combination of units. When anybody is solely concerned with the single skill, however complex it may be, without regard to what precedes or follows it, time means nothing to him, however much it may signify to anybody who may be watching his behaviour. But he can fit one unit to another in fully adaptive performance only by the aid of a formulated time schedule. This is a late achievement of the brain and very unstable. When a man gets tired the skill units dissociate, the time schedule, if, as in the experiment, one is provided, slips back into the time standard and if, during its progress or when the unit is finished, he is required to estimate its length in a formulated time order, he goes wildly wrong.

It is very tempting to believe that the fitting of units of skill into combined action first becomes urgent in connexion with concerted behaviour, where what one man does in a complex skilled production must harmonize with what another does. Then, while the time standard is an individual phenomenon, the time schedule is a social discovery, as many have held to be the case. But of this there is, of course, no proof.

The splitting of the stimulus field, and the order of its disintegration, are merely the environmental sides of all this. It is a character of all skill stimuli to be patterned, with certain central features dominant. The threshold range, rising for the central signals, gives less time for all the others, and those in the extreme margin get crowded out, while the others have to be dealt with in a hurry.

The fact that sensations of bodily origin become both more insistent and less attached to the skill is exactly what would be expected if this general picture is correct. There are two important points.

The proprioceptive impulses concerned are, in this case, additional stimuli, not, in fact, directly required by the skill, but set up in the course of the performance and capable of being used to improve the performance. When the stimuli and the skill split up, under the influence of increasing fatigue, the proprioceptive signals, like all the other stimuli, get accepted less and less in their relations to all the others, and more and more as individual occurrences. They then move in the direction of becoming veritable distractions, for they are not to be found among the original stimuli that set the skill going. If this were all that happened they would tend to become more and more marginal and, in accordance with the general rule, they might be expected to be increasingly ignored. But it is not all that happens. All the time the general drift in the operator is towards a less closely organized and effective central control. He is moving back towards a stage of behaviour which has many of the characters of an early phase in the history of increasing neuromuscular guidance. Evidence from many other sources shows that in this early stage sensations of bodily origin play a large part in directing behaviour. With the increase of weariness they get back their character of being pressing, interesting, very inadequately understood, less tied up with specific performance and more individual occurrences, attractive on their own account. They are not, therefore, easily ignored, but their function is persistently limited to their occurrence.

It seems possible to make a generalization about distractions and fatigue, though this must await more exact experimental confirmation. If distractions, or additional stimuli, can be woven into the general stimulus context the alert nervous system will use them and after a very brief initial disturbance, the skill will improve. With the onset of fatigue they fall apart from the performance once more, but if they represent important general factors in the acquisition of special forms of muscle control they cannot be ignored. Their threat is met with the characteristic increased effort of the early phases of central fatigue, but this effort will not be maintained. They then become hampering, obsessive and disagreeable.

At first sight the subjective symptoms of the fatigue characteristic of long continued skill all seem highly paradoxical. The widening of threshold range, the increasing inaccuracy of timed response, the dissociation of performance and of stimulus units – all these proceed or may proceed unwittingly. Yet the operator becomes more and more unreliable about the facts of his situation, he is more worried and possessed by physical discomfort and his irritability grows. He is at once more optimistic about his performance and pessimistic about his state. He asserts that he is doing well and at the same time he blames something or somebody else for making him do badly. The explanation perhaps is simple. He does not know *how* his bodily mechanisms are operating to achieve the required skill. Hardly anybody ever does, for skill does not depend on that kind of knowledge. He does know or suspect, however, that the task is not proceeding in quite the same way as at first and so he must have his excuses.

This is the beginning of the story of fatigue following highly skilled work. It is only the beginning and only the broad outlines are as yet available. If the details are to be filled in there must be more and more experiments. At least we know how to shape these experiments. We know that we must look less at what the fatigued man does, and more at how he does it. We must adopt as our criteria, not some measure of total effort, and not any necessary deterioration of specific and repeated reaction, but the widening of the threshold of range, the loss of accurate timing, the splitting up of stimulus and response patterns.

Perhaps it is not unfair to suggest also that this experiment has applications far beyond the limits of its own immediate purpose. For generations investigators have sought a fuller understanding of the functions of central nervous control. Frequently they have upset such control by fatigue, by drugs, by cutting out bits of brain structure and then have looked to see what is lost in the way of behaviour. Perhaps this is wrong. Perhaps we should try first and foremost, not to see what is lost or even what is left, but how that which is held is maintained.

The experimental investigations upon a study of which this lecture is mainly based was carried out at the request and with the support of the Flying Personnel Research Committee.

23 D. E. Broadbent

Differences and Interactions between Stresses

D. E. Broadbent, 'Differences and interactions between stresses', *Quarterly Journal of Experimental Psychology*, vol. 15, 1963, pp. 205–11.

Introduction

During the past twenty years or so, it has been demonstrated that each of a number of unpleasant environments affects human behaviour. High temperatures (Mackworth, 1950; Pepler, 1958), noise (Grimaldi, 1958; Jerison, 1957) and deprivation of sleep (Wilkinson, 1960; Williams, Lubin and Goodnow, 1959) are typical of the variables that have been studied and proved harmful. It has been usual, however, to consider each variable alone, and very often the investigation has enquired only whether the effects were undesirable, without analysing the type of effect more closely. Nevertheless it is desirable that one should understand the mechanism by which the effects of stress are produced. If that mechanism is the same for different stresses, the disorders of performance should be the same in the different cases. If they are different, the nature of the differences may shed some light upon the various mechanisms in play.

There is also a considerable practical problem of combined stresses. An environment which is hot may also be noisy: although there appears to be a critical temperature in the region of 81° F above which performance deteriorates, ought this to be set at a lower level when noise is also present? Are the effects of different stresses multiplicative, additive, or do they perhaps even cancel each other?

Systematic research on this point has been rare, presumably because there are even more combinations of stresses than there are simple stresses, and therefore the time required for investigation becomes considerable. Even if single stresses are being compared, the same task and the same type of subjects must be used in each case, and thus the whole research must normally take place in one laboratory. The following results are therefore a summary only of Cambridge research, and are correspondingly incomplete. It seems reasonable to conclude already, however, that different stresses do affect different mechanisms, and even to suggest the nature of some of the mechanisms.

Comparisons of Stresses

There are certain tasks which have been studied in several different stresses and on similar populations of naval ratings. The first of these is a serial-choice task, which lasts half an hour. The subject sits before a panel, on which there are five brass contacts arranged in an equilateral pentagon. There are also five lights, one corresponding to each of the contacts. (In some cases the lights are next to the contacts and in some cases mounted on a vertical panel in front of the subject. Although this later condition may perhaps require more practice, the particular results to be mentioned are not affected by it.) At the start of the period, one of the lights is on and the others are off. The subject touches the appropriate contact with a stylus and the light goes out. Another light immediately comes on, receives its response and so on. Thus the rate of work depends on the man himself, and provides a score. His errors also can be counted.

On this task the average rate of work remains constant during a period of half an hour under normal conditions (Broadbent, 1953; Pepler, 1959; Wilkinson, 1959). It is also the same in noise as in quiet (Broadbent, 1953, 1957) and in heat as at normal temperature (Pepler, 1959). But it is slower after loss of sleep (Pepler, 1959; Wilkinson, 1959).[1] Furthermore, the size of the effect of loss of sleep increases as the work-period goes on and may be entirely absent in the first five minutes.

The incorrect responses, on the other hand, become more frequent towards the end of a work period (Broadbent, 1953; Pepler, 1959). They are increased in noise, but this effect is greater at the end of the period and may be reversed in the first 5 minutes

1. By 'heat' in this context is meant an environment of 105° F dry-bulb and 95° F wet-bulb temperature. By 'noise' is meant continuous wide-band noise of 100 dB re. 0·0002 dynes/sq. cm; and by 'loss of sleep' one complete night's deprivation.

(Broadbent, 1953, 1957). They are not increased by loss of sleep (Pepler, 1959; Wilkinson, 1959), but do become more frequent in heat (Pepler, 1959). The latter effect remains constant in size throughout the work period.

Thus each stress has its own pattern of behaviour: loss of sleep affects speed but not errors and only does so at the end of the task, noise affects errors but not speed and does so at the end, while heat affects errors but not speed and does so at the beginning. It must immediately be said that these results do not imply that scores on other tasks, which may also be called 'speed' and 'errors', will be similarly affected. But since the task has been held constant, it is at least clear that the stresses differ in their effects.

A second task which has been used in several experiments is a pursuit-meter, in which the subjects followed a target pointer with another pointer controlled through a lever. The target oscillated with a mean frequency of 0·5 c.p.s., and the whole display was viewed through a diffuser which made it very difficult to see. On this task the discrepancy between the two pointers was integrated over time and provided a score which may be called 'error', although it is, of course, quite different from error in the serial-choice task: in the latter the subject had to do something to make an error, whereas in the pursuit-meter he would score highly in error if he did nothing at all. A second score was provided by the number of times the controlled pointer changes its direction of movement; this provides some indication of the extent to which the subject was in fact attempting to follow the target and is called the 'movement' score.

On this task the error score increases in heat (Pepler, 1959, 1960), after a loss of sleep (Pepler, 1959), in glare (Pepler, 1960) and under the distracting condition of hearing a faintly spoken passage from a thriller (Pepler, 1960). Thus this score does not appear to differentiate between the stresses, except perhaps in that the effect of loss of sleep shows more tendency to increase during the run than does the effect of heat. (This, it will be remembered, was also true on the serial-reaction task.) Heat and sleeplessness differ most markedly, however, in the movement score; whereas in heat there is an increase in that score, loss of sleep produces no such increase (Pepler, 1959). Glare and distracting speech give a definite decrease (Pepler, 1960). Thus in this task also, different stresses give different patterns of behaviour.

The interpretation of these patterns is, however, not completely clear. In the case of glare and distraction, it seems likely that there is an interference with perceptual processes and therefore the subjects not only do badly but also fail to perceive the extent of their error and do not try to correct it. By analogy one might suppose that the effect of sleeplessness is also perceptual but that the effect of heat is not. Therefore the latter stress is the only one in which increased error is accompanied by increased attempts to correct that error. Unfortunately, the pursuit-meter task has not been used in noise of intensity and duration similar to that employed as a stress on the serial-reaction task. Thus it remains unknown whether noise would resemble heat or loss of sleep on the movement score of the pursuit-meter.

Despite these uncertainties, it is clear that different stresses have quite different effects; and in general that loss of sleep gives an inert type of behaviour while high temperatures and noise give active but inaccurate types.

Interactions of Stresses

These differences in type of breakdown must imply that the stresses either affect different mechanisms or else that they affect the same mechanism to different extents: say in opposite directions. If two stresses act by quite different mechanisms, their effects should be independent of each other; and if they operate by manipulating the same mechanism in two opposite directions (say, one by raising and one by lowering a general level of arousal), then their effects should tend to cancel out. Thus by applying the two stresses together we should be able to separate these possibilities. In fact as will be seen, the present evidence suggests that heat affects an independent mechanism of its own whereas loss of sleep and noise affect the same mechanism in opposite directions. It might be for instance that one of them reduces and the other raises the general level of arousal.

To consider first the evidence for the independence of heat and loss of sleep, Pepler (1959) applied both stresses together and was unable to show any statistically significant interaction of their effects on either the serial-choice task or the pursuit-meter. Furthermore, there is some evidence that the two stresses are differently affected by incentives. In all the experiments using the serial-reaction task which have been described so far, the man performing the task had no information about his own success beyond that which he obtained from realization of his own errors and rate of work. It is possible to raise the subject's level of motivation by telling him every five minutes the number of correct and incorrect responses which he has made. When this stimulating and informative treatment is applied the man performs almost equally well whether sleepless or not (Wilkinson, 1961a). It is noteworthy that other forms of incentive, which do not inform the subject about his own performance, reduce the effect of loss of sleep (Corcoran, 1963b). Thus it is truly the motivating effects of knowledge of results, rather than the informative ones which oppose those of loss of sleep.

If now the effect of heat was mediated by the same mechanism as that of loss of sleep, it too should be reduced by incentives. Most unfortunately this experiment has not been carried out using the serial-reaction task but it has several times with other tasks (Mackworth, 1950; Pepler, 1958) and in no case has there been any sign of a reduction in the effect of heat by incentives. They improve performance, but they do so by the same amount whether the temperature is high or normal. Thus here again there is no evidence that the effects of heat have anything in common with those of loss of sleep.

When we compare the interaction of effects of noise with those of loss of sleep, however, the picture is quite different. Experiments on the application of both stresses together (Corcoran, 1962; Wilkinson, 1963) show that the effect of loss of sleep is less when loud noise is present; and a study of the effects of knowledge of results upon performance of the serial reaction task in noise (Wilkinson, 1963) shows that the effect of noise is greater when incentives are applied than when they are not. Thus the effects of noise and of loss of sleep oppose each other, at least in part.

Some authors, such as Hebb (1955), have suggested that men may be inefficient not only because of too low a level of arousal, but also because of too high a level (see Broen and Storms, 1961, for a recent review and discussion of this possibility). Since sleep is certainly connected in some way with the general level of arousal of the nervous system, it is possible that one of the stresses raises the level too high whereas the other reduces it too low. While a case might in the abstract be made for regarding continuous noise as de-arousing (because it masks out the usual varied background of auditory stimulation), and loss of sleep as over-arousing (because it means more exposure to stimulation), this view encounters various difficulties. First, the effects of incentives already mentioned would be surprising on such a theory. Incentives surely ought to be arousing, and therefore the stress which they cancel out should be de-arousing; and that is loss of sleep. Secondly, for similar reasons we would expect the effect of an over-arousing stress to be greater when the number of stimuli per minutes increases in a task which otherwise remains the same. But Corcoran (1963a) has shown that loss of sleep affects a task less when the rate of stimulation is greater. Thirdly, Wilkinson (1961b) has found that individuals with relatively high muscle tension are those who show less effect of loss of sleep: and this would be surprising if sleeplessness were de-arousing. Fourthly, in unstimulating tasks it has been found by Corcoran (1963b) that physiological measures show signs of lowered arousal after loss of sleep, even though in stimulating tasks the reverse may be the case (Malmo, 1959).

It is therefore a more plausible hypothesis that loud noise is over-arousing because it represents too high a level of stimulation; and that this effect is greater when incentives are applied since they may be supposed to bring the level of arousal up to its optimum even in the absence of noise. Loss of sleep on the other hand reduces the level of arousal to a dangerous extent, but is less likely to do so when incentives are present. Such a view is also consistent with the type of breakdown which occurs on the serial-reaction task under the two stresses; with loss of sleep the man does badly by doing little whereas in noise he does badly by doing the wrong thing.

Some Difficulties and Omissions

The most major difficulty in the foregoing account is that both sleeplessness and noise have their greatest impact at the end of a work period than the beginning. If noise were hyper-arousing, it surely ought to have its main effect at the start of work before the task becomes familiar and monotonous. Some addition is therefore needed to the simple theory that sleeplessness and noise are opposite in their effects: there might perhaps be some other consequence of continuous work which makes the man inefficient and then sleeplessness or noise determines the way in which the inefficiency shows itself.

Another point which requires more examination is the relationship of heat to the other stresses. From everyday experience one would have thought that very high temperatures made it difficult to sleep, but moderately high ones were distinctly soporific: and it may therefore be only the particular condition of 105° dry-bulb and 95° wet-bulb that is independent of the arousal mechanism. Furthermore, although the experiment of Pepler (1959) shows quite clearly that, for instance speed on the serial-reaction task shows no interaction between heat and loss of sleep, yet there was an interaction (even though statistically insignificant) on the movement score of the pursuit-meter. Thus there may possibly be some marginal effects of heat which do interact with those of loss of sleep even though we can be sure of a large area of independence. It would also be desirable to study the combined effects of heat and noise, which ought to show no interaction if our other conclusions are sound. Indeed, Viteles and Smith (1946) did study various combinations of noise and temperature and concluded that there was no interaction between them. Their noise levels were all lower than those in the other experiments cited, and their tasks and subjects were, of course, different but at least it can be said that their conclusions raise no difficulty for our view that noise and sleeplessness are polar opposites while heat is a stress of a different kind.

It would also be desirable, as has been noted, to study the interaction of knowledge of results and heat on the serial reaction task, since so far this combination has only been used with other tasks. The interaction of incentives with noise should also be examined using incentives other than knowledge of results: although as already indicated other incentives have been shown by Corcoran to reduce the effect of loss of sleep, it is likely that different types of incentives are different in their nature. Williams,

Lubin and Goodnow (1959) did not find an interaction of loss of sleep and knowledge of results, perhaps, as they say, because their knowledge of results did not possess a very strong incentive character: or possibly, of course, because of differences in task and subject sample from those used in Cambridge.

Other studies which should be done in noise concern the individual differences, and the effect of varying the frequency of signals in the task. If the general view of sleeplessness as under-arousing and noise as over-arousing is not an over-simplification, those men with the highest muscle tension in noise should be the most impaired in efficiency; since in sleeplessness the reverse is true. (This point was drawn to my attention by Air Comdr W. K. Stewart, R.A.F.) Furthermore we would expect a task with a high signal frequency to show bigger effects than a task with a low frequency. To some extent the latter comparison has been made and the prediction confirmed by Jerison (1957, 1959). There were, however, other differences between his tasks, and he himself considered that the necessity for division of attention was the crucial variable in making a task vulnerable to noise. Further work on this point is in progress.

Another profitable field for further study would be the use of drugs to raise and lower arousal, in combination with other stresses. To put the point crudely, it might be that sedatives will reduce the ill effects of noise on efficiency. It is noteworthy that a study of the effects of a tranquillizer on the serial-reaction test (Steinberg, 1959) has shown that the ill effects are much less when knowledge of results is given, so that the action of the drug appears similar in this respect to that of sleeplessness. Admittedly the effects in this case were on errors rather than speed, and this points to a difference between the two variables. On the other hand, the sample of subjects was very different from those used in the other experiments cited and this might be the reason for the difference.

All these areas of research clearly require investigation, and any of them may yield results inconsistent with the simple theory based on the concept of arousal which has been put forward in this paper. Perhaps the main weakness in such a theory is already evident, however: it can explain both rises and falls in efficiency with equal ease when almost any treatment is applied to a man.

This point has already been discussed (Broadbent, 1963); it obviously means that very stringent precautions must be taken to tie down the exact level of arousal at which particular predictions are supposed to apply. So far, little has been done in

Table 1

The Summarized Effects of Three Stresses on the Serial-Reaction Test as far as Present Evidence Goes

	Speed	Errors	Place in work period where effect appears	Effect of incentives	Interaction with	
					Heat	Noise
Heat	no effect	increased	throughout	(no change in effect*)	—	(none)
Noise	no effect*	increased*	end*	increases effect	(none)	—
Loss of sleep	reduction*	no effect*	end*	decreases effect*	none	reduced effect*

Results in brackets are not from the serial-reaction test and are therefore not strictly comparable.

*These results are from more than one experiment and are therefore particularly trustworthy.

this way. Whatever the fate of the concept of arousal, however, it does seem clear that heat, noise and sleeplessness are not to be lumped indistinguishably together under the single label of stress; for each produces distinctive effects. Heat on the whole seems to impair performance by a mechanism of its own, while noise and sleeplessness act on some common mechanism in opposite directions.

References

BROADBENT, D. E. (1953), 'Noise, paced performance, and vigilance tasks', Brit. J. Psychol., vol. 44, pp. 295–303.

BROADBENT, D. E. (1957), 'Effects of noise and low frequency upon behaviour', Ergonomics, vol. 1, pp. 21–9.

BROADBENT, D. E. (1963), 'Possibilities and difficulties in the concept of arousal', in Vigilance: a Symposium, McGraw-Hill.

BROEN, W. F., and STORMS, L. H. (1961), 'A reaction potential ceiling and response decrements in complex situations', Psychol. Rev., vol. 68, pp. 405–15.

CORCORAN, D. W. (1962), 'Noise and loss of sleep', Quart. J. exp. Psychol., vol. 14, pp. 178–82.

CORCORAN, D. W. (1963a), 'Doubling the rate of presentation in a vigilance task during a long sleep deprivation', *J. appl. Psychol.*, vol. 47, pp. 412–15.

CORCORAN, D. W. (1963b), Individual differences in the effect of loss of sleep, *Ph.D. Thesis, University of Cambridge.*

GRIMALDI, J. W. (1958), 'Sensori-motor performance under varying noise conditions', *Ergonomics*, vol. 2, pp. 34–43.

HEBB, D. O. (1955), 'Drives and the C.N.S. (Conceptual Nervous System)', *Psychol. Rev.*, vol. 62, pp. 243–54.

JERISON, H. J. (1957), 'Performance on a simple vigilance task in noise and quiet', *J. acoust. Soc. Amer.*, vol. 29, pp. 1163–5.

JERISON, H. J. (1959), 'Effects of noise on human performance', *J. appl. Psychol.*, vol. 43, pp. 96–101.

MACKWORTH, N. H. (1950), Researches in the measurement of human performance. *M.R.C. Report Series, no. 268,* H.M.S.O.

MALMO, R. B. (1959), 'Activation: a neuropsychological dimension', *Psychol. Rev.*, vol. 66, pp. 367–86.

PEPLER, R. D. (1958), 'Warmth and performance: an investigation in the tropics', *Ergonomics*, vol. 2, pp. 63–88.

PEPLER, R. D. (1959), 'Warmth and lack of sleep: accuracy or activity reduced', *J. comp. physiol. Psychol.*, vol. 52, pp. 466–50.

PEPLER, R. D. (1960), 'Warmth, glare and a background of quiet speech: a comparison of their effects on performance', *Ergonomics*, vol. 3, pp. 68–73.

STEINBERG, H. (1959), 'Effects of drugs on performance and incentives', in D. R. Laurence (ed.), *Quantitative Methods in Human Pharmacology and Therapeutics*, Pergamon.

VITELES, M. S., and SMITH, K. R. (1946), 'An experimental investigation of the effect of change in atmospheric conditions and noise upon performance', *Trans. Amer. Soc. Heat. Vent. Engrs.*, vol. 52, pp. 167–82.

WILKINSON, R. T. (1959), 'Rest pauses in a task affected by a lack of sleep', *Ergonomics*, vol. 2, pp. 373–80.

WILKINSON, R. T. (1960), 'The effect of lack of sleep on visual watch-keeping', *Quart. J. exp. Psychol.*, vol. 12, pp. 36–40.

WILKINSON, R. T. (1961a), 'Interaction of lack of sleep with knowledge of results, repeated testing and individual differences', *J. exp. Psychol.*, vol. 62, pp. 263–71.

WILKINSON, R. T. (1961b), 'Effects of sleep deprivation on performance and muscle tension', in *The Nature of Sleep*, Ciba Foundation Symposium, Churchill.

WILKINSON, R. T. (1963), 'The interaction of noise with loss of sleep and knowledge of results', *J. exp. Psychol.*, vol. 66, pp. 332–7.

WILLIAMS, H. L., LUBIN, A., and GOODNOW, J. J. (1959), 'Impaired performance with acute sleep loss', *Psychol. Monogr.*, vol. 73, no. 14.

24 G. C. Drew, W. P. Colquhoun and H. A. Long

Effect of Small Doses of Alcohol on a Skill Resembling Driving

G. C. Drew, W. P. Colquhoun and H. A. Long, 'Effect of small doses of alcohol on a skill resembling driving', *British Medical Journal*, vol. 5103, 1958, pp. 993–9.

Since the drinking of alcohol in one form or another is so common a characteristic of the social life of man in a variety of cultures, it would seem important that as much as possible should be known both of its physiological effects and of its effects on behaviour. In fact, at the present time, very little precise information is available, in spite of an extensive literature on the subject. This literature has been reviewed, more or less comprehensively, periodically since the early part of this century (Darrow, 1929; Drew, 1950; Emerson, 1933; Fisk, 1917; Jellinek and McFarland, 1940; M.R.C. Alcohol Investigation Committee, 1938).

The most striking feature to emerge from any such review is the marked lack of agreement between authors, amounting in many instances to direct contradiction of one another. This is especially true of the effects of smaller doses. Perhaps not surprisingly, doses of intoxicating strength have generally resulted in deterioration in efficiency in almost all aspects of behaviour tested. For doses below this level, however, the picture is not clear.

Some authors have reported deterioration in performance however small the dose, some have failed to find any effects, while several have shown actual improvements following doses of the order of one single whisky.

In part these discrepant findings reflect the unreliability of many of the results in this field but in part they arise from the complexity of the effects of alcohol.

For moderate and intoxicating levels it has been established that the effect of alcohol is related to its concentration in the blood and that the blood/alcohol concentration obtained from a given ingested dose depends both on the body weight of the recipient and on the rate at which the alcohol is absorbed into the blood (Winton and Bayliss, 1948). The rate of absorption, in turn, has been found to be dependent on the amount, type, and dilution of alcohol, the contents of the stomach, and the drinking habits of the individual (Goldberg, 1951).

Previous reports further suggest that, apart from a slowly developed tolerance to alcohol from repeated exposure to it over a number of years, known as habituation, there is also a more rapid adaptation to each dose consumed, so that it has a greater effect when the blood alcohol level is rising than when it is falling (Eggleton, 1955; Goldberg, 1951; Mellanby, 1919; Miles, 1924).

The nature of the task used is also important. Goldberg (1943) has shown that some tasks are more readily impaired by a given dose than are others. Familiar tasks, too, deteriorate less than ones that are unfamiliar (Jellinek and McFarland, 1940). The method of measuring change in performance is often of great importance. The additional stimulation provided by a new task frequently enables the subject to compensate, for a short time, for conditions which have produced an over-all reduction in his efficiency. For this reason, short interpolated tests may fail altogether to measure this deterioration and may show normal or even above normal efficiency (Drew, 1942). Reasonably long-lasting tests seem necessary unless the deficiency is a gross one. Welford (1951) has stressed the importance, for the analysis of skilled behaviour, of measuring different aspects of performance, since relatively gross measures may obscure changes in the way in which different actions are integrated in the final performance.

The wide individual variations in performance in response to alcohol remaining when the above factors are taken into account have been attributed to temperamental differences, and especially to those differences related to extraversion–introversion.

Differences along this dimension have been noted in other contexts. Extraverts have been shown to be relatively less concerned with accuracy of performance (Himmelweit, 1946), to deteriorate more rapidly during continuous work (Broadbent, 1956; Eysenck, 1957a) and to be less consistent in performance (Venables, 1956). It has, furthermore, often been noticed, when giving depressant drugs to psychiatric patients, that a given dose has a greater effect on patients with hysterical disorders than on anxiety and depressive patients. A theory postulating a greater amount of cortical control for introverts and a greater suscepti- bility of extraverts to depressant drugs due to the reduction of cortical control was first put forward by McDougall (1929) and has recently been extended by Eysenck (1957b). Experimental confirmation of the greater susceptibility of extraverts to the depressant action of amylobarbitone sodium has been published by Shagass (1954, 1956).

The aims of this experiment were to investigate the effect of small doses of alcohol on a complex skill, resembling driving; to relate any changes found to the level of blood alcohol; to see whether individual differences in response to alcohol could be explained in terms of previous experience or of temperamental differences, when every effort had been made to minimize differ- ences in blood alcohol level; and, finally, to investigate the accuracy with which blood alcohol level could be estimated by measuring the alcohol excreted in urine and in breath. This article is a preliminary report of the main results of the experiment which was carried out on behalf of the Road Users' Committee appointed jointly by the Medical Research Council and the Road Research Board (Department of Scientific and Industrial Re- search). Full details will be published later by the Medical Research Council.[1]

Experimental Method

In deciding upon the task to be used, two considerations had to be borne in mind: that the task would need to be a continuous one of reasonably long duration and that such a task runs the risk of becoming extremely boring for subjects. It was finally decided that an apparatus known as the 'Miles motor driving trainer' provided the best compromise between a task, perfor- mance on which could be scored adequately, and one which had the motivating capacity of a real-life situation.

1. G. C. Drew, W. P. Colquhoun and H. A. Long, *Effect of Small Doses of Alcohol on a Skill Resembling Driving*, H.M.S.O., 1959. [*Ed.*]

In this apparatus the subject sits in a dummy car, facing a translucent screen in a darkened room. Behind the screen is a 'perspex' disk with a road scene painted on it. This road scene is projected, very much magnified, on the screen by a lamp on the perspex surface. As the driver operates the accelerator and steering-wheel to change his speed and direction of movement, the car appears to progress along the road. The effect is reasonably realistic, and the task bears some resemblance to driving in that non-drivers find the machine difficult to control without considerable practice, whilst experienced drivers have little difficulty with it. Though the central task is very similar to driving, it differs from it in being completely devoid of danger and emergencies. The track used was a continuous winding circuit, the equivalent of slightly over one mile in length. Its repetitive nature was not very apparent to the subjects and had considerable advantages for scoring in presenting the same objective task to the subjects at all stages of the trial.

The main aspects of performance to be scored were accuracy of tracking, speed of driving and the control movements of steering-wheel, accelerator, brake, clutch and gear lever. Of the latter, only steering-wheel and accelerator pedal movements proved worth considering. Accuracy of tracking, measured in terms of deviations from a course parallel to the left-hand kerb, and steering-wheel and accelerator pedal movements were recorded graphically and simultaneously scored on counters, photographed once each lap. Separate recording was made of the number of collisions of the car with the side of the road; 'hunting' movements of the steering-wheel too small to change the car's direction; gear changes; identification marks for lap completion and major corners; and a time mark.

The subjects were forty volunteers from the staff of the Road Research Laboratory. Their ages ranged from 23 to 40 years, except for one subject aged 58. The mean age was 31 years. Five of the subjects were women. All were in good health and held a current driving licence. The majority reported that they took alcohol only occasionally.

The alcohol was administered orally as analar grade absolute alcohol, diluted to a 20 per cent solution and flavoured to disguise the alcohol content. Haggard, Greenberg and Cohen (1943)

G. C. Drew, W. P. Colquhoun and H. A. Long

found that the toxic effect of alcohol varied considerably even within the same kind of spirit owing, apparently, to the presence, in minute quantities, of substances related to the original distilling. They found that, after very careful distilling, absolute alcohol was less toxic than any of the other forms tried. As analar grade absolute alcohol was used in this experiment, it seems probable that the results reported here represent minimum effects for these quantities and concentrations. Equivalent amounts of alcohol taken as beer or spirits could be expected to have somewhat greater effects.

This investigation was concerned with blood alcohol concentrations of less than 100 mg per 100 ml of blood, since this is the figure recommended by the National Safety Council of America (1953) as the limit of 'safe' and only 'possibly under the influence'. To achieve these concentrations, doses were given of 0·00 (placebo), 0·20, 0·35, 0·50 and 0·65 g of alcohol per kg of body weight. In terms of the concentrations used by Cohen, Dearnaley and Hansel (1958) these doses represent approximately 18, 31, 44 and 57 ml of absolute alcohol for an 11-stone (70-kg) man. The largest dose is the approximate equivalent of 3 pints (1700 ml) of 'average' beer or 5 fl. oz (142 ml) of whisky for an 11-st (70-kg) man.

In view of the expected wide individual variations, and of the difficulty of defining a 'correct' performance on such a task as this, it was decided to use each subject as his own control. That is, the effect of alcohol was measured as the degree of change in performance of each subject against his own performance without alcohol. To minimize practice effects, a latin square design was used, each square containing five subjects and five doses. This square was repeated eight times with different subjects. The women subjects were assigned to one square. Each subject was tested on the same day of the week for five consecutive weeks. Thus each subject received every dose.

Subjects were given preliminary practice to familiarize them with the task, and information was obtained on body weight, age, driving experience and drinking habits. (They were asked not to drink on the evening before a trial.) On the morning of the trial the subject took a fat-free breakfast and 2 to 2½ hr later, at 10 a.m., the first urine sample was collected to provide a check on ketones and residual alcohol and to empty the bladder. (In a subsidiary experiment, urine samples were taken with a full bladder.) He was then given his drink and requested to finish it within 10 min. After a further 10 min he entered the apparatus and was instructed to drive as he normally would in a real car and not to stop until told to do so, unless an emergency arose. The subject drove for 20 min and then had a 10-min break, during which the blood, urine and breath samples were collected. There followed three further 20-min periods of driving, and 10-min rest pauses during which samples were taken. Each experimental series lasted $2\frac{1}{2}$ hr.

Approximately 0·5 ml of blood was taken from the thumb on each sampling occasion and the blood and urine samples were analysed at the South-Western Forensic Science Laboratory, at Bristol, by the microanalytic modified Cavett method recommended by the B.M.A. Committee (Kent-Jones and Taylor 1954). Samples taken on the alcohol-free days were usually discarded but occasionally were used as a check on the analytic procedure. Readings from three instruments for the measurement of breath alcohol were recorded at the time of blood sampling on a number of occasions. The breath analysis instruments used were the 'alcometer' (Greenberg and Keator, 1941), the 'drunko-meter' (Harger, Lamb, and Hulpieu, 1938) and the 'breathalyser' (Borkenstein).

The subjects were given a battery of personality tests, from which only the measures of extraversion are considered in this paper. Tests included the Minnesota Multiphasic Personality Inventory, the Maudsley Personality Inventory and the Bernreuter Personality Inventory.

Alcohol Concentration

Blood analysis

The means and standard deviations of each dose, in mg per 100 ml of blood, are given in Table 1. It will be observed that peak concentrations for the four doses were roughly 20, 40, 60 and 80 mg per 100 ml of blood. The doses used, therefore, have been effective in producing concentrations normally regarded as low or 'safe'. It will be seen from the standard deviations that there is relatively little overlap between the concentrations following different doses, implying that the technique of adjusting the absolute quantity of alcohol given to total body weight produces reasonably consistent blood alcohol values. The change in the mean blood alcohol values for each dose through time is shown in Figure 1. Following each dose, blood alcohol rises steeply to a

Table 1

Mean Blood Alcohol Levels and Standard Deviations, Following Four Doses of Ingested Alcohol

Dose	Time After Drinking in Minutes							
	30		60		90		120	
	Mean	S.D.	Mean	S.D.	Mean	S.D.	Mean	S.D.
1. (0·20 g/kg)	23	10	19	9	13	8	6	5
2. (0·35 g/kg)	36	15	37	10	30	9	20	9
3. (0·50 g/kg)	58	14	59	11	51	12	39	10
4. (0·65 g/kg)	74	19	77	12	71	14	62	15

maximum, reached somewhere between 30 and 60 min after drinking, and then falls off in an approximately linear way. There is a tendency for the peak concentration to occur slightly later as the dose increases. That following the largest dose gives a mean time of nine minutes later than that for the smallest. For some subjects, measurements were taken up to 6 hr after drinking. Dose 1 fell to near zero concentration by the end of 2 hr, dose 2 at about 4 hr, dose 3 at rather over 5 hr, and at 6 hr the mean concentration following dose 4 was still 20 mg per 100 ml. Once the peak was passed blood alcohol levels fell, on average, by approximately 10 mg per 100 ml per hr.

Urine analysis

Full details of the urine and breath analysis will be given in the main report. The concentration of alcohol in urine built up more slowly, reaching a peak concentration between 20 and 25 min later than that in the blood. After the peak was passed the fall-off paralleled that in the blood, the value at any given time being

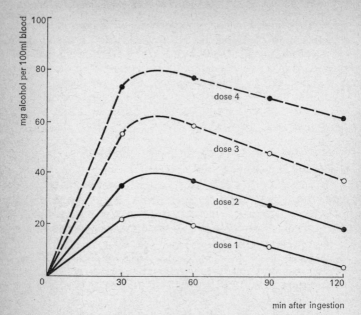

Figure 1 Relation between the level of alcohol in the blood and time after ingestion, for four levels of alcohol. Each point is the mean of forty subjects

proportionately higher. The over-all ratio of urine to blood alcohol was 1·252 : 1. When the samples were taken with the bladder full, values were slightly more variable, but did not differ significantly from those taken after the bladder had been emptied. Correlating the urine alcohol level with that in the blood 30 min earlier, to make an approximate correction for the time lag, gives a product–moment correlation of $r = +0.92$.

Breath analysis

Of the instruments used to analyse alcohol in expired breath, the breathalyser proved most satisfactory. It proved highly reliable and gave values corresponding closely to the blood alcohol values, having a constant error of $+2$ mg per 100 ml. Some difficulties were experienced with the other instruments used. In 95 per cent of the comparisons the breathalyser values lay within ± 21 mg per 100 ml of the blood alcohol readings, the drunkometer within ±22 to 26 mg per 100 ml, depending on the operating technique used, and the alcometer within ±34 mg per 100 ml.

Performance Changes

The aspects of performance measured concerned the accuracy of tracking, the speed at which the task was taken and the operation of the controls.

The accuracy measures consisted, firstly, of tracking error (the amount of deviation across the road surface from a track parallel to the left-hand kerb) and kerb-bumpings (the more serious error of colliding with the side of the road). Secondly, two detailed accuracy measures were obtained – positioning of the car relative to the left-hand side (this was measured on a sample of ten subjects for no-alcohol and dose 4), and consistency in car positioning at a corner in the circuit (measured, for thirty-five subjects, as the range of differences in negotiating the same corner on six successive occasions in the second driving period under each dose condition).

Speed was recorded as the number of seconds taken to complete one lap. The total amount of steering-wheel movement made will be the only aspect of control movements considered here.

All scores were expressed as a summed score per lap, and were then averaged over 5 min. The 5-min averages were then summed over 20 min. They were subjected to a variety of statistical treatments, including analysis of variance. Regression lines and coefficients of correlation are used here.

The results are presented in terms of group effects, followed by some discussion of individual differences in response to alcohol and their relationship to other personal characteristics. A table of the mean effects of alcohol for each scoring category is given in the Appendix.

Group Effects

Practice effects varied in the different performance measures. Tracking error showed very little change with practice, but there was a progressive increase in speed of driving throughout the experiment. Time per lap and tracking error were negatively correlated ($r = -0.39$), but correction of error scores for increased speed makes little difference to the over-all picture. Steering-wheel movement shows a pronounced practice effect in a progressive and marked reduction in the amount of movement throughout the experiment.

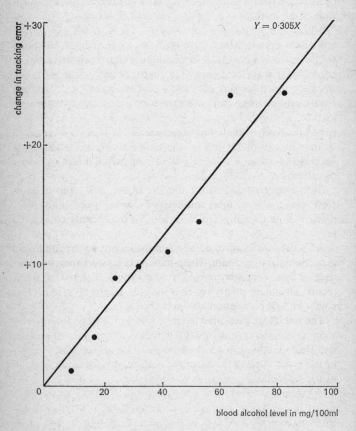

Figure 2 Regression of tracking error on blood alcohol level. Each point is the mean of eighty paired values

Effect of alcohol on accuracy

Accuracy of steering, in a complex task of this kind, decreases progressively as blood alcohol increases, even with the low concentrations used in this experiment. Furthermore, there is, from the group effects, no evidence of a threshold. Instead, there is a measurable increase in mean error as soon as there is a measurable quantity of alcohol in the blood. The relation between accuracy, expressed as tracking error, and blood alcohol is shown in Figure 2. This shows the regression of error on blood alcohol. The regression is highly significant ($p < 0.001$). This is confirmed by an analysis of variance, which shows a relation of error and blood alcohol significant at better than the 0.01 level of probability. The mean increase in error for the 80 mg per 100 ml concentration compared with no-alcohol performance is about 16 per cent.

It has been noted above that blood alcohol concentration shows a characteristic change with time after drinking, showing, first, a steep rise to a maximum value, followed by a slow return to normal. Tracking error shows a very similar pattern with time after drinking. The close correspondence of the rise and fall through time of blood alcohol and tracking error is shown in Figure 3. In this figure, tracking error scores are expressed as the mean score for each driving period. Blood alcohol concentrations have therefore been expressed in the same way. The rise and fall of urine alcohol, expressed similarly, have been included. The figure for urine alcohol has been reduced by one-fifth (in view of the ratio of $1.252 : 1$) to enable it to be presented on the same scale. Although only the largest dose has been plotted, the data for the other doses follow the same pattern.

It can be seen that urine alcohol reaches a maximum about 20 min later than blood alcohol. The error curve looks as though its peak would occur somewhere between the two. The calculation of lag correlations confirms this. Maximum correlations are obtained when error scores are correlated with blood values some 10 min earlier and with urine values some 10 min later. From this it would appear that maximum error slightly lags in time behind the maximum blood alcohol and slightly precedes maximum urine alcohol.

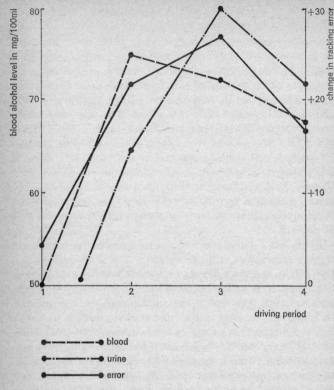

Figure 3 Rise and fall of blood alcohol, error score and urine alcohol with time after drinking. (Urine alcohol levels reduced by one-fifth.) Each point is mean of forty subjects

Product–moment correlation of the rise and fall of blood alcohol and the rise and fall of error is positive and significant. The mean correlation of the four paired values, calculated separately for each individual, is $r = +0.271$, with p lying between 0.01 and 0.02. The size of this correlation, though significant, seems small. It will be seen from Figure 3 that there is a time lag between the two variables with an inverted relationship in periods 2–3. This, and the clustering of points in the second, third and fourth driving periods, probably have reduced the size of the correlation. When blood alcohol values at 5-min intervals, obtained by interpolation from the individual curves, are correlated with the 5-min error scores, allowing a much smaller lag than the 20-min scores, the correlation rises to $r = +0.89$. Because the test ends before blood alcohol has dropped very markedly, it is not possible from these scores to say whether error scores recover more quickly than blood alcohol levels, though inspection of Figure 3 shows that the slope of error scores in the last half hour is steeper than for blood alcohol. The frequency of kerb-bumping rises steeply to a maximum, for each dose, with blood alcohol, and falls almost equally steeply after the maximum has been passed.

In an attempt to interpret the increased error with increased blood alcohol, records were sampled for mean position on the road surface, amount of swing about this position and consistency of behaviour on corners. Significant differences were found. Without alcohol, subjects tended to drive on the left-hand side of the road, to remain on that side for relatively long periods – that is, with relatively little 'wobble' – and rapidly to correct swings to the right by moving back to the left once more. The effect of alcohol appears to be to produce a shift of the mean driving line from the left towards the crown of the road ($p < 0.01$). With increasing dosage there is an increasing swing or 'wobble' about this new, more central position ($p < 0.01$), together with a tendency to tolerate swings to the right but rapidly to correct swings to the left ($p < 0.01$). There was, furthermore, greater variability in the positioning of the car in negotiating a corner ($p < 0.01$).

Effect of alcohol on speed

In this experiment there were no clear-cut group effects on speed of driving. Mean driving speeds are insignificantly different for all doses. Variability in speed around a mean shows a tendency to rise and fall through time with blood alcohol rise and fall, but this again is not significant. It is possible that the large effect of practice on speed is camouflaging any alcohol effect for the group. Changes in speed of driving after alcohol were found to be closely related to personality characteristics. These are discussed below.

Effect of alcohol on steering-wheel movement

Like error, steering-wheel movement increases progressively as blood alcohol increases. The regression of amount of change of steering-wheel movement on blood alcohol is shown in Figure 4. This regression is linear and is highly significant ($p < 0.001$).

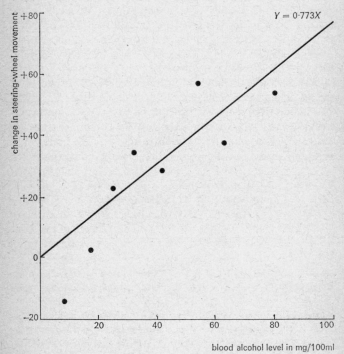

Figure 4 Regression of steering-wheel movement on blood alcohol level. Each point is the mean of eighty paired values

There is also a decrease in the consistency of steering-wheel movement after alcohol ($p < 0.01$). The decrease in consistency appears to be due to a greater variability in the timing of responses to a corner.

As might be expected, the amount of steering-wheel movement is related to the amount of tracking error made. The relationship is U-shaped, such that there is an optimum amount of movement for controlling the car, both less and more movement resulting in increased error. Following alcohol there is an increasing tendency to make either too little or too much movement in negotiating a particular corner, though the predominant effect is to make too much.

Individual Differences in Response to Alcohol

Although the latin square design used makes comparison of the performances of individuals difficult, certain features nevertheless emerge. There is undoubtedly a considerable range of individual variation in response to alcohol. This is summarized in Table 2

Table 2

Number of Subjects Showing Different Percentage
Change in Scores After Alcohol (Dose 4)

Measure	Percentage Change of Score											
	Decrease				Increase							
	−50	−40	−30	−20	−10	+10	+20	+30	+40	+50	+60	+70
Error	1	0	2	2	5	10	12	4	2	2	—	—
Steering-wheel movement	—	—	—	3	5	12	13	3	3	—	—	1
Time	—	—	5	11	13	5	2	—	—	—	—	

which gives the number of subjects changing their score after alcohol by varying amounts. The changes are expressed as percentage change from their own no-alcohol score. Tracking error shows a wide scatter. Though the distribution is fairly heavily skewed towards increased error after alcohol, ten of the forty subjects show reduced error, one as much as 50 per cent reduction. This subject, however, showed also one of the largest reductions in speed and achieved a high degree of accuracy by driving extremely slowly. Time scores, on the other hand, are distributed fairly normally around the 'no change' position.

An attempt has been made to relate these individual differences in response to alcohol to various personal characteristics. No relationship was found between response to alcohol and differences in initial level of skill, previous driving experience, age, sex or drinking habits. The subjects varied widely in their initial level of skill and in previous driving experience, so the lack of relationship between these variables and alcohol effect may be stated with some confidence. The range of drinking habits, however, was small, so that the comparison was between the few individuals who drank once or twice a week and those who drank very rarely. The range was therefore too small to draw conclusions on the lack of relationship.

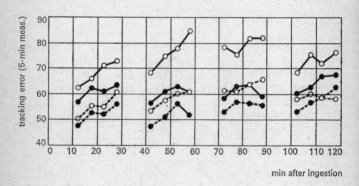

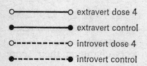

Figure 5 Comparison of the tracking error of extraverts and introverts under no alcohol and dose 4 conditions (extraverts, $n = 7$; introverts, $n = 9$)

Scores obtained, for thirty-five subjects, on the extraversion scale of the Maudsley Personality Inventory were well distributed. The mean was 10·24 (sigma 4·53) as compared with the standard norm of 10·94 (sigma 4·74). Performance scores were compared for a group of subjects scoring high in extraversion and a group scoring low. Figure 5 shows the mean differences in tracking performance between the resulting seven extraverts and nine introverts. The extravert group made more error ($p < 0.05$), were less consistent in car positioning ($p < 0.05$), and showed a bigger increase in error during each period of driving ($p < 0.01$). The effect of alcohol on error was greater for the extravert group ($p < 0.05$), the extraverts having an average increase of 23 per cent and the introverts of 6 per cent.

The extraverts responded to alcohol in a similar manner, but the introverts showed more varied responses. For example, the extraverts all increased their tracking error after alcohol, whereas two of the introverts made less error. This is especially clearly shown in the effect of alcohol on speed of driving. The extraverts showed very little change of speed after alcohol, but the introverts changed considerably. The nearer the introvert end of the scale they were, the more speed changed. They subdivided, however, into two distinct groups, one of which speeded up very considerably and the other slowed down. It has not so far been possible to relate this to any personal characteristics. Figure 6 shows the regression of change of speed on extraversion–introversion as measured by the Bernreuter Neurotic Inventory. This regression is linear and is significant at the 5 per cent level. Comparing those scoring more than 50 on the Bernreuter with those scoring less than this in terms of whether they change speed by more or less than 8 units gives χ^2 significant at better than 0.01. It would appear that personality characteristics – at least those of the extravert–introvert dimension – are related to the effects of alcohol.

Discussion

It is now generally agreed that a relationship exists between the concentration of alcohol in the blood and the appearance of clinical signs of intoxication. The definition of intoxication based on clinical evidence is, however, a variable one. Lijestrand (1940) gives evidence of a considerable variation in diagnoses made by different clinicians on people who all had blood alcohol concentrations between 100 and 150 mg per 100 ml. Moreover, the range of blood alcohol concentrations at which people are

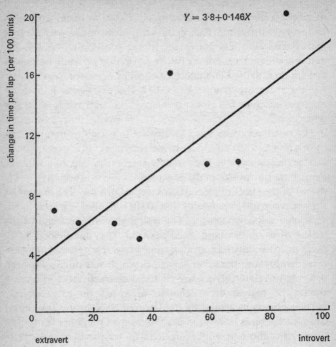

Figure 6 Regression of change of speed after alcohol on extravert–introvert score. Each point plotted is the mean of five subjects

judged intoxicated is very wide. Goldberg (1951) has shown that the level at which 50 per cent of people are judged clinically to be intoxicated varies with the legal definition in different countries. In America it has been defined by the National Safety Council as 150 mg per 100 ml in Sweden it is 100–120 mg per 100 ml, and in Denmark and Norway 80 mg per 100 ml.

The level of alcohol in the blood at which people are diagnosed clinically to be intoxicated, besides being variable, tends to be high in comparison with the concentrations used here. This is not surprising, since an estimate of impaired behaviour is made in the absence of any criterion of normal behaviour for that individual, so that the impairment must be obvious before it is detected, and since it is known that people can compensate for their reduced efficiency over the short periods of time during which they are examined. It does not follow, however, that, because no impairment is found in clinical tests, more complex skills, like driving, will also be unaffected.

The present study shows that performance begins to deteriorate with very low blood alcohol concentrations, certainly of the order of 20–30 mg per 100 ml, and that the deterioration is progressive and linearly related to blood alcohol level. There is, in this study, no evidence of a threshold effect.

The impairment of performance was shown most clearly in the operation of the controls. As the aim of the task was primarily to track, it is perhaps not surprising that in attempting to retain a level of accuracy the operation of the steering-wheel should be most affected. Efficiency in using the steering-wheel is indicated by the amount of tracking error which results. With practice the amount of steering-wheel movement made goes down without a reduction in the accuracy of tracking, whereas after alcohol tracking error increases despite an increase in steering-wheel movement. This suggests that timing of the steering-wheel movement was upset. The decrease in consistency of the movements required to negotiate a corner supports this view. The importance of timing of control movements in a complex skill has been stressed previously by Bartlett (1943), and adverse conditions such as fatigue have been shown to have a marked effect on timing (Drew, 1942; Russell Davis, 1948).

The work of Cohen, Dearnaley and Hansel (1958) is interesting additional evidence. While the task used in this present study reasonably reflects the tracking aspect of driving, it is almost completely free of hazard and risk taking. These authors have shown that an amount of alcohol not much larger than the biggest dose used in this experiment produced a significant increase in the hazards in which drivers became involved. From the two studies it is reasonable to assume that not only will drivers become involved in greater hazards with this amount of alcohol but they will be less efficient in dealing with them.

It is suggested, furthermore, that the results reported here show that the level of alcohol in the blood is a good indicator of the extent of impairment of performance. It may be pointed out that the blood alcohol levels reported by Cohen *et al.* (1958) seem surprisingly low. Assuming their drivers to weigh rather more than 11 st (70 kg), on average, their two doses correspond fairly closely to the smallest and biggest used here. Their blood samples, however, would appear to have been taken almost 2 hr after subjects began to drink. If this is so, the blood alcohol levels correspond very closely to those found here. They report a concentration of 4 mg and 58 mg per 100 ml for the two doses. At 2 hr comparable figures in this experiment were 6 mg and 62 mg per 100 ml.

While this in no way affects the conclusions reached by these authors about the effect of such doses on performance, it does affect their discussion about 'safe' levels of blood alcohol. At the time of the tests the blood alcohol levels in their drivers would almost certainly be at least 10–20 mg per 100 ml higher than those reported. Even so, their experiments, and these, suggest a marked impairment of performance on such tasks with blood alcohol levels of 60–80 mg per 100 ml.

In view of the known difficulty of clinical estimates of impairment in such situations and of the individual's capacity, if he is capable of realizing that he is under test, to compensate temporarily for loss of efficiency, estimation of blood alcohol level would seem the most direct way of assessing impairment. Estimation of the alcohol excreted in urine and in breath allows a close approximation to blood alcohol. In these experiments, urine alcohol agreed very closely with blood alcohol. Breath analysis, which has enormous administrative advantages over both blood and urine analysis, can, from these results, given a suitable instrument, also give a very close approximation.

It would seem fairly clear, from these results, that the efficiency with which a task like driving is performed is likely to decrease progressively as blood alcohol rises. At some point the loss of efficiency is likely to be large enough to constitute a danger in a practical driving situation. As this experiment has been carried out in a laboratory, necessarily free of the hazards and many of the motivating features of a real-life situation, it is not possible, from these results, to say at what level of blood alcohol the increased risk of accident would become unacceptable. Some evidence on this is available from the experience of the U.S.A.,

Denmark, Norway and Sweden, where rather different cut-off levels are used.

Individual differences in response to alcohol appear to be related, at least in part, to personality characteristics, especially those of extraversion–introversion. Eysenck (1953) has collected the evidence for the existence of this dimension of personality and has postulated (Eysenck, 1957a) that extraverts would be more susceptible to the effects of depressant drugs like alcohol. The extraverts in this experiment behaved as a group, and tend to confirm Eysenck's hypothesis. The introverts do not behave as a group. It is of interest that all the scales used agreed on the extravert end but did not agree on the introverts. It is possible that the almost bimodal effect noted on change of speed for introverts reflects the intrusion of some other personality characteristic not tested in this experiment. The test which showed this bimodal effect most clearly was the Bernreuter, which uses a more 'neurotic' criterion of introversion than the Maudsley.

In this experiment extraverts appear not to be bothered by the extra stress imposed by alcohol. They drive at much the same speed as before, make very little additional corrective movements, but make much greater error, are less consistent, and deteriorate more rapidly during 20-min driving periods. Introverts, on the other hand, appear to be striving to compensate for the alcohol effect, and to be anxious to demonstrate their efficiency. They over-react to the situation, make more corrective movements of the steering-wheel, and change their speed markedly. Some slow right down, presumably in an attempt to achieve accuracy, though they do not necessarily do so, while others appear to be attempting to demonstrate how quickly they can drive, again not always with a proportionate loss of efficiency.

Summary

An experiment has been carried out to investigate the effects of small doses of alcohol on a complex skill.

Four alcohol doses and a placebo dose were used. The peak blood alcohol concentrations from the doses were approximately 20, 40, 60 and 80 mg /100 ml of blood.

Urine and breath analyses were compared with direct blood

analysis. Urine alcohol peaked later and higher than blood, but breath alcohol followed blood alcohol in time. The ratio of urine alcohol to blood alcohol was $1·252 : 1$.

Three kinds of breath-testing apparatus were used. Best results were obtained from the 'breathalyser'. The others either showed high constant errors or were unreliable. The results from the breathalyser were good enough to warrant its consideration from a practical point of view.

Mean error showed an increase, with increase in blood alcohol, amounting to about 16 per cent deterioration with a blood alcohol concentration of some 80 mg/100 ml. Part at least of the increase in error is to be explained by a significant tendency for subjects to move towards the right-hand side of the road after alcohol and also by less consistent positioning. Error scores and control movement scores also showed a variation in time, rising and falling in a way similar to that of blood alcohol.

Mean speed showed no significant change, but marked individual differences in speed after alcohol were found.

Control movements, as measured by steering-wheel movement, showed significant increases and a significant reduction in consistency.

Age, sex, previous driving experience and previous drinking habits, within the limits available, showed no relation to individual differences in response to alcohol.

Personality ratings, especially those relating to extraversion–introversion, showed a definite relation to behaviour changes. Extraverts did not change either speed or control movements very much, though they were less consistent in control movements, but showed large increases in error. Introverts changed speed considerably, though it is not possible to differentiate between those who slowed down and those who speeded up. Control movements also increased, but were relatively consistent. Error may or may not increase, but the mean error score was significantly less than that for extraverts.

Appendix. Average Scores for Various Aspects of the
Tracking Task, After Each Alcohol Dose

Performance Variable	Dose 0	Dose 1	Dose 2	Dose 3	Dose 4
Tracking error	227	230	235	246	246
Kerb bumpings	209	255	350	260	359
Inconsistency in tracking	4·82	5·08	5·63	5·78	5·53
Time per lap	403	390	386	393	398
Steering-wheel movement	674	673	690	708	764
Inconsistency in steering-wheel movement	3·61	3·51	3·61	4·03	4·15

References

BARTLETT, F. C. (1943), *Proc. roy. Soc. B.*, vol. 131, p. 247.

BROADBENT, D. E. (1956), *Bull. Brit. psychol. Soc.*, vol. 29, p. 13.

COHEN, J., DEARNALEY, E. J., and HANSEL, C. E. M. (1958), *Brit. med. J.*, vol. 1, pp. 1438.

DARROW, C. W. (1929), *Psychol. Bull.*, vol. 26, p. 527.

DREW, G. C. (1942), *Flying Personnel Research Committee Report*.

DREW, G. C. (1950), *Department of Scientific and Industrial Research, Road Research Laboratory, Research Note*, no. RN/1291.

EGGLETON, M. G. (1955), in *Proc. II int. Conf. Alcoh. Road Traff.*, Toronto, 1953.

EMERSON, H. (1933), *Alcohol and Man: the Effects of Alcohol on Man in Health and Disease*, Macmillan.

EYSENCK, H. J. (1953), *The Structure of Human Personality*, Methuen.

EYSENCK, H. J. (1957a), *The Dynamics of Anxiety and Hysteria*, Routledge & Kegan Paul.

EYSENCK, H. J. (1957b), *J. ment. Sci.*, vol. 103, p. 119.

FISK, E. L. (1917), *Alcohol: its Relation to Human Efficiency and Longevity*, Funk and Wagnalls.

GOLDBERG, L. (1943), *Acta physiol. Scand.*, vol. 5, suppl. 16, p. 1.

GOLDBERG, L. (1951), *Proc. I int. Conf. Alcoh. Road Traff.*, Stockholm, 1950.

GREENBERG, L. A., and KEATOR, F. W. (1941), *Quart. J. Stud. Alcohol*, vol. 2, p. 57.

HAGGARD, H. W., GREENBERG, L. A., and COHEN, L. H. (1943), *Quart. J. Stud. Alcohol*, vol. 4, p. 3.

HARGER, R. N., LAMB, E. B., and HULPIEU, H. R. (1938), *J. Amer. med. Ass.*, vol. 110, p. 779.

HIMMELWEIT, H. (1946), *Brit. J. Psychol.* (general section), vol. 36, p. 132.

JELLINEK, E. M., and MCFARLAND, R. A. (1940), *Quart. J. Stud. Alcohol*, vol. 1, p. 272.

KENT-JONES, D. W., and TAYLOR, G. (1954), *Analyst*, vol. 79, p. 121.

LIJESTRAND, G. (1940), *Tirfing*, vol. 34, p. 97.

MCDOUGALL, W. (1929), *J. abnorm. soc. Psychol.*, vol. 24, p. 293.

MEDICAL RESEARCH COUNCIL, Alcohol Investigation Committee (1938), *Alcohol, Its Action on the Human Organism*, H.M.S.O., 3rd edn.

MELLANBY, E. (1919), *Spec. Rep. Ser. med. Res. Coun. (Lond.)*, H.M.S.O.

MILES, W. R. (1924), *Alcohol and Human Efficiency*, Carnegie Institute of Washington, publ. no. 333.

NATIONAL SAFETY COUNCIL (1953), *Committee on Tests for Intoxication*, Chicago.

RUSSELL DAVIS, D. (1948), *Pilot Error: some Laboratory Experiments*, H.M.S.O.

SHAGASS, C. (1954), *EEG clin. Neurophysiol.*, vol. 6, p. 221.

SHAGASS, C. (1956), *Psychosom. Med.*, vol. 18, p. 400.

VENABLES, P. (1956), *J. appl. Psychol.*, vol. 40, p. 21.

WELFORD, A. T. (1951), *Skill and Age*, Oxford University Press.

WINTON, F. R., and BAYLISS, L. E. (1948), *Human Physiology*, Churchill, 3rd edn.

25 A. T. Welford

Changes in Speed of Performance with Age and Their
Industrial Significance

A. T. Welford, 'Changes in the speed of performance with age and their
industrial significance', *Ergonomics*, vol. 5, 1962, pp. 139–45. (Incorporating
the author's amendments to Figure 2.)

1. Introduction

The approach customarily adopted to the question of how people
can best be employed in later years is to look at the work which
older people tend to do at present and to consider ways and
means whereby certain jobs can be earmarked for them and they
can be eased into these jobs when their present work proves to
be beyond their capacities. Such an approach has several obvious
disadvantages both for older workers themselves and for industry, and for some years past the need has been recognized for
the alternative approach of considering the characteristics of
older people and of jobs in the same terms, of pinpointing
features of jobs which cause trouble as age advances and of
trying to modify the jobs accordingly. Such an approach is undoubtedly difficult, but researches over the last 15 years have
brought us to the point at which a number of changes with age
and their implications for modification of jobs seem fairly clear.
The purpose of the present paper is to consider one of the most
important of these, namely, *slowing of performance*, and to point
to some of its ramifications and industrial consequences.

With increasing age slowing is found in the performance of
many tasks, and a considerable research effort had been made to
ascertain its nature and locus within the chain of processes leading from the sense organs through various central mechanisms
to the effectors. While much remains to be done, it is clear from
what has been achieved so far that several different mechanisms
are involved. It is therefore an understandable question to ask
whether slowness should be regarded as a single unitary phenomenon of ageing, or whether a number of distinct types should be
recognized. It may be said at once that studies comparing the

same individuals at several tasks have suggested that age changes in different performances are correlated. How far there are genuinely unitary factors underlying the various changes, and how far the correlations are merely due to a concurrence of several discrete factors, is not at present clear. Discrete factors must, however, be of substantial importance since the correlations are usually rather small unless the tasks are closely related (Birren and Botwinick, 1951; Césa-Bianchi, 1955; Goldfarb, 1941; Pacaud, 1960).

Experiments, comparing performances at several related tasks having different degrees of difficulty, have shown three rather distinct patterns of slowing with age. In some, the extra time taken by older subjects could be represented by the addition of a *constant* to the time taken by younger people for both simple and more difficult tasks. In others, the times taken by older people have risen in fairly strict *proportion*. In yet others older subjects have taken quite *disproportionately* longer over the more difficult tasks.

Obviously these three patterns have different implications for the placement of older people in industry. With the first, the *relative* slowing with age is least for the most difficult tasks, with the second it is equal for all tasks, and with the third it is least for the easiest tasks.

2. Constant and Proportional Increases of Time

An important clue to the definition of the conditions producing a constant as opposed to a proportional increase is contained in an experiment by Botwinick, Brinley and Robbin (1958). Pairs of lines were exposed side by side in a tachistoscope, the longer (x_1) always 80 mm and the shorter (x_2) from 1·32 to 20 per cent less. The longer line was in half the presentations on the right and in half on the left. The subject had to say which line was longer as quickly as possible. The experiment was tried under two conditions: one with an exposure of 2 s so that on virtually all occasions the lines remained on view until after the subject had given his judgement. In the other condition the exposure was only 0·15 s.

The results are shown in Figure 1. The 20 per cent points need

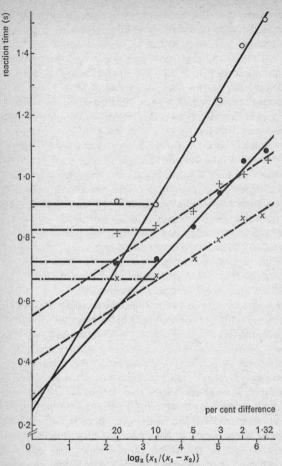

Figure 1 Example of constant and proportional rises with age of time to perform a discrimination task. Data of Botwinick *et al.* (1958). The times are plotted against an 'information' formula (see Welford, 1961). Results are indicated as follows:

age range	65–79	65–79	18–35	18–35
exposure time (s)	2·00	0·15	2·00	0·15
symbol	O	+	●	×

Each point is the mean of the medians of thirty-four older or twenty-six younger subjects. The medians were each based on eight readings not concern us: it was clear from a previous experiment by Birren and Botwinick (1955) using the same apparatus but presenting differences of up to 50 per cent, that points from 20 per cent upwards fall above any regression lines which are a reasonable fit to the points from 1·32 to 10 per cent. Birren and Botwinick found that the reaction times for differences of 15 to 50 per cent were all approximately equal, suggesting that when discrimination is very easy, reaction time is determined by the time needed not for discrimination but for choice of which response to make.

Turning first to the points for the 2-s exposures, it can be seen that the regression lines for the two age groups meet approximately at the zero line: the age difference can be described as a difference of slope from a common origin, i.e. as proportional. Reaction times with the 0·15-s exposures are all shorter than with the corresponding 2·0-s exposures and, surprisingly, show no difference of slope with age: the age effect is a constant added to the times taken by the younger subjects. Since all the conditions except length of exposure were the same under the two conditions, it seems clear that the change from one age effect to the other was due to a change from long to short exposure.

We can only speculate on the reason why the different conditions of exposure affected the age effect in the ways they did, but we may note that the constant extra time taken by older subjects with short exposures cannot have been spent in making the choice of response, since this would have raised the time required by older subjects for easy discriminations but left more difficult ones unaffected. The age effect must therefore have been in some process of receiving the signal prior to the discrimination of longer from shorter. With brief exposures, once the signal had been received, there seems to have been no difference between older and younger in the speed of discrimination, but the accuracy achieved with the more difficult discriminations was very poor for both age groups. With longer exposures accuracy was much greater and we may therefore suppose that, when the signal remained on view, subjects collected further data from it with a view to greater accuracy. If so, the collection of this extra data appears to have been proportionally slower among the older subjects, but to have overlapped with the time taken to receive the signal so that it masked the constant rise of time shown with short exposures. The same two distinct patterns of results have also been shown in experiments by other authors for choice reaction times with varying degrees of choice, and for making tapping movements between targets of different sizes at different distances. In each case the hypothesis appeared reasonable that the age effect is a constant rise of time if action has to be taken on data gathered in a brief glance, and a proportional rise if action follows a more prolonged inspection (for a review, see Welford, 1961, and for a direct test on a slightly different type of task, Griew, 1959).

Both types of slowing may reasonably be explained in terms of the theory put forward by Crossman and Szafran (1956) and by Gregory (1959) that signals to the brain from sense organs and within the brain itself have to exert their effects against a background of ambient, random neural activity ('neural noise'). This makes it necessary to 'sample' a signal over an appreciable period (albeit a fraction of a second) for it to be distinguished from the 'noise'. Various neurological changes in the brain and falls in the sensitivity of the sense organs, such as are known to occur in older people, would tend to lower the signal level, and suggestions have been made by the authors mentioned that ambient 'noise' level tends to rise with age (see also Axelrod, 1960). In either case the *signal-to-noise ratio* would be lowered and the information transmission capacity thereby reduced.

3. Disproportionate Increases of Time

Disproportionate rises of performance time with age have so far been shown for two types of task. The first of these is where a fairly complex sequence of actions is required. It may be illustrated by two examples:

1. Clay (1954, 1957) required subjects of different ages to place numbered counters on chequer boards to add up to given marginal totals on both rows and columns simultaneously. She found the times to rise a little with age on a board with 3 × 3 squares and progressively more with larger boards up to 6 × 6. The results were complicated by the fact that times suddenly fell again in later age ranges accompanied by an increase of errors,

but this appeared to indicate that when problems became excessively difficult, older subjects realized early that they would not be able to complete them satisfactorily and 'gave up'.

2. Several experiments have shown disproportionate slowing with age when complications are introduced into the relationships between display and control. A simple example is when actions are guided by a display seen in a mirror as opposed to one seen directly (Szafran, see Welford, 1958). Perhaps the most striking demonstration, however, is in a set of five tasks studied by Kay (1954, 1955). All these used a box containing a row of twelve light bulbs and a corresponding box of twelve keys. The subject's task was to press the corresponding key as quickly as possible when a light came on. The arrangements of box and keys in the several tasks were as follows:

A. Each light was immediately above its corresponding key.

B. The same as A, but with the box of lights set 3 ft away across the table from the box of keys, so that in order to relate light to key the subjects had to align across a 3-ft gap.

C. The same as B, but with the lights related to the keys by means of a number code instead of by straightforward spatial correspondence. Subjects had to imagine the lights as numbered and to find the number of the light on a card bearing the numbers 1–12 in random order and placed immediately above the keys.

D. The same as C, but with the card placed mid-way between the lights and keys, so that subjects had both to use the number code and to align across a 1½-ft gap.

E. The same as C, but with the card by the lights, so that both use of the number code and alignment across a 3-ft gap were required.

The disproportionate rise of time with age as the tasks became more difficult, which is shown in Figure 2, is very striking. The pattern of errors was similar so that there is no question of the older subjects having been slower because of having been more accurate.

Two points should be noted about both these examples. Firstly, the times include time taken to correct errors and are of a quite

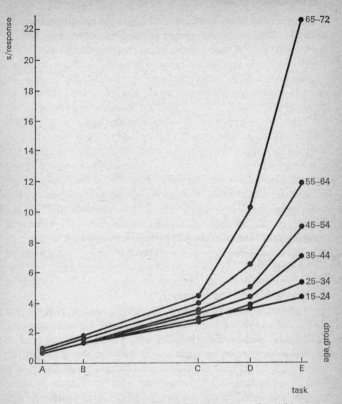

Figure 2 Example of an accelerating rise of performance time with age as difficulty of task increases. The times for older age groups rise more steeply as the tasks become more complex (from A to E). Data from Kay (1954, 1955). Each reading for tasks A and B is based on thirty responses by ten subjects in each age group (fourteen in the 55–64 age group). Each reading for tasks D, E and F is based on twenty responses by the same subjects. For tasks A and B the points of the 15–24, 25–34, 35–44 and 45–54 age groups are virtually identical and have not been distinguished.

The tasks are plotted at such distances along the abscissa that the performance times for the youngest age groups fall on a straight line. If the increase in the performance time with age was linear, the times for the other age groups would also fall on straight lines. If, however, the times increase in an accelerating manner the curves for the higher age groups will be concave upward, as indeed they are different order from those of reaction time experiments; and secondly, difficulty in both types of task appeared to depend upon failure with age in some form of short-term retention. This is known on other grounds to become more liable as age advances to disruption from other activity by the subject during the period of retention (Cameron, 1943; Kirchner, 1958). The main cause of difficulty in Clay's tasks lay in correcting errors. Since the total of the counters provided was the same as that of all the rows (or columns), each error made at least two rows or columns wrong. Correcting an error thus involved finding a row or column which was wrong and remembering which it was until another which was also wrong was found and an exchange of counters worked out to correct both. Subjects, especially the older ones, tended to forget the first while searching for the second, or one counter while checking another. In Kay's more complex tasks D and E the older subjects tended to find the 'rule of translation' from light to key difficult to 'carry' while actually performing the task, and most of their errors appeared to be due to attempts (probably unconscious) to simplify the task to that of conditions B or C. The laboratory results seem to be reflected in the industrial findings by Murrell, Griew and Tucker (1957) that older people tend not to be working on the most complex skilled jobs, and by Murrell and Tucker (1960) that they tend to be under-represented on jobs which demand the following of elaborate instructions. Certainly the laboratory results suggest that very substantial advantages are likely to accrue to older people from building devices into machines to obviate the need for short-term memory, and from simplification of layouts and procedures: just as adding one complication to another has a disproportionately adverse effect for older people, so any simplification is likely to be disproportionately beneficial.

The second kind of disproportionate slowing with age is of an entirely different nature. It is not a matter of longer time from the appearance of a signal to the taking of appropriate action, but of the length of time for which material has to be viewed for accurate identification to be achieved. Wallace (1956), for example, found that in order to identify designs and pictures seen in a tachistoscope, subjects in their sixties required an exposure about six times as long as did those in their twenties when material was very simple, and up to about twenty times as long with more complex material. The types of wrong identification made in a number of experiments when exposure was inadequate, or conditions of viewing otherwise difficult, suggest that older subjects tend to be unduly bound by their immediate associations and therefore search in an unduly restricted area of possible identifications for any object presented (Korchin and Basowitz, 1956; Verville and Cameron, 1946; O'Doherty, see Welford, 1958). The corollary of this is that they are often unable to keep separate objects which need to be treated separately but are placed in close spatial contiguity (Axelrod and Cohen, 1961; Clay, 1956). Both facets of this problem emphasize the importance for older people of good layout of items such as control panels, keeping items which are functionally related close together and separated from other items. They also point to the need for clear and logical presentation of data in such a way that each item leads on from the last with as few major leaps as possible from one class of item to another.

4. Effects of Slowing

The causes of various types of slowing with age appear to be very different, and it is in a sense artificial to bring them together. From the industrial point of view, however, they share a number of implications in common.

The direct effects of slowness with age are that older people tend to drop out of work which makes severe demands for speed or fine visual discrimination. It is now becoming recognized that because of such demands much light work is less suitable for people over the age of fifty than many moderately heavy jobs. This is understandable in view of the fact that declines of speed from the twenties to the sixties in continuous tasks studied in the laboratory are usually about 50 per cent or more, whereas declines of muscular strength between the same ages are, on average, only about 25 per cent (Fisher and Birren, 1947).

Slowing with age has also a number of indirect effects which appear especially when performance is carried out with some actual or implied time limits. Often the first sign of slowing at an industrial job is that a man works more continuously, taking fewer short rests for a smoke or conversation. More severe cases may result in items being missed or in hurrying which leads to errors and perhaps to chronic feelings of being harassed. An interesting effect of slowing is the tendency, sometimes conscious but often quite unconscious, to simplify the task being done: one example has already been noted in Kay's experiments, another has been shown by Griew and Tucker (1958) who found older workers to use fewer of the displays on the machines they were operating, and to look at those they did use for a shorter time in spite of the fact that they were working more continuously than younger men.

By far the most important factor tending to mitigate the effects of slowing with age is increased experience, which can provide ready answers to problems which might otherwise have to be thought out from scratch and, even more important, build up *routines* of action and the ability to recognize sequences in events. The 'coding' of sequences of events and series of actions greatly lightens the load of decision: instead of separate decisions being required about each detailed event or action, the perception of one event enables several others to be assumed, and short programmes of action can be initiated as single 'units'. Coding of this kind has the danger that the ready-made sequences and routines may not be entirely appropriate to particular situations, and that over-use of them may lead to 'rigidity' and lack of adaptability. They do, however, seem to be an important means of handling situations on a large scale and essential to all except the simplest conceptual thought. A possible method of avoiding rigidity in some cases was suggested in a chance remark made recently to the writer by an eminent management selection consultant. He had observed in the course of his work that ability to adapt in later middle age seemed to be better among businessmen than among those engaged in industrial management. It seems fair to argue that those in commerce and trade tend to have much more immediate and definite knowledge of the results of their actions than do those in higher industrial management. It has been known for a long time in laboratory studies that knowledge of results given quickly after an action improves both accuracy and willingness to exert onself. We may reasonably suppose that routine would often be less rigidly followed if clear evidence of its inadequacy was forthcoming in time for modification to be made, and that such evidence would make those concerned much more ready to look for the need for change.

One of the difficulties of applying ergonomics in industry is that many of the demands of industrial work do not normally stretch a man's capabilities to an extent which causes obvious breakdown or impairment of performance. They may, however, come near to doing so and thus cause strain, dissatisfaction and, sometimes, accidents. Older people, having less margin of capacity in hand, are likely to show the onset of undue demand more clearly than younger and thus make easier the identification of points about a job which are in need of attention. If so, the ergonomics of ageing is not an 'extra' or speciality to be added to other studies of industrial work by human biologists. Rather it is the avenue through which initial approaches can with advantage be made.

References

AXELROD, S. (1960), Some observations on cognitive tasks in several modalities, and suggestions for psychophysiological research, *Paper to International Research Seminar on Social and Psychological Aspects of Aging*, Berkeley.

AXELROD, S., and COHEN, L. D. (1961), 'Senescence and embedded-figure performance in vision and touch', *Percept. mot. Skills*, vol. 12, pp. 283–8.

BIRREN, J. E., and BOTWINICK, J. (1951), 'Rate of addition as a function of difficulty and age', *Psychometrika*, vol. 2, pp. 219–32.

BIRREN, J. E., and BOTWINICK, J. (1955), 'Speed of response as a function of perceptual difficulty and age', *J. Gerontol.*, vol. 10, pp. 433–6.

BOTWINICK, J., BRINLEY, J. F., and ROBBIN, J. S. (1958), 'The interaction effects of perceptual difficulty and stimulus exposure time on age differences in speed and accuracy of response', *Gerontolog.*, vol. 2, pp. 1–10.

CAMERON, D. E. (1943), 'Impairment of the retention phase of remembering', *Psychiat. Quart.*, vol. 17, pp. 395–404.

CESA-BIANCHI, M. (1955), 'Contributi allo studio delle modificazione psichiche in rapporto con l'età', *Publicazioni dell' Università Cattolica del Sacro Cuore, Milan*, vol. 49, pp. 1–61.

CLAY, H. M. (1954), 'Changes of performance with age on similar tasks of varying complexity', *Brit. J. Psychol.*, vol. 45, pp. 7–13.

CLAY, H. M. (1956), 'An age difficulty in separating spatially contiguous data', *J. Geront.*, vol. 11, pp. 318–22.

CLAY, H. M. (1957), 'The relationship between time, accuracy and age on similar tasks of varying complexity', *Gerontolog.*, vol. 1, pp. 41–9.

CROSSMAN, E. R. F. W., and SZAFRAN, J. (1956), 'Changes in age in the speed of information intake and discrimination', *Exper. Suppl.*, vol. 4, pp. 128–35.

FISHER, M. B., and BIRREN, J. E. (1947), 'Age and strength', *J. appl. Psychol.*, vol. 31, pp, 490–97.

GOLDFARB, W. (1941), 'An investigation of reaction time in older adults and its relationship to certain observed mental test patterns', *Teachers Coll. Contr. Educ.*, no. 831, Columbia University.

GREGORY, R. L. (1959), 'Increase in "neurological noise" as a factor in ageing', *Proc. 4th Cong. intern. Ass. Geront. Merano, 1957*, vol. 1, pp. 314–24.

GRIEW, S. (1959), 'A further note on uncertainty in relation to age', *Gerontolog.*, vol. 3, pp. 335–9.

GRIEW, S., and TUCKER, W. A. (1958), 'The identification of job activities associated with age differences in the engineering industry', *J. appl. Psychol.*, vol. 42, pp. 278–82.

KAY, H. (1954), 'The effects of position in a display upon problem solving', *Quart. J. exp. Psychol.*, vol. 6, pp. 155–69.

KAY, H. (1955), 'Some experiments on adult learning', in *Old Age in the Modern World*, Livingstone, pp. 259–67.

KIRCHNER, W. K. (1958), 'Age differences in the short-term retention of rapidly changing information', *J. exp. Psychol.*, vol. 55, pp. 352–8.

KORCHIN, S. J., and BASOWITZ, H. (1956), 'The judgement of ambiguous stimuli as an index of cognitive functioning in ageing', *J. Personal.*, vol. 25, pp. 81–95.

MURRELL, K. F. H., GRIEW, S., and TUCKER, W. A. (1957), 'Age structure in the engineering industry: a preliminary study', *Occup. Psychol.*, vol. 31, pp. 150–68.

MURRELL, K. F. H., and TUCKER, W. A. (1960), 'A pilot job-study of age-related causes of difficulty in light engineering', *Ergonomics*, vol. 3, pp. 74–9.

PACAUD, S. (1960), 'The structure of psychological and psychomotor functions with age in the light of multiple factor analysis', *Proc. 5th. Cong. intern. Ass. Geront.*, San Francisco, 1960.

VERVILLE, E., and CAMERON, N. (1946), 'Age and sex differences in the perception of incomplete pictures by adults', *J. genet. Psychol.*, vol. 68, pp. 149–57.

WALLACE, J. G. (1956), 'Some studies of perception in relation to age', *Brit. J. Psychol.*, vol. 47, pp. 283–97.

WELFORD, A. T. (1958), *Ageing and Human Skill*, Oxford University Press.

WELFORD, A. T. (1961), 'Age changes in the times taken by choice, discrimination and the control of movement', *Gerontolog.*, vol. 5, pp. 129–45.

Further Reading

J. A. Adams, 'Human tracking behavior', *Psychol. Bull.*, vol. 58 (1961), pp. 55–79.

F. Attneave, *Applications of Information Theory to Psychology*, Holt, 1959.

F. C. Bartlett, 'The measurement of human skill', *Brit. med. J.*, i (1947), pp. 835–8, 877–80.

S. H. Bartley and E. Chute, *Fatigue and Impairment in Man*, McGraw-Hill, 1947.

G. H. Begbie, 'Accuracy of aiming in linear hand-movements', *Quart. J. exp. Psychol.*, vol. 11 (1959), pp. 65–75.

E. Belbin, R. M. Belbin and F. Hill, 'A comparison between the results of three different methods of operator training', *Ergonomics*, vol. 1 (1957), pp. 39–50.

C. Berry, M. G. Gelder and A. Summerfield, 'Experimental analysis of drug effects on human performance using information theory concepts', *Brit. J. Psychol.*, vol. 56 (1965), pp. 255–65.

E. A. Bilodeau (ed.), *Acquisition of Skill*, Academic Press, 1966.

P. Bertelson, 'Central intermittency twenty years later', *Quart. J. exp. Psychol.*, vol. 18 (1966), pp. 133–63.

D. E. Broadbent, *Perception and Communication*, Pergamon, 1958.

D. E. Broadbent and M. Gregory, 'Psychological refractory period and the length of time required to make a decision', *Proc. roy. Soc.*, B, vol. 168 (1967), pp. 181–93.

I. D. Brown, 'Subjective and objective comparisons of successful and unsuccessful trainee drivers', *Ergonomics*, vol. 9 (1966), pp. 49–56.

L. Buck, 'Reaction time as a measure of perceptual vigilance', *Psychol. Bull.*, vol. 65 (1966), pp. 291–304.

D. N. Buckner and J. J. McGrath (eds.), *Vigilance: a Symposium*, McGraw-Hill, 1963.

J. A. Carpenter, 'Effects of alcohol on some psychological processes', *Quart. J. Stud. Alc.*, vol. 23 (1962), pp. 274–314.

A. Chapanis, W. R. Garner and C. T. Morgan, *Applied Experimental Psychology*, Wiley and Chapman & Hall, 1949.

R. A. Chase, 'An information-flow model of the organization of motor activity. I: Transduction, transmission and central control of sensory information', *J. nerv. ment. Dis.*, vol. 140 (1965), pp. 239–51; 'II: Sampling, central processing and utilization of sensory information', ibid., pp. 334–50.

D. W. J. Corcoran, 'Personality and the inverted-U relation', *Brit. J. Psychol.*, vol. 56 (1965), pp. 267–73.

B. J. Cratty, *Movement Behaviour and Motor Learning*, Lea & Febiger, 1964.

Further Reading

E. R. F. W. Crossman, 'Information processes in human skill', *Brit. med. Bull.*, vol. 20 (1964), pp. 32–7.

G. C. Drew, W. P. Colquhoun and H. A. Long, *Effect of Small Doses of Alcohol on a Skill Resembling Driving*, H.M.S.O., 1959.

O. G. Edholm, *The Biology of Work*, Weidenfeld & Nicolson, 1967.

P. M. Fitts and J. R. Peterson, 'Information capacity of discrete motor responses', *J. exp. Psychol.*, vol. 67 (1964), pp. 103–12.

P. M. Fitts and M. I. Posner, *Human Performance*, Brooks/Cole, 1967.

P. M. Fitts and C. M. Seeger, 'S–R Compatibility: spatial characteristics of stimulus and response codes', *J. exp. Psychol.*, vol. 46 (1953), pp. 199–210.

E. A. Fleishman, 'Psychomotor tests in drug research', in L. Uhr and J. G. Miller (eds.), *Drugs and Behavior*, Wiley, 1960.

E. A. Fleishman and S. Rich, 'The role of kinaesthetic and spatial-visual abilities in perceptual–motor learning', *J. exp. Psychol.*, vol. 66 (1963), pp. 6–11.

W. F. Floyd and A. T. Welford (eds.), *Human Factors in Equipment Design*, H. K. Lewis for Ergonomics Research Society, 1954.

J. P. Frankmann and J. A. Adams, 'Theories of vigilance', *Psychol. Bull.*, vol. 59 (1962), pp. 257–72.

R. M. Gagné and E. A. Fleishman, *Psychology and Human Performance*, Holt, Rinehart & Winston, 1959.

C. B. Gibbs, 'The continuous regulation of skilled response by kinaesthetic feedback', *Brit. J. Psychol.*, vol. 45 (1954), pp. 24–39.

R. Gottsdanker, 'The effect of superseding signals', *Quart. J. exp. Psychol.*, vol. 18 (1966), pp. 236–49.

S. Griew, 'Age, information transmission and the positional relationship between signals and responses in the performance of a choice task', *Ergonomics*, vol. 7 (1964), pp. 267–77.

M. Hammerton and A. H. Tickner, 'An investigation into the comparative suitability of forearm, hand and thumb controls in acquisition tasks', *Ergonomics*, vol. 9 (1966), pp. 125–30.

D. O. Hebb, 'Drives and the C.N.S. (conceptual nervous system)', *Psychol. Rev.*, vol. 62 (1955), pp. 243–54.

W. E. Hick, 'On the rate of gain of information', *Quart. J. exp. Psychol.*, vol. 4 (1952), pp. 11–26.

D. H. Holding, *Principles of Training*, Pergamon, 1965.

S. W. Keele, 'Movement control in skilled motor performance', *Psychol. Bull.*, vol. 70 (1968), pp. 387–403.

J. I. Laszlo, 'The performance of a simple task with kinaesthetic sense loss', *Quart. J. exp. Psychol.*, vol. 18 (1966), pp. 1–8.

D. Legge, 'Analysis of visual and proprioceptive components of motor skill by means of a drug', *Brit. J. Psychol.*, vol. 56 (1965), pp. 243–54.

J. F. Mackworth, 'Performance decrement in vigilance, threshold, and high speed perceptual motor tasks', *Canad. J. Psychol.*, vol. 18 (1964), pp. 209–23.

N. H. Mackworth, *Researches on the Measurement of Human Performance*, H.M.S.O., 1950.

A. W. Melton (ed.), *Categories of Human Learning*, Academic Press, 1964.

G. A. Miller, E. Galanter and K. H. Pribram, *Plans and the Structure of Behavior*, Holt, 1960.

K. F. H. Murrell, *Ergonomics*, Chapman & Hall, 1965.

J. D. North, 'Manual control as a stochastic process', *Ergonomics*, vol. 6 (1963), pp. 247–54.

J. M. Notterman and D. E. Page, 'Evaluation of mathematically equivalent tracking systems', *Percept. mot. skills*, vol. 15 (1962), pp. 683–716.

R. W. Obermayer, W. F. Swartz and F. A. Muckler, 'Interaction of information displays with control system dynamics and course frequency in continuous tracking', *Percept. mot. Skills*, vol. 15 (1962), pp. 199–215.

J. B. Oxendine, *Psychology of Motor Learning*, Appleton-Century-Crofts, 1968.

R. B. Payne and E. W. Moore, 'The effects of some analeptic and depressant drugs upon tracking behaviour', *J. Pharmacol. exp. Therapeut.*, vol. 115 (1955), pp. 480–84.

R. D. Pepler, 'Warmth and performance: an investigation in the tropics', *Ergonomics*, vol. 2 (1958), pp. 63–88.

E. C. Poulton, 'Measuring the order of difficulty of visual-motor tasks', *Ergonomics*, vol. 1 (1958), pp. 234–9.

E. C. Poulton, 'On increasing the sensitivity of measures of performance', *Ergonomics*, vol. 8 (1965), pp. 69–76.

W. T. Powers, R. K. Clark and R. L. McFarland, 'A general feedback theory of behavior', *Percept. mot. Skills, Monogr. Suppl.*, nos. 1–VII and 3–VII.

K. A. Provins, 'Handedness and skill', *Quart. J. exp. Psychol.*, vol. 8 (1956), pp. 79–95.

A. F. Sanders (ed.), *Attention and Performance*, North-Holland Publishing Co., 1967.

W. T. Singleton, R. S. Easterby and D. J. Whitfield, 'The human operator in complex systems', *Ergonomics*, vol. 10 (1967), pp. 99–292.

E. E. Smith, 'Choice reaction time: an analysis of the major theoretical positions', *Psychol. Bull.*, vol. 69 (1968), pp. 77–110.

K. U. Smith, S. Ansell and W. M. Smith, 'Sensory feedback analysis in medical research. I. Delayed sensory feedback in behavior and neural function', *Amer. J. phys. Med.*, vol. 42 (1963), pp. 228–62.

M. C. Smith, 'Theories of the psychological refractory period', *Psychol. Bull.*, vol. 67 (1967), pp. 202–13.

M. A. Vince, 'Intermittency of control movements and the psychological refractory period', *Brit. J. Psychol.*, vol. 38 (1948), pp. 149–57.

A. T. Welford, *Ageing and Human Skill*, Oxford University Press for the Nuffield Foundation, 1958.

A. T. Welford, *Fundamentals of Skill*, Methuen, 1968.

Further Reading

K. F. Wells, *Kinesiology*, Saunders, 1960.

R. T. Wilkinson, 'Effects of up to 60 hours' sleep deprivation on different types of work', *Ergonomics*, vol. 7 (1964), pp. 175–86.

L. S. Woodburne, 'Partial analysis of the neural elements in posture and locomotion', *Psychol. Bull.*, vol. 68 (1967), pp. 121–31.

Acknowledgements

Permission to reproduce the Readings in this volume is acknowledged from the following sources:

Reading 1 Oxford University Press and the Nuffield Foundation
Reading 2 John Wiley & Sons, Inc.
Reading 3 American Psychological Association and Dr A. Fleishman
Reading 4 Wadsworth Publishing Company, Inc.
Reading 5 Taylor & Francis Ltd and Dr A. T. Welford
Reading 6 American Psychological Association and Dr E. A. Alluisi
Reading 7 American Psychological Association and Dr E. Poulton
Reading 8 *Quarterly Journal of Experimental Psychology* and Dr E. R. F. W. Crossman
Reading 10 The British Psychological Society
Reading 11 *Quarterly Journal of Experimental Psychology* and Dr A. T. Welford
Reading 12 American Psychological Association and Dr H. P. Bahrick
Reading 13 The British Psychological Society and Dr C. B. Gibbs
Reading 14 *Perceptual and Motor Skills* and Dr A. J. Dinnerstein
Reading 15 American Physiological Society and Dr J. Paillard
Reading 16 Professor C. B. Gibbs
Reading 17 Free Press of Glencoe
Reading 18 Holt, Rinehart & Winston, Inc.
Reading 19 Pergamon Press Ltd
Reading 20 Pergamon Press Ltd
Reading 21 Taylor & Francis Ltd and Dr E. R. F. W. Crossman
Reading 22 The Royal Society and Sir Frederic Bartlett
Reading 23 *Quarterly Journal of Experimental Psychology* and Dr D. E. Broadbent
Reading 24 *British Medical Journal*, Professor G. C. Drew, Dr W. P. Colquhoun and Hazel Frank
Reading 25 Taylor & Francis Ltd and Dr A. T. Welford

Author Index

Subject Index

Penguin Modern Psychology Readings

Other titles in this series are:

Published simultaneously with *Skills:*

Perceptual Learning and Adaptation
Ed. P. C. Dodwell

While indicating the origins of the problem of perceptual learning in the Empiricist–Nativist controversy, Professor Dodwell in his selection of Readings shows how to a considerable extent psychologists have unravelled the tangled threads of the subject. In doing so he illustrates the importance of perceptual learning for comparative, developmental and cognitive psychology. These areas are represented by the work of Tinbergen, Hebb and Riesen on early experience in animals, and by Piaget and Fantz in children. Detailed theoretical considerations are also included, amongst them important papers by the Gibsons, Postman and Selfridge.

Penguin Modern Psychology Major Texts

Behaviour Therapy
Victor, Meyer, and Edward S. Chesser

A thorough, balanced account of the theory, practice and
effectiveness of behaviour therapy. This form of treatment, derived
from experimental psychology, plays a growing role in the treatment
of many illnesses, such as phobic anxieties, alcoholism, sexual
deviations, stammering, tics and enuresis. Its techniques have at
times also been successfully employed in psychoses, psychosomatic
disorders, obsessional neuroses and childhood behaviour disorders.

After a brief introduction to psychiatric disorders for readers
unfamiliar with clinical psychiatry, chapter 2 gives a full account of
the relevant theories of conditioning and learning, and chapter 3
considers how well experimental psychology can account for
psychiatric disorders. Chapter 4 reviews the main methods of
treatment in behaviour therapy such as desensitization, aversion
therapy, 'flooding' or implosive therapy, and operant conditioning,
while chapter 5 looks very carefully at the empirical evidence for the
effectiveness of these methods. After two chapters that offer a
wide-ranging view of current research, chapter 8 confronts the
practical world of the clinic – the problems that arise in the selection
of patients, selection of symptoms to be treated, method of
treatment, selection of therapist and in the conduct of treatment.
'An attempt is made', the authors explain, 'to discuss these topics
in a constructive manner based on our experience with a variety of
behaviour therapy methods employed in the treatment of 150
patients, the majority of whom were suffering from psychoneurotic
disorders with a preponderance of phobic anxiety states.'

A short conclusion looks to the prospects of treatment and
research in behaviour therapy units.

This text should be of interest to those already engaged in clinical
practice or research and those undergoing training who may choose
to enter this field. It should therefore be of value to those training or
practising in clinical psychology, psychiatry, psychiatric social work
and occupational therapy.

Introducing Psychology:
An Experimental Approach

D. S. Wright, Ann Taylor, D. R. Davies, W. Sluckin, S. G. M. Lee and J. T. Reason

The authors select a number of the main problem areas in psychology and deal with them in some depth. These include the biological determinants of behaviour, the analysis of perceiving, remembering and thinking, the structure of intelligence and personality, and the social influences which shape behaviour. After an introductory Part One on the scope of the book and on observational and experimental method in psychology ('the strongest unifying bond of the present book'), Part Two relates heredity, maturation and physiology to behaviour. A discussion of perceptual processes is followed by chapters on the effects of early experience, learning processes, the development of skills, and remembering. This last chapter leads on to the discussion of symbolic processes, which is the concern of the chapters on language and thinking in Part Four. In Part Five the authors explore methods of measuring individual differences, and discuss the notions of intelligence, personality and normality. In Part Six a chapter on some mechanisms of social influence describes recent work, in which basic principles of learning have been extended to the two-person situation. This is followed by a review of certain aspects of socialization, and the book ends with a chapter on persuasive communications and the determining influence of group membership upon an individual's behaviour.

Clear illustrations, an extensive bibliography (keyed back to page numbers in the text) and a full index complete the volume. Here for the general reader and the student of allied subjects is an introduction that really faces up to the challenges of the subject. For the student of psychology the authors' readability, their concentration on method, and their emphasis on key concepts and problems make *Introducing Psychology* a thoroughly useful companion, not just for the first year, but for much of the degree course.

Penguin Science of Behaviour
A series of short unit texts

Brain Damage and the Mind
Moyra Williams

One of the aims of the Penguin Science of Behaviour series is to serve both the study of psychology and the needs of workers in applied fields. Dr Moyra Williams's analytical summary of our present knowledge of brain damage and the mind precisely fulfils this aim.

The effects of brain damage provide valuable information about the working of the healthy mind and also give clues to further progress in the clinical field. Dr Williams's survey presents this information clearly and usefully under the familiar categories of consciousness and mood, memory, perception, motor skill and verbal expression, and intelligence and personality. An interesting conclusion offers a tentative model of mental activity.

Vigilance and Attention:
A Signal Detection Approach
Jane F. Mackworth

In this companion volume to *Vigilance and Habituation: A Neuropsychological Approach* the author concludes her important review of performance decrement: '. . . repetition and monotony produce habituation of physiological responses, particularly neural ones . . . as a result of such habituation it becomes increasingly difficult for the subject to continue to pay attention . . . he will cease to make responses of any kind, right or wrong, or he will react more slowly to obvious changes that do attract his attention.'

The human importance of this pioneering review of the interaction of physiology and psychology is made very clear by the author: 'We are faced with vigilance tasks for a greater part of the day than we realize. Driving is one example. Operating a calculating machine, typing, inspecting endless parts for a flaw, even listening to an unending stream of patients, all these and many other familiar and monotonous tasks may lead to devastating consequences, when a small error or failure to catch the small but vital symptom may be disastrous.'